Dental

Biochemistry

Dental Biochemistry

EUGENE P. LAZZARI, Ph.D., Editor

Professor, Department of Biochemistry
University of Texas Dental Branch
Houston, Texas

SECOND EDITION

Lea & Febiger • *Philadelphia* • *1976*

Library of Congress Cataloging in Publication Data

Lazzari, Eugene P.
    Dental biochemistry.

    Includes bibliographies and index.
    1. Teeth.   I. Title.   [DNLM: 1. Oral health.   2. Tooth—Anatomy and
histology.   WU101   D414]   QP88.6.L39   612'.311   76–11786
ISBN 0–8121–0552–4

Published in Great Britain by Henry Kimpton Publishers, London

Print number: 3   2   1

PRINTED IN THE UNITED STATES OF AMERICA

Preface

"You ask me one question," cried the old man; "let me answer by asking another: Which is the most durable, a hard or a soft thing; that which resists, or that which makes no resistance?"

"A hard thing, to be sure," replied the mandarin.

"There you are wrong," returned Shingfu. "I am now four score years old; and, if you look in my mouth, you will find that I have lost all my teeth, but not a bit of my tongue."*

This same quotation began the preface to the first edition of this book. In that, I wrote of the time having arrived when giving "tongue" to biochemical considerations of the oral cavity had to make way for the written word. Hopefully, the warm coals of experience scattered among the cooling embers of time have cast some enlightenment on the subjects selected for inclusion in this volume.

The deficiencies of the past were noted at their conception but in the rush for early parentage, necessity and ignorance coupled to spawn a physically scrawny, knowledgeably inadequate offspring. The new arrival is larger, wiser, and more adoptable; still its many faults leave it barely adequate. Like man, his works also suffer imperfection.

As editor, it was again my decision that guided the course, intent, and character of the information presented. The contributors have ably delivered what I requested for which they have earned and deserve my deepest gratitude. My warmest regards are extended also to all the secretaries, illustrators, and proofreaders who gave of their valuable time and expertise to capture sometimes elusive thoughts and fragile ideas, imprisoning them permanently in print. My special thanks go to Mrs. Eleanor Edmonds for her generous aid in multiple tasks and to our secretary Mrs. Lillie Jean.

This book is intended for teachers and students who desire information about the fundamental structure and biochemical processes of the soft and hard tissues of the oral cavity. It presupposes that the reader has at least

* Goldsmith, Oliver: *The Citizen of the World* (1762), reprinted J. Dent. Educ., *28*, 378, 1964.

the elementary knowledge of organic and biochemistry usually acquired in basic courses.

The facts contained herein have resulted from arduous investigations by many scientists who mined those biological minerals seeking to unearth their many mysteries. We deeply appreciate the many gems which they have uncovered and await those still to be found.

> For I would have you know Sancho, that a mouth without molars is like a mill without a stone and a tooth is more precious than a diamond.*

Houston, Texas   EUGENE P. LAZZARI

---

* Miguel De Cervantes: *Don Quixote*, Part 1, Chapter 18.

Contributors

ERNEST BEERSTECHER, JR., PH.D.,
Chairman, Department of Biochemistry, The University of Texas Dental Branch, Houston, Texas

NICOLA DI FERRANTE, M.D., PH.D.,
Department of Biochemistry, Baylor University College of Medicine, Houston, Texas

THOMAS R. DIRKSEN, D.D.S., PH.D.,
Department of Biochemistry, School of Dentistry, Medical College of Georgia, Augusta, Georgia

SAMUEL DREIZEN, D.D.S., M.D.,
The University of Texas Dental Science Institute, Houston, Texas

J. P. KENNEDY, PH.D.,
Director, The University of Texas Environmental Science Park, Houston, Texas

EUGENE P. LAZZARI, PH.D.,
Department of Biochemistry, University of Texas Dental Branch, Houston, Texas

KENNETH O. MADSEN, PH.D.,
Department of Biochemistry and Nutrition, University of Texas Dental Branch, Houston, Texas

EDWARD H. MONTGOMERY, PH.D.
Department of Pharmacology, University of Texas Dental Branch, Houston, Texas

DON M. RANLY, D.D.S., PH.D.,
Department of Physiology and Pedodontics, University of Texas Dental Branch, Houston, Texas

PAUL B. ROBERTSON, D.D.S., M.S.,
Department of Periodontics, University of Texas Dental Branch, Houston, Texas

IRA L. SHANNON, D.D.S., M.S.,
> Director, Oral Physiology Research Laboratory, Veterans Administration Hospital, Houston, Texas

JOHN W. SIMPSON, PH.D.,
> The University of Texas Dental Science Institute, Houston, Texas

RICHARD P. SUDDICK, D.D.S., PH.D.
> Department of Physiology, Medical University of South Carolina, Charleston, South Carolina

JAMES J. VOGEL, PH.D.,
> The University of Texas Dental Science Institute, Houston, Texas

ROBERT R. WHITE, PH.D.,
> Department of Microbiology, University of Texas Dental Branch, Houston, Texas

STUART ZIMMERMAN, PH.D.,
> Department of Biomathematics, The University of Texas System Cancer Center, M. D. Anderson Hospital and Tumor Institute, Houston, Texas

Contents

Chapter 1

Chemical Composition of Teeth

EUGENE P. LAZZARI, Ph.D.

Vertebrate tooth-like projections and jaws first appeared in the fossil record about 405 million years ago in a class of bony Paleozoic fishes called the Placodermi.

All vertebrates, except the Agnatha, jawless fishes, either possess teeth or have evolved from toothed ancestors. There also exist many deceptively tooth-like structures such as the horny tubercles of the lamprey, the serrations on the beaks of some turtles and the enamel-coated, bony ridges on the jaws of Sphenodon, or Tuatara, a primitive reptile living on New Zealand.

The primitive ancestors of the vertebrates were polyodont, many toothed, as would be expected since teeth originated from numerous, small dermal denticles. The general trend in all vertebrates has been toward fewer teeth, oligodonty, larger in size and with firmer attachment. Man has but eight teeth on each side of his jaw (Fig. 1–1) and has not become as extreme in oligodonty as some mammals such as the female norwhal, a type of toothless whale. The male norwhal is only slightly better provided in that he has a single large left incisor protruding tusk-like forward from his head. The dentition of man, like that of most mammals, is heterodont, having two or more types or tooth forms. Because he has an incomplete set of deciduous teeth and a secondary permanent set he is also a hemidiphyodont.

True teeth (Fig. 1–2) can be defined as individual structures consisting of an outer thin layer of enamel derived from ectoderm, a thicker middle layer of dentine derived from mesoderm and an inner pulp.

Enamel is a non-living, exceedingly hard, almost totally inorganic material. Dentine is very bone-like in inorganic and organic composition and contains fine protoplasmic strands of living matter originating from the odontoblasts. Odontoblasts lie in a layer near the inner wall of the dentine in the pulp cavity which also contains connective tissue, blood vessels, and nerves.

1

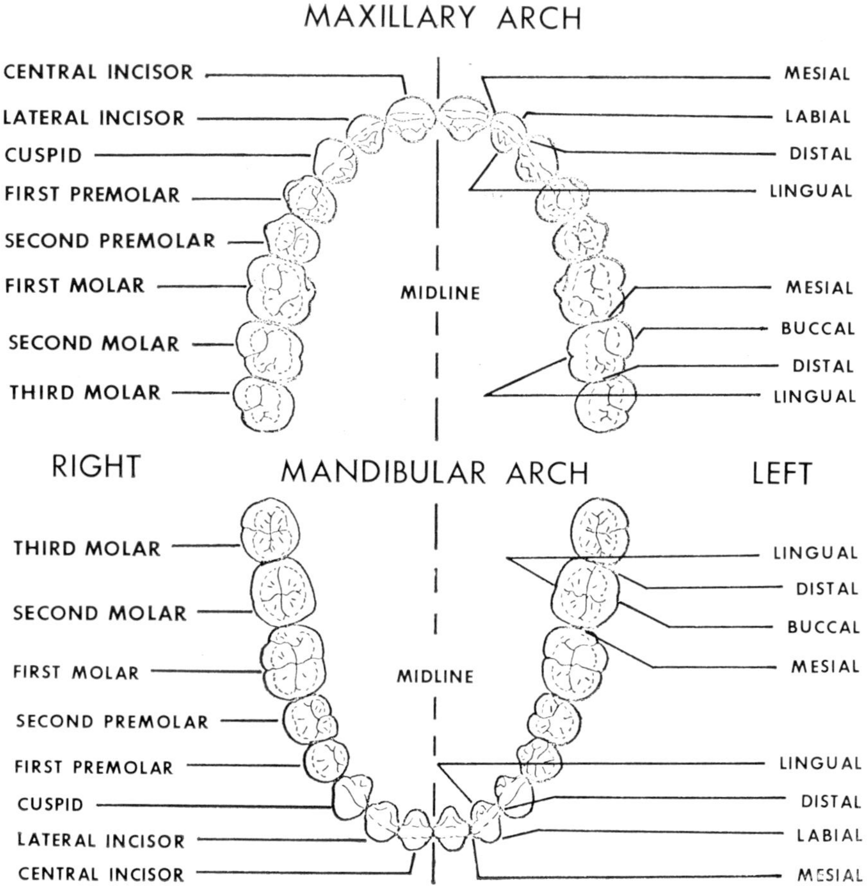

MAXILLARY ARCH

CENTRAL INCISOR —

LATERAL INCISOR —

CUSPID —

FIRST PREMOLAR —

SECOND PREMOLAR —

FIRST MOLAR —

SECOND MOLAR —

THIRD MOLAR —

MESIAL

LABIAL

DISTAL

LINGUAL

MIDLINE

MESIAL

BUCCAL

DISTAL

LINGUAL

RIGHT   MANDIBULAR ARCH   LEFT

THIRD MOLAR —

SECOND MOLAR —

FIRST MOLAR —

SECOND PREMOLAR —

FIRST PREMOLAR —

CUSPID —

LATERAL INCISOR —

CENTRAL INCISOR —

MIDLINE

LINGUAL

DISTAL

BUCCAL

MESIAL

LINGUAL

DISTAL

LABIAL

MESIAL

FIG. 1–1. A diagram of the permanent human dentition. Buccal (toward cheeks), Distal (away from midline), Labial (toward lips), Lingual (toward tongue), Mesial (toward midline). (Drawn by Gary W. Johnston.)

SAMPLE PREPARATION

Due to the anatomy of the tooth it is difficult to obtain dentine-free enamel for exact chemical analysis. In attempts to overcome this sampling problem three methods and/or combinations of these methods have evolved which, although still not perfect, are the best presently available.

Mechanical Methods

A blunt dental chisel can be used to remove the enamel or dentine. This is a tedious and painstaking procedure.

A diamond saw or cutting disc is usually used to obtain layers of enamel or dentine or thin sections of longitudinal or horizonal planes for use as slides in light microscopy or electron probe analysis.

Larger amounts of dentine or enamel material are usually prepared by using a diamond grinding wheel with great care to avoid contaminating the desired material. It is possible that the heat generated from the grinding and the material lost from the wheel may cause some undesirable changes through pyrolysis or contamination in the samples being prepared.

Flotation Technique of Manly and Hodge

Once the tooth has been pulverized, the more dense enamel particles can be separated from the dentine by using a flotation or centrifuge-flotation technique. The particles are introduced into a solution of acetone-bromoform having a specific gravity of 2.70. Enamel having a density of 2.92 ± 0.1 settles during centrifugation or flotation, while the lighter dentine with a density of about 2.40 floats on the surface permitting either fraction to be readily collected (Fig. 1-3). A single separation gives enamel and dentine of 99% purity as determined by a refractive index method. Cementum, density 2.03, can also be separated by this technique.

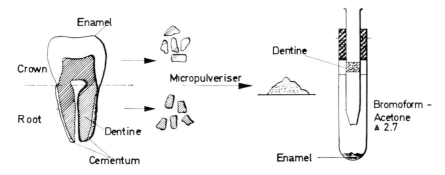

FIG. 1-3. Procedure involved in the separation methods of the dental tissues.
(Courtesy of W. C. Armstrong.)

Chemical Methods

Acids have been used to etch away successive layers of enamel and dentine to give either solutions of the desired soluble material or pure residues of wanted material. By adjusting the strength of the acid and the etching time, any thickness from as low as 10 microns may be achieved.

HARDNESS

The Knoop hardness numbers (KHN) on sections of mature, freshly extracted, human, noncarious teeth gave an overall average of 343 ± 23 kg/mm^2 for enamel and 68 ± 3 for dentine. These would be comparable to the mineral magnesia, MgO, or periclase (a good refractory material), and metallic silver respectively. No definite trend was detected in the hardness of the enamel from the dentino-enamel junction to the outer surface or from the crown to the cervical margin. The dentine showed no change in hardness from one area to another.

Recent studies show that sound enamel is mechanically isotropic for microhardness tests as long as the impression covers several enamel rods. Hardness has also been correlated with the local calcium content and can be used as an indication of mineralization, demineralization, and remineralization. The well-known softness of carious enamel indicates that the densely packed crystallites have probably been affected by acid dissolution or that a partial transformation of the normal calcified material into one of similar composition but different physical properties has occurred.

CHEMICAL COMPOSITION

A tooth, unlike a shaker full of recrystallized salt, has no single, constant chemical stoichiometry. It has been constituted and shaped by a unique genetic and biochemical individual and therefore can be as varied as nature will permit. On reporting the composition of a tooth one must constantly keep in mind the effects of diet, position in the mouth, geographical locality, age, condition of the tooth and medical history of the contributing individual. In the instances where these facts and their effects are known, they will be noted.

INORGANIC CONSTITUENTS

Certainly one of the earliest descriptions of the composition of mineralized tissues was made by Empedokles of Akragas (492–432 B.C.), founder of the Sicilian School of Medicine, who described mineralized tissue as consisting of 2 parts water, 4 of fire, and 2 (or 8) of earth. Later, Aristotle (384–322 B.C.), the Greek philosopher and educator, decided bone was 3 parts fire and 2 parts earth.

In the spring of 1770, C. W. Scheele discovered the presence of calcareous earth ($CaCO_3$) and an unknown substance combined with lime (CaO) in hartshorn. J. G. Gahn, acting on the information, found that the unknown substance was phosphoric acid, thus they both share the credit for the discovery that the phosphate of lime was the principal component of bone. By 1799, Hatchett (1756–1847) was able to show that the three different structures of an elephant's tooth were composed of lime and phosphoric acid and the differences are probably due to "a small change in the proportions of their constituent principles and by a different arrangement." Hatchett also reported that shells of eggs and marine animals were made up of a carbonate of lime.

By 1803, W. H. Pepys, Jr., reported the first quantitative analyses of human tooth enamel in Joseph Foxes "The Natural History of the Human Tooth." His analysis gave 78% phosphate of lime, 6% carbonate of lime, and a 16% loss which was "chiefly water."

Later, analytical chemists in the middle of the 19th century knew that tooth consisted mainly of "phosphate of lime" with lesser amounts of "phosphate of magnesium, carbonate of lime, soda, salts, water and organic matter." By the end of the century, Tomes reported an average of 72.5% lime salts in dentine. Carious teeth had 1% fewer lime salts, and molars and bicuspids were more highly calcified than incisors and canines, 73.2 versus 71.5%. More recent studies show that incisors possess about 30% enamel with the percentage increasing gradually from the canines to the molars which contain about 40% enamel. By 1906, a complete and accurate analysis of the inorganic and organic elemental composition of the enamel and dentine of pooled teeth was reported.

After the first quarter of this century, Armstrong and others decided that a comprehensive study of the analysis of enamel and dentine by "modern methods" was necessary to understand the calcification process. They concluded that the mineral phase of enamel and dentine were not identical, that carious and sound teeth do not differ in the elements determined, that no correlation of enamel composition with susceptibility to decay or with an eruption age existed and that variations in enamel composition are as great in the teeth of one person as in teeth from several individuals.

Contrary to Armstrong, in the following year French and her co-workers found that the average calcium to phosphorus ratio (Ca/P) for dentine was the same as for enamel and the mineral, hydroxyapatite. They concluded that the dentine and enamel consisted principally of "particles of hydroxyapatite with occluded, absorbed or interstitially crystallized carbonates and other salts."

Tooth Analysis

In 1937, Lefevre and Hodge reported the values in Table 1–1 for the chemical analysis of teeth. Their data permitted the following conclusions:

Table 1–1. Inorganic Composition of Human Teeth, Enamel, and Dentine

Chemical	Teeth %	Enamel, Dry Wt.% Sound	Enamel, Dry Wt.% Carious	Dentine, Dry Wt.% Sound and Carious
Mineral Cont.		95		70
H_2O	8.98 ± 2.23	2.02 ± 0.04	3.07 ± 0.05	3.57 ± 0.103
Ca	35.2 ± 0.76	36.75 ± 0.17	35.95 ± 0.21	28.2 ± 1.2
P	16.8 ± 0.36	17.4 ± 0.04	17.01 ± 0.06	13.5 ± 2.8
Mg	0.32 ± 0.25	0.54 ± 0.01	0.40 ± 0.01	0.83 ± 0.083
CO_2	3.45 ± 0.26	2.42 ± 0.02	1.56 ± 0.03	3.57 ± 0.103
Ca/P	2.10 ± 0.03	2.09 ± 0.02	2.08 ± 0.03	2.05

(1) deciduous teeth have more moisture, less inorganic residue, Ca and P, and about the same carbonate content as permanent teeth, (2) there is little difference, except in moisture content, between sound and carious teeth, (3) age causes no change in the chemical constitution of teeth, (4) there is little chemical difference between teeth from male and female patients, (5) increasing severity of pyorrhea may cause a decrease in the carbonate content of teeth, and (6) the composition of tooth substance is remarkably constant.

Calcium and Phosphorus

The latest studies show that Ca, P and Ca/P ratio are slightly lower in carious than in sound enamel (Table 1–1). Sound enamel from age groups beyond 30 years has a lower Ca/P ratio (1.97) than sound enamel from the younger age group (2.07).

Electron probe microanalysis of sound human dental enamel shows that the concentration of Ca and P slightly increases from the dentino-enamel junction (DEJ) towards the enamel surface.

As can be seen in Table 1–1, the Ca/P ratio of enamel and dentine lies between that of octacalcium phosphate, $Ca_8H_2(PO_4)_6+_5H_2O$, 1.72, and hydroxyapatite, $Ca_{10}(PO_4)_6(OH)_2$, 2.15. Possible intermediate compounds include hydrated tricalcium phosphate. Two theories have been formulated to explain the continuous series of apatitic calcium phosphate:

1. The absorption theory, in which acid phosphate groups absorb to microcrystalline hydroxyapatite.
2. The defect theory, which proposes that hydrogen ions in hydroxyapatite are substituted for Ca ions.

A recent study by Winand involving the physicochemical techniques of infrared spectroscopy, x-ray diffraction, differential thermal analysis, thermogravimetry, and chemical analysis resulted in the derivation of a general formula for the apatitic calcium phosphate series: $Ca_{10-X}H_X(PO_4)_6$-$(OH)_{2-X}$, where x can vary between 0 and 2. In this calcium defect concept it was suggested that adjacent orthophosphate groups of the apatitic lattice are linked by hydrogen bonds. In this dynamic crystalline system, magnesium can substitute for calcium and carbonate can replace the phosphate radical to a limited extent.

Electron probe microanalyses of individual human enamel rods gave a Ca/P ratio of 2.16 ± 0.07 for the sheath area compared to 2.07 ± 0.06 for the core. Therefore, the bulk of the enamel core material is composed of calcium-deficient hydroxyapatite, whereas the peripheral or sheath area has an almost exact stoichiometry.

Levine, using a micropuncture sampling technique, was able to show a lower calcium (0.45 ± 0.11 mg/mm^3) and phosphorus (0.20 ± 0.07 mg/mm^3) level in the dentine near the pulp chamber than that at the DEJ. The mean Ca/P ratio was 2.04 ± 0.31 with no detectable trend in the ratio demonstrable throughout the dentine. When it is assumed that dry dentine has a density of 2, the mean calcium and phosphorus concentrations of 0.520 ± 0.11 mg/mm^3 and 0.255 ± 0.05 mg/mm^3, respectively, are equal to 26% Ca and 12.7% P on a dry weight basis.

Levine was unable to show a significant difference between the dentine in sound teeth and the sound dentine from carious teeth. The wide variations in the Ca/P ratio suggest that dental mineral may be more heterogeneous than heretofore suspected. This variation may occur by ionic substitution within the crystal lattice, such as carbonate for phosphate or magnesium for calcium, and/or absorption of calcium ions. Low ratios could arise from a defective apatite lattice in which tertiary phosphate ions (PO_4^{3-}) are replaced by secondary phosphate ions (HPO_4^{2-}) which require fewer calcium ions to effect electroneutrality.

Progressing dentinal lesions were divided into four defined zones:

Zone of Sclerosis. Usually, this zone is more radiopaque than adjacent sound dentine, however, it is not significantly different in calcium and phosphorus concentration or Ca/P ratio from the sound dentine.

Demineralization Front. An average mineral loss was about 50% with a slightly lower Ca/P ratio.

Body of the Lesion. A mean maximum reduction in calcium concentration of 70% and in phosphorus concentration of 60% per unit volume was obtained for active and slowly progressing lesions.

Surface Zone. Generally, there is a higher level of calcium concentration without an accompanying increase in the phosphorus level resulting in high Ca/P ratios. The extra calcium may result partly from material such as calcium carbonate from the oral fluid. Calcium oxalate precipitation or phosphate replacement by carbonate ions may also provide a possible explanation.

The inorganic composition of arrested carious dentine was investigated by an x-ray diffraction technique and shown to be predominantly hydroxyapatite. Non-apatitic phosphate-containing compounds such as octacalcium phosphate, whitlockite, and brushite were found in amounts from 2–5%. Whewellite and weddellite, hydrated calcium oxalates, and a calcium carbonate, as calcite, were also detected occasionally.

Water

Enamel humidified to a 100% relative humidity loses 1.7% and 2.1% by weight of water at 61 and 100° C, respectively. The use of nuclear magnetic resonance (NMR) techniques revealed that heating to 200° C was insufficient to dehydrate dental enamel. Bone, dentine, synthetic mixtures of hydroxy- and fluorapatite with casein and apatite mineral did not display this phenomenon. In addition, enamel water does not show signs of freezing until it reaches −40° C, and over a 3-hour period only 10% of the water exchanges with D_2O. Possible explanations for these reactions are that the water is contained in capillaries with an average pore radius of 25 Å or that the water is associated with the hydroxyl groups of the apatite lattice.

The NMR results indicate the presence of two types of enamel water, hydrate water and water represented by a narrow line on the tracing. The difficulty in removing the latter type of water component by heating has led to its being called "unbound" but "trapped." It is probably semi-crystalline water associated with the crystallite edges and internal enamel surfaces that act as sites for hydrogen bonding. It has been approximated to be 6% of the total weight of enamel. Others report lower amounts of 4%.

Crystalline hydrate water may be associated with either octacalcium phosphate (OCP) or dicalcium phosphate dihydrate (DCPH). If enamel contains 5–7% total water, the hydrate component is equivalent to 0.35–0.50% corresponding to 1.74–2.40% DCPH or 4.0–5.45% OCP, if it is assumed that all of the hydrate water is associated with either of these compounds.

The internal surface area of enamel has been measured as high as 14–20 m^2/gm estimated from electron microscopy. Krypton adsorption studies demonstrate a system of enamel pores measuring 10 to 300 Å with an average pore radius of 60 Å. The same measurements indicate a volume of 0.25% with a surface area of 0.4 m^2/gm. These figures, which are much lower than predicted from the water content, may result from a nonpenetration of the organic matrix by the krypton. Gravimetric studies of water adsorption on sound enamel have suggested a porosity of about 5%.

Preliminary results on demineralized enamel show a 30-fold increase in surface area after a 14-day lactic acid treatment at pH 4.

Autoradiographs of serial sections of teeth have shown that ^{14}C-labeled glucose quickly penetrates throughout carious lesions and the defective structures and lamellae of enamel. Enamel can imbibe quinoline which has a molecular size slightly larger than glucose; however glucose penetration occurs slowly. The whole dentine is permeable to glucose except for the "calcific" barriers around the dead tracts.

Acriflavin has been found to diffuse more rapidly into enamel than potassium fluoride. The penetration appeared to be along the prism boundary of the enamel rod and was approximately 10 times as fast *in vivo* as *in vitro*. The differential rate of diffusion would result from (1) the usual negative electrical charge carried by the "pore" of the enamel membrane and (2) the reaction of the fluoride ion with the apatite crystal to form fluorapatite. After a 6-hour diffusion, the dye penetrated the entire *in vitro* enamel, whereas it penetrated only 10–20% of the thickness of the *in vivo* enamel after 30 minutes.

Altered enamel increases 150% in water by weight, indicating a loss of inorganic crystals and a replacement by water. Enamel from older persons appears to have a lesser amount of water than that of persons under 30 years of age.

Carbonate

Carbon dioxide (carbonate), unlike zinc, lead or fluoride, has a reverse distribution pattern. An earlier study gave the content of the outer enamel surface to be about 1.5% by weight increasing in a smooth (concave) curve to about 2.9% by weight at the dentino-enamel junction (DEJ). A later study illustrates density and carbonate maps for the same enamel section (Fig. 1–4). The surface region of enamel is extremely variable with respect

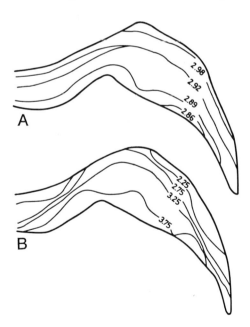

FIG. 1–4. Distribution of density (A) and carbonate (B) variations in the same section of premolar enamel. (Robinson, C., Weatherell, J. A., and Hallsworth, A. S.: Variation in composition of dental enamel within thin ground tooth sections. Caries Res., 5, 44–57, 1971.)

to density and carbonate concentration. An increased carbonate concentration increases the ease of enamel acid dissolution. Carbonate concentrations in the external enamel tend to decrease with age, whereas no changes are observed in the body of the enamel. This compositional pattern may result from a decreasing ameloblastic activity towards the end of enamel formation. The lowered pCO_2 in the crystallizing milieu might result in smaller amounts of carbonate incorporation in the forming crystallites. Dentine and bone carbonate levels of about 3.5% have been reported.

In his arguments against the presence of an amorphous phase in any biological precipitate, McConnell suggests that carbon dioxide is contained in all vertebrate bones and in the minerals resulting from vital processes. Therefore, he believes that the calcified product should not be called hydroxyapatite but dahllite or carbonate hydroxyapatite (CarHap).

Magnesium

Brudevold and his co-workers showed that the surface enamel has a lower Mg content than the body of intact enamel, 30 to 60 versus 60 to 74 μM per gm. Electron microprobe analysis shows that the magnesium concentration is low at the enamel edge (EE) increasing through the enamel to the

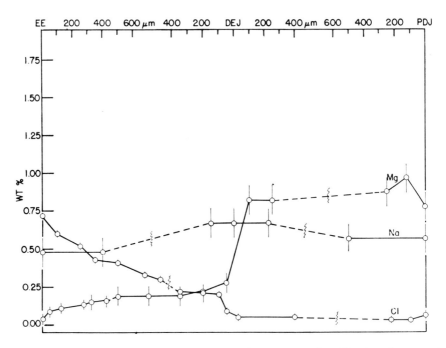

Fig. 1–5. Sodium, magnesium, and chlorine (trace elements) wt% values for enamel and dentin. Specimen 1 (Chicago native). (Besic, F. C., Knowles, C. R., Wiemann, M. R., Jr., and Keller, O.: Electron probe microanalysis of noncarious enamel and dentin and calcified tissues in mottled teeth. J. Dent. Res., *48*, 131–139, 1969.)

DEJ and continuing upward throughout the dentine (Fig. 1–5). Unlike bone, there is no apparent effect on the magnesium composition of enamel related to the presence of fluoride, carbonate, or citrate. Johansen postulates that the reduced content of carbonate and magnesium in carious enamel might reflect a low concentration of these substances in the lesion environment during recrystallization and/or a preferential loss of the substances during demineralization.

Fluoride

Most investigators agree that the caries-inhibiting effect of fluoride is due to its relatively high concentration in the surface layer of the enamel. Brudevold and his co-workers reported their extensive study of this distribution in 1956 (Fig. 1–6). The continuous drinking of water containing 0.1 to 0.5 ppm of fluoride by persons under 20 years of age caused the level of surface enamel fluoride to rise from 419 to 3,370 ppm. A high degree of caries protection occurs when one hydroxyl group of hydroxyapatite ions is replaced by a fluoride per surface unit cell. The rate of fluoride uptake in teeth is much greater preeruptively and accessible tooth surfaces take up more fluoride than inaccessible tooth surfaces posteruptively. This latter

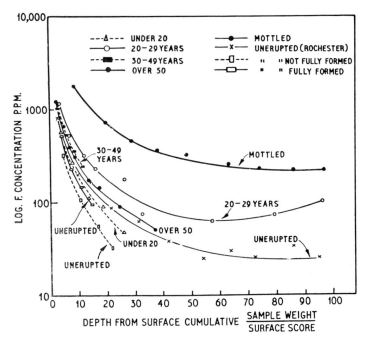

Fig. 1–6. Layer samples pooled from groups of 20 or more unerupted teeth in different stages of development, and of erupted teeth from persons under 20, 20–29, 30–49 and over 50 years of age. All the teeth except the mottled group came from a low fluoride area. (Brudevold, F., Gardner, D. E., and Smith, F. A.: Distribution of fluoride in human enamel. J. Dent. Res., 35, 420–429, 1956.)

fact limits the effectiveness of fluoride exposure on caries reduction since the inaccessible tooth areas are most caries susceptible. Unlike bone, there appears to be no relationship between enamel fluoride and carbonate, citrate or magnesium. Therefore, the inhibition of caries found in fluoride areas is due to the presence of fluoride alone and not to changes in other enamel components.

Fluoride concentration in deciduous teeth follows a pattern similar to that in permanent teeth, although the levels in the enamel surface to approximately 30 microns in depth are lower than in the permanent teeth.

Fluoride concentration shows a consistent increase from the dentino-enamel junction to the pulp. Junction dentine contains 3 or 4 times more fluoride than junction enamel and crown dentine near the pulp shows a marked increase with age, while the remainder shows no change.

The distribution of fluoride in the roots is high in the cementum, decreasing to a minimum in the mid-root regions and again increasing near the pulp to a level equaling the cementum.

Chloride

Chloride is capable of exchanging with the hydroxyl group of hydroxyapatite but is not fixed in calcified tissues. The distribution profile of chloride concentration obtained by electron probe microanalysis shows a gradual decrease from the enamel surface to the DEJ. The surface area showed levels of 0.6% decreasing to 0.1% in the deepest enamel. The distribution of chloride is similar in the enamel of erupted and unerupted teeth. It does not appear to be associated with the water spaces nor does it follow sodium, which is evenly distributed in enamel (Fig. 1–5).

Strontium

The uptake of strontium occurs prior to eruption, probably during tooth formation, since there is no change in concentration with age. The level of strontium concentration is about constant in the surface and subsurface enamel. Residents in areas having water and vegetables with a high strontium concentration have consistently higher levels in their bones and teeth. Whole enamel has been found to have a range of 14–280 ppm with a mean of about 70–115 ppm in three studies of geographic areas having a low strontium level. Whole teeth from inhabitants of an area with high strontium levels in the drinking waters have a concentration range of 485–565 ppm.

Vanadium

Until recently, vanadium was not considered as one of the essential trace elements but, after showing that it is necessary for the growing rat, in 1972 it was added to the list of elements essential for life. It has been reported to promote the mineralization of bones and teeth and to offer a high degree of protection against caries in rodents. Past studies on human dental caries and the vanadium present in the drinking water had been inconclusive, but more recent studies in monkeys indicated a lowering of the caries rate when the element was added. A 1974 study of enamel samples from caries-free premolars from persons younger than 20 years of age and 50 widely differing geographic areas showed a mean concentration of 0.036 ppm (S.D. ±0.037). No relationship between enamel concentration and geographic origin or high and low caries areas was demonstrated.

Lead

It is estimated that lead poisoning affects 400,000 children each year. Ghetto children between the ages of one and six who eat flaking lead-based paint, bits of painted plaster, or putty are usually involved. Convulsions, cerebral palsy, mental retardation, and other disorders—even death—can result from lead ingestion. As much as 85% of the lead entering the gastrointestinal tract is eventually stored in the calcified tissue. Analysis of lead blood levels does not indicate the previous lead intake since there is a drop when ingestion ceases. Deciduous teeth have been found to give an excellent indication of the lead accumulation in individual children.

Preliminary studies on whole teeth from residents of Baltimore and rural Delaware indicate that (1) the amount of lead increases at a fairly uniform rate through age 50 (11 to 27 ppm), when a rapid increase occurs that levels off (50–55 ppm) until age 79; (2) there is little difference in assimilation by males and females; (3) urban residents had lower levels than those of suburban or rural residents; (4) ancient teeth (A.D. 200–600) had low metal levels and no age correlation (5.3 to 2.0 ppm); and (5) cadmium (3.1 to 5.8 ppm) and zinc (1.6 to 3.6 ppm) levels showed no correlation with age.

Previous studies, showing a difference in lead concentration levels in teeth of urban and suburban Philadelphia residents, were not substantiated by these results. An explanation of this contradiction awaits further study.

An investigation on teeth from persons in Birmingham, England, was conducted using the technique of activation analysis, which permits a scan of the distribution of lead in the different regions of the tooth. The exterior and interior enamel gave 38.5 ± 1.7 and 29.4 ± 1.7 ppm, respectively, contrasting with 50.6 ± 1.9 and 41.0 ± 1.8 ppm for the dentine. These results may be explained by (1) differences due to the original mineralization, (2) porosity of the structures and ionic exchange phenomena, (3) rate of diffusion and absorption from the saliva or blood, and (4) the ingestion schedule of the individual.

Trace Elements

Hardwick and Martin, in 1967, reporting on the results of a pilot study using mass spectrometry stated that, "trace elements can be divided into three categories:

Table 1–2. Trace Elemental Composition of Sound Human Enamel and Dentine in Micrograms/Gram (PPM) (Numbers Indicate Mean ± Standard Error)

Elements	Symbol	Enamel 1	Enamel 2	Dentine 3
Aluminum	Al	12.5 ± 2.94	86.13 ± 4.54	68.6 ± 22.5
Antimony	Sb	0.13 ± 0.01	0.96 ± 0.69	0.69 ± 0.41
Barium	Ba	4.2 ± 0.60	125.11 ± 23.68	129.05 ± 54.69
Boron	B	5.0 ± 1.51		94.33 ± 11.47
Bromine	Br	1.12 ± 0.12	33.79 ± 5.71	114.37 ± 2.80
Cadmium	Cd	0.51 ± 0.12		
Chloride	Cl	6022 ± 723	3200 ± 100	350 ± 30
Chromium	Cr	3.2 ± 0.80	1.02 ± 0.51	1.99 ± 0.84
Cobalt	Co		0.13 ± 0.13	1.11 ± 0.27
Copper	Cu	4.20 ± 3.01		
Fluorine	F	293 ± 34		
Gold	Au		0.11 ± 0.07	0.07 ± 0.04
Iron	Fe	4.4 ± 0.95	118.27 ± 71.65	93.38 ± 35.05
Lead	Pb	3.6 ± 0.24		
Lithium	Li	1.13 ± 0.13		
Magnesium	Mg	1670 ± 120	2800 ± 100	8700 ± 300
Manganese	Mn	0.28 ± 0.03	0.59 ± 0.05	0.63 ± 0.05
Molybdenum	Mo	7.2 ± 1.35		
Niobium	Nb	0.28 ± 0.03		
Potassium	K	401 ± 31		
Rubidium	Rb	0.39 ± 0.03		
Selenium	Se	0.27 ± 0.02		
Silver	Ag	0.35 ± 0.07	0.56 ± 0.29	2.19 ± 0.84
Sodium	Na		7000 ± 100	5500 ± 300
Sulfur	S	281 ± 20		
Strontium	Sr	81 ± 11	111.19 ± 9.86	94.33 ± 11.47
Tin	Sn	0.21 ± 0.04		
Vanadium	V	0.036 ± 0.037[3]		
Zinc	Zn	293 ± 34		

1. Losee, F. L., Cutress, T. W., and Brown, R., Caries Res., 8, 123–134, 1974.
2. Retief, D. H., and Cleaton-Jones, P. E., Arch. Oral Biol., 16, 1257, 1971.
3. Curzon, M. E. J., Losee, F. L., Brown, R., and Taylor, H. E., Arch. Oral Biol., 19, 1161–1165, 1974.

(1) Those which appear to have no biological role and which are present in tissues only as adventitious contaminants from the environment.

(2) Those elements which appear to be essential to the enzymatic processes of living cells (*e.g.* Fe, Zn, Cu, Mo, I, Co, Mn, Se).

(3) Elements which are probably essential nutrients but whose metabolic action is not clear (*e.g.* F, Br, Ba, Sr)."

Trace elements may assist in reducing caries incidence by altering tooth solubility, by changing tooth morphology, or by altering the size and/or shape of the crystallites and, ultimately, the enamel structure. Investigators have attempted the difficult analytical task of determining the normal distribution of the various elements prior to attempting to interpret their function or concentration changes.

Losee and his coworkers, in a study designed to determine the occurrence and variation of many minor elements in enamel, and also to ultimately enable interpretation of their influence on the enamel carious process, used a spark source mass spectroscopy technique to analyze 66 minor inorganic elements in human enamel. Their investigation deleted the seven major and most abundant elements in living organisms (C, H, O, N, Na, P, and Ca), the inert gases (He, Ne, Ar, Kr, Xn, and Rn), and the eight naturally occurring radioactive elements (Po, At, Fr, Ra, Ac, Th, Pa, and U). In the analysis for the remaining elements conducted on whole enamel obtained from bicuspid teeth (<20 yr.), 35 elements were present in measurable concentrations while 31 elements, if present, were below the detectable limits of the procedure (Table 1–2). At least 41 elements of the periodic table are incorporated into human dental enamel.

A more recent, thorough study from the same laboratory reported that the elements F and Sr were in significantly higher concentration in the enamel of individuals from low versus high caries areas (DMFT 2.9 ± 0.31 vs 6.1 ± 0.38). Twenty-eight other elements tested were not found to be significantly different in the communities selected.

ORGANIC CONSTITUENTS

Citrate

Citrate occurs in greater concentration in the surface and junction enamel than in the body of the enamel going from values of 3.5 μM/gm to 1.1 and back to about 4.4 μM/gm. Whether the distribution varies with age has not yet been determined.

Citrate, which has been found in all mineralized tissues, may be (1) an accidental coprecipitation component of calcium phosphates, (2) in a citrate-containing arginine-rich peptide, and/or (3) in the form of phospho- or pyrophosphoric-citrate. The foregoing speculations, based on incomplete evidence, indicate that citrate may be an intimate part of the mineralized structure.

Lactate

Lactate follows almost the same distribution and content as citrate and it is possible that both are located primarily in the water in the enamel since a comparison shows similar curves. Lactate, unlike citrate, does not coprecipitate with apatite at physiological pH and its role in mineralized tissue is even more conjectural than that of citrate.

Nitrogen

The amount of nitrogen can be used as a measure of the concentration of organic material in areas of the tooth. Brudevold and his co-workers found that there is no change with age in the N concentration in enamel except that occurring in the last decades of life when measured on a weight basis. There is no theoretical basis to expect that the organic material in a tooth should change with age. Possible alterations may occur from external sources through cracks and voids which would be more numerous in the older tooth due to wear and tear. Teeth over 50 years old differ from younger teeth by having: (1) greater N concentrations in the surface enamel, 0.15% versus 0.1%; (2) greater N concentration at the dentino-

Table 1-3. Organic Constituents of Human Sound and Carious Enamel, Dentine and Bone

	Enamel Dry %		*Dentine Dry %*	*Bone*
	Sound	*Carious*	*Sound and Carious*	*Dry %*
Lactic	0.01 −0.03		0.15	
Citrate	0.10 ± 0.02		0.8 − 0.9	0.82–1.25
Total Organic	1.53 −3.80	3.65–6.98	19–21	24–27
N	0.073–0.077		3.4 − 3.5	4.15–4.97
Protein	0.194–0.275	0.64–1.89	18.2	15–27
Collagen	0.09		17–18	23
Insoluble Protein			0.2	1–2
Carbohydrate	0.015 ± 0.005	0.18	0.2 − 0.6*	0.04
Mucopoly-saccharide	0.1		0.2	0.24–0.4
Lipid	0.6	0.04–0.18	0.2	0.1

* In carious dentine this value is 4%

enamel junction, 0.2% versus ca. 0.12% and (3) lower N concentration in the body of the enamel for a greater depth, ca. 0.04% versus ca. 0.07% N.

Dentine has a nitrogen content between 3.4 and 3.5% which is about 1% less than that reported for human femur (Table 1–3).

Protein

The presence of protein in enamel and dentine has been known for about 100 years. However, the amino acid content of these proteins has been reported only in the last 10 years.

Although much thought and care have been given to overcoming the problem of obtaining pure samples of enamel or dentine, it becomes critically important when discussing the organic composition of the tooth and its separate areas. Since the dentine has about 20% protein which is at least 100 times that found in enamel, an enamel sample contaminated with just 1% dentine, or 99% pure enamel, will have equal amounts of dentinal as well as enamel protein. Any quantitative value reported on such a sample would be the result of a pooling of dentinal and enamel material.

The protein associated with the "tufts," as seen in thin transverse sections of enamel, appears to possess a consistent composition and universal presence in early and mature human enamel. This protein fraction is present in unerupted permanent human molars, mature deciduous human molars, mature permanent human incisors, and mature permanent human molars. Each has a similar amino acid composition. The tuft-like protein is highest in concentration near the DEJ but probably extends throughout the enamel constituting a fine network. As a large part of the interprismatic organic material, it could provide some resilience to the rigid inorganic structure, help to retain water, and aid in the movement of fluid.

As shown in Figure 1–7a, the nonmineral enamel volume varies to a high of 20%, assuming all of the mineral to be pure hydroxyapatite. This space may be occupied by fluid and organic material, mostly protein. The data do not support the possibility of the space being occupied solely by protein or water but is probably an association of both. The protein concentration is high beneath enamel fissures where the density is low and low in the mid-buccal and mid-lingual enamel, which are pockets of high mineral concentration (Fig. 1–7). Disagreement in the literature values, which range from a total enamel protein content of 0.05 to 0.5%, may be due to the area sampled for analysis. Other investigators report a concentration of protein in enamel of $1.03 \pm 0.483\%$ at a depth of 25 μm plateauing to a value of $0.33 \pm 0.156\%$ at a depth of 100 μm. This study also suggests the possibility that a different protein is present in the surface versus bulk enamel. The amino acid composition of human enamel protein differs from both collagen and keratin and bears little relation to them either chemically or physically. The terms "enamelin" and "amelogen" have been suggested as possible names for enamel protein instead of the less accurate "eukeratin."

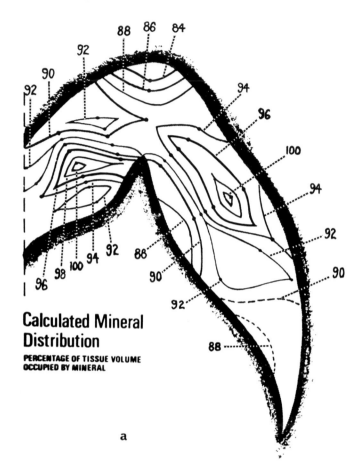

Calculated Mineral Distribution

PERCENTAGE OF TISSUE VOLUME
OCCUPIED BY MINERAL

a

FIG. 1-7. Legend on facing page.

A measure of the concentration of hydroxyproline, assumed to be constant for the dentinal collagen, was found to be about 53 μg/mm^3 near the pulp, increasing in a fairly smooth curve to about 80 μg/mm^3 at the DEJ. The mean concentration for all samples tested was 52.7 μg/mm^3, which would give a calculated value of about 18% by weight of collagen in sound dry dentine. The high collagen concentration near the DEJ may be associated with the von Korff fibers in the outer or mantle dentine, although the origin, composition, and role of these fibers are in dispute. Consistent with the increase of organic matrix and especially collagen near the DEJ is the fall of the mineral content in the same area as revealed by microradiography.

A similar type of study on the distribution of hydroxyproline in carious dentine gave the results depicted in Figure 1–8. The sound dentine in this

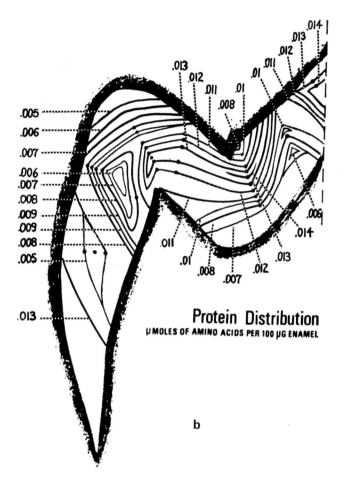

Fig. 1–7. Contour map of percentage of tissue occupied by mineral calculated from calcium per weight data (a). Contour map of protein distribution (b). (Robinson, C., Weatherell, J. A., and Hallsworth, A. S.: Variation in composition of dental enamel within thin ground tooth sections. Caries Res., *5*, 44–57, 1971.)

study shows lower amounts of hydroxyproline than in the previous one; whether there is any significance in the difference is unknown. The increased collagen content in zones B and C may be due to the much more dense organic matrix seen occasionally within some occluded tubules. In carious dentine, a collagenous intertubular matrix is seen with an increase in the granular organic material in the lumen of peritubular dentine. Thus, it appears that, as part of the sclerotic reaction to caries, a collagenous fibrous matrix is deposited in the peritubular and intratubular regions.

The total non-collagenous, non-dialyzable matrix (NCM) of human dentine is about 9% of the total organic matrix, the other 90% being

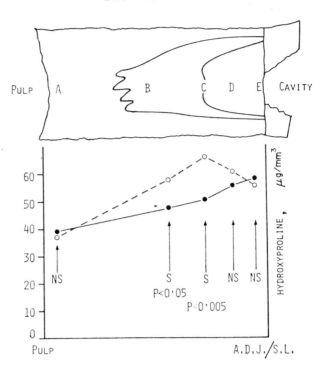

Fig. 1–8. Mean hydroxyproline distribution in carious dentine and corresponding sound dentine related to topographical zones. S—significant difference. NS—difference not significant. O—Carious dentine, series I. ●—Corresponding sound dentine, series II. (Levine, R. S.: The distribution of hydroxyproline in the dentine of carious human teeth. Arch. Oral Biol., *17*, 127–135, 1972.)

collagen. This fraction does not include the smaller peptides, organic acids (citric and lactic), or any molecular entity having a molecular weight less than about 20,000. Human dentine NCM contains a minimum of 20 different components including two anionic glycoproteins, one containing 25% sialic acid and the other being sialic acid free, and a chondroitin-4-sulfate containing proteoglycan in which the protein amounted to 6%. There exists a considerable difference between the minor organic components of bone and dentine.

Carbohydrate

An analysis of the carbohydrates found in human enamel gave the results reported in Table 1–4. Bovine enamel treated in the same way gave similar results. It could not be determined conclusively whether glucuronic and galacturonic acids were present. Clear-cut evidence for the presence of the hexosamines, galactosamine and glucosamine, could not be obtained in the reported study. The insoluble enamel organic fraction contained over 80% protein revealing that the aldoses must be part of a carbohydrate-protein complex. The carbohydrate and protein moieties of the soluble organic fraction could not be separated by electrophoresis indicating the presence of protein-bound aldose sugars or mucopolysaccharide.

Armstrong determined the carbohydrate content in sound and carious dentine hydrolysates prepared by an EDTA demineralization and partial formic or sulfuric acid hydrolysis. The carbohydrate content was arbitrarily expressed in "glucose" units using the α-naphthol, anthrone and cysteine methods. The hexosamine content was expressed in "glucosamine" units of color developed with Ehrlich's reagent. The results are shown in Table 1–5.

Attempts to separate and identify the possible hexosamines by paper chromatography were unsuccessful.

The carbohydrate material in carious dentine may be due to contaminants absorbed from the environment, bacterial polysaccharides, salivary muco-polysaccharides or other external sources.

A study in 1965 on the dentine-cementum and enamel of human teeth used similar colorimetric procedures. The total hexosamine content of dentine-cementum and enamel is 0.08 and 0.03% respectively. The enamel contained 10 times the amount of chondroitin-4- and/or -6-sulfate than hyaluronic acid, whereas the dentine-cementum had 20 times the amount. However, these accounted for about one-half of the hexosamines and the remainder most probably have a glycoprotein rather than a glycosamino-glycan source.

An unidentified component separated from the dentine-cementum hydrol-ysate by a strong cation exchange column made up 15% of the total hexos-amine. The unknown hexosamine, present in dentine-cementum but not in enamel, is thought to be 20 to 30% of the total hexosamine in sheep wool and human hair.

It was concluded that the dentine-cementum and enamel contain chon-droitin-4-sulfate and/or chondroitin-6-sulfate as the major glycosaminoglycan in human teeth.

Carious dentine and enamel are reported to have a carbohydrate content 10 to 12 times that of the sound material. Whether the carbohydrate increase is an important cause or an unfortunate consequence of the carious process is unknown. It is believed that carbohydrates are lost during calcification; the possibility exists that a reverse process may occur during demineraliza-tion.

Glycogen has a wide distribution in the developing tooth and is believed to play a part in the production of mineralized tissue. It has been sug-gested that the glycogen stored in the ameloblasts and the stratum inter-

Table 1-4. Approximate Concentration of Aldose Sugars in Human Enamel

	Galactose	Glucose	Mannose	Fucose	Xylose	Rhamnose	Total Aldose
Mg Sugar per 100 gm Enamel	0.83	0.63	0.23	0.04	0.05	trace	1.78
% of total Aldose Sugar	46.8	32.4	15.1	3.2	2.5	—	100

Table 1-5. Carbohydrate Determination of Sound and Carious Dentine

Dentine Sample	Percentage			
	α-Naphthol	Anthrone	Cysteine	Hexosamine
Sound	0.05	0.4	0.3	0.3
Carious	1.8	4.0	3.7	2.0

medium is the initial source of hexosephosphate which is hydrolyzed by alkaline phosphatase. The phosphate released may be utilized in bone salt formation or utilized in the synthesis of the mucopolysaccharide component of hard tissue. The absence of glycogen from the odontoblasts may be due to the adequate supply of hexosephosphate from the ameloblasts making an accumulation of glycogen by the odontoblasts unnecessary.

SELECTED REFERENCES

ARMSTRONG, W. G.: Modifications of the Properties and Composition of the Dentine Matrix Caused by Dental Caries, Adv. Oral Biol., 1, 309, 1964.

BRUDEVOLD, F., McCANN, H. G., and GRØN, P.: Caries Resistance as Related to the Chemistry of the Enamel in Caries-Resistant Teeth, CIBA Foundation Symposium, Wolststenholme, G. E. W., and O'Connor, Maeve, Editors, Little, Brown and Company, Boston, 1965.

BRUDEVOLD, F., STEADMAN, L. T., and SMITH, F. A.: Inorganic and Organic Components of Tooth Structure, Ann. N.Y. Acad. Sci., 85, 110, 1960.

FRENCH, E. L., WELCH, E. A., SIMMONS, E. J., LEFEVRE, M. L., and HODGE, H. C.: Calcium, Phosphorus and Carbon Dioxide Determinations of All the Dentine from Sound and Carious Teeth, J. Dent. Res., 17, 401, 1938.

JENKINS, G. N.: The Physiology of the Mouth, F. A. Davis Co., Phila., Pa., 3rd Ed. 1966.

JOHANSEN, E.: Comparison of the Ultra Structure and Chemical Composition of Sound and Carious Enamel from Human Permanent Teeth in Tooth Enamel, Stack, M. V., and Fearnhead, R. W., Editors, Williams and Wilkins Co., Baltimore, 1965, p. 177.

LEFEVRE, M. L. and HODGE, H. G.: Chemical Analyses of Tooth Samples Composed of Enamel, Dentine and Cementum, II, J. Dent. Res., 16, 279, 1937.

LEVINE R. S.: The Differential Composition of Dentine within Active and Arrested Carious Lesions, Caries Res., 7, 245, 1973.

LOSEE, F. L., CUTRESS, T. W., and BROWN, R.: Natural Elements of the Periodic Table in Human Dental Enamel, Caries Res., 8, 123, 1974.

McCONNELL, D.: Apatite, its Crystal Chemistry, Mineralogy, Utilization, and Geologic and Biologic Occurrences, Springer-Verlag, New York, 1973.

MILES, A. G. W., Editor: Structural and Chemical Organization of Teeth, Academic Press, New York, 1967, Vol. I and II.

SMITH, H. M.: Evolution of Chordate Structure, Holt, Rinehart and Winston, Inc., New York, 1960, p. 265–278.

ZIPKIN, I.: Biological Mineralization, John Wiley and Sons, New York, 1973.

Chapter 2

Proteins in Teeth

JOHN W. SIMPSON, Ph.D.

Recent development of more sophisticated techniques in protein chemistry has permitted more intensive study of the proteins of teeth. In spite of this, our knowledge is limited principally because of the difficulty in obtaining sufficient quantities of pure material. The proteins of the teeth reside in a highly mineralized environment and their investigation requires careful separation and demineralization of the three calcified layers of the solid tooth—enamel, dentine, and cementum.

Isolation of Cementum

Cementum is the calcified layer which covers the submerged root of the tooth and, in at least one species (bovine), extends over the crown. Cementum has been separated by differential density flotation or removed mechanically either by revolving steel burrs or by a rotating carborundum disc under a jet of water. Recently, Glimcher dissected cementum from the underlying layers following partial demineralization of the whole tooth.

Separation of Enamel and Dentine

Mature enamel is the most highly mineralized vertebrate tissue and in the human tooth contains about 0.05 to 0.2% protein. Dentine interdigitates with enamel, making it difficult to obtain clean separation between the two.

Two major approaches have been utilized to effect separation and purification of enamel and dentine: differential density flotation and mechanical separation under the dissecting microscope utilizing the dentino-enamel junction as a landmark.

AMINO ACID COMPOSITION

As a step in the study of the intact native proteins, investigation of the amino acid composition of the enamel, dentine, and cementum has been carried out.

Amino acids are the fundamental structural units of proteins and are sequentially linked together through peptide bonds, thereby constituting the primary structure of the protein. Hydrolysis of the linkages allows identification and quantitation of the resulting free amino acids.

Preparation of Sample

The calcified tissue usually is demineralized prior to hydrolysis of the peptide bonds to avoid possible excessive destruction of the constituent amino acids during hydrolysis and to avoid inferior resolution during the subsequent analysis. Demineralization is achieved at physiological pH with the chelating agent, ethylenediaminotetraacetic acid (EDTA). The demineralized sample then is hydrolyzed. The common method of hydrolysis involves heating the sample at 100 to 110° C for 20 to 24 hours in a sealed tube containing excess 6N hydrochloric acid (HCl) in a low oxygen environment. After removal of HCl, the protein hydrolysate is dissolved in a sodium citrate buffer (pH 2.2) and further analyzed for amino acid content by ion exchange column chromatography.

Amino Acid Analysis

Ion exchange column chromatography generally has superseded the gravimetric and microbiologic methods of amino acid analysis. Sulfonated polystyrene, a synthetic cation exchange resin bearing many sulfonic acid groups $(-SO_3H)$, is employed for quantitative separation of the amino acids. The resin is placed in a column and is converted to the sodium salt $(-SO_3^-Na^+)$. Amino acids in the cationic form (pH ∼2) are introduced at the top of the column. The cationic amino acid molecule is attracted to the resin principally through ionic forces and displaces Na^+. Each amino acid moves down the column in an individual and independent zone depending on the strength of the forces between the amino acid and the resin. A colorimetric method using ninhydrin reagent is employed for the detection and quantitation of the amino acids in the effluent from the column. Under controlled conditions, the position of emergence from the column and the color response are constant for each amino acid. The method has been automated.

ENAMEL PROTEINS

The organic matrix of enamel is synthesized by cells (ameloblasts) derived from the stratified epithelium of the primitive oral cavity. Developing dental enamel matrix contains a heterogeneous system of proteins which possess some unique features, such as amino acid composition, structural conformation, and aggregation properties. Therefore, the enamel proteins are a separate class of structural proteins referred to as "enamelins" or "amelogens."

Table 2-1. Amino Acid Composition of Some Enamel Proteins

Amino Acid	Mature Enamel		Developing Enamel					
	Bovine[1]	Human[2]	Bovine[3]	Human[4]	Rhesus Monkey[5]	Horse[5]	Canine[5]	Pig[5]
	residues of amino acids/1000 residues							
3-Hydroxyproline	0	0	trace	0	—	—	—	—
4-Hydroxyproline	0	8	trace	0	trace	—	—	—
Aspartic acid	94	57	37	30	28	40	58	39
Threonine	48	42	29	38	42	30	32	39
Serine	102	120	63	62	50	63	58	50
Proline	90	146	213	251	264	221	221	218
Glutamic acid	128	107	156	142	156	153	153	152
Glycine	195	199	70	65	55	61	61	69
Alanine	59	54	22	20	21	20	32	24
Valine	36	36	37	40	42	36	41	35

		1	2				
Half-cystine	11			—	—	—	—
Methionine	5	49	42	51	44	47	54
Isoleucine	28	30	33	25	38	36	38
Leucine	67	61	96	91	92	103	83	95
Tyrosine	7	49	53	52	58	43	51
Phenylalanine	39	31	36	23	16	25	24	25
Hydroxylysine	21	2.5	0	—	trace	—	—
Lysine	35	19	18	17	17	26	16
Histidine	26	62	65	66	56	69	71
Arginine	29	27	23	16	18	18	20

[1] From Glimcher, M. J., Friberg, U. A., and Levine, P. T.: The Isolation and Amino Acid Composition of the Enamel Proteins of Erupted Bovine Teeth, Biochem. J., 93, 202, 1964.
[2] From Weidmann, S. M., and Eyre, D. R.: Amino Acid Composition of Enamel Protein in the Fully Developed Human Tooth, Caries Res., 1, 349–355, 1967. (Partial Amino Acid Analysis.)
[3] From Glimcher, M. J., Mechanic, G. L., and Friberg, U. A.: The Amino Acid Composition of the Organic Matrix and the Neutral-Soluble and Acid-Soluble Components of Embryonic Bovine Enamel, Biochem. J., 93, 198, 1964.
[4] From Eastoe, J. E.: The Amino Acid Composition of Proteins from Oral Tissue, Arch. Oral Biol., 8, 633, 1963.
[5] From Levine, P. T., Seyer, J., Huddleston, J., and Glimcher, M. J.: The Comparative Biochemistry of the Organic Matrix Protein of Developing Enamel, Arch. Oral Biol., 72, 407, 1967.

In discussing the enamel proteins, attention must be given to the age of the tooth because of major differences observed between the developing (immature) and the mature tooth. These differences include (1) total protein content, (2) solubility, and (3) amino acid composition.

The total protein content of human enamel diminishes from approximately 15 to 20% in the developing tooth to about 0.05 to 0.2% at maturity. A similar large decrease in the enamel protein content of the maturing bovine tooth has been observed. An absolute loss of 90% in the weight of enamel protein during maturation has been demonstrated. The process responsible for the loss is unknown.

In the erupted mature human and bovine tooth, the major portion of the enamel protein is soluble in ethylenediaminotetraacetic acid (EDTA) and is dialyzable. Eastoe found that 85% of human fetal enamel was insoluble in water and in EDTA.

Detailed analysis of the structure of enamel proteins has been hampered by the great difficulty in obtaining sufficient quantities of purified material. Several studies on the amino acid composition of enamel organic matrix have been reported, but even in this type of study, the purity of the sample has not been uniform. The principal problem involves preventing contamination of the isolated enamel protein sample with collagenous proteins which reside in the contiguous dentinal and cemental layers. Many analyses of mature enamel have revealed varying but significant amounts of hydroxyproline, an amino acid which is characteristic of collagen.

Recent careful isolation techniques have been carried out by Glimcher and his colleagues using mature bovine teeth. They separated mature enamel from the overlying coronal cemental collagen and from the underlying dentinal collagen. Analysis of the mature bovine enamel revealed an amino acid composition different from that of collagen. It was characterized by a relatively high content of serine, glutamic acid, and glycine (Table 2–1). Furthermore, several fractions with differing amino acid compositions were isolated, suggesting heterogeneity of enamel proteins.

Methods utilized to prepare pure bovine enamel (flotation and microdissection) were found to be unsuitable to prepare mature human enamel, since human teeth are smaller and possess a more convoluted form than the relatively large and flat bovine incisors. By using an acid etching procedure, Weidmann and Eyre have prepared enamel samples of more than 99.99% purity (using hydroxyproline content as a criterion of purity).

Most of the amino acid values of human enamel protein are of the same order of magnitude as those of mature bovine enamel protein (Table 2–1). One notable difference is the higher proline value for human enamel protein. A high serine value is found in both human and bovine teeth, which is apparently characteristic of mature enamel protein. Small amounts of hydroxyproline are present in human enamel protein hydrolysates. Whether hydroxyproline is a pure component of these proteins or represents a slight contamination by dentinal collagen has not been resolved.

Analysis of enamel isolated from human fetal central incisors revealed an amino acid composition different from that of mature enamel protein (Table 2–1). Noteworthy was the high content of the amino acid proline, accounting for about one-quarter of the total number of amino acid residues. This represents the highest proline content thus far reported for any vertebrate protein. Additional important features included the high content of glutamic acid, leucine and histidine. Similar analyses have been carried out on the enamel of developing teeth from 15 different species and a clear pattern has emerged. All the analyses revealed high contents of proline and relatively high contents of glutamic acid, leucine, and histidine. These 4 amino acids constituted approximately 60% of the total amino acid residues in 14 of the 15 species.

The higher protein content of enamel from developing teeth has permitted more extensive studies. X-ray diffraction analysis of enamel isolated from developing bovine teeth revealed a pattern (cross-β configuration) distinct from the characteristic one produced by the triple helical fibrous collagen, thereby establishing the fact that enamel protein is not a collagen. Another apparent characteristic of proteins from fetal enamel matrix is their reversible aggregating properties. In aqueous systems, fetal enamel protein components exist primarily as high molecular weight aggregates. The degree of protein interaction is dependent on several factors such as ionic strength, temperature, and H^+ concentration.

On the basis of solubility, the proteins of the organic matrix of developing bovine enamel have been divided into two major fractions: proteins that are soluble at neutral pH at 4° C and the insoluble residue, most of which can be dissolved in dilute acid at 4° C. Proteins soluble at neutral pH comprise 80 to 90% of the organic matrix and have been characterized as a multicomponent system involving different aggregate complexes of approximately the same size. Available evidence suggests that the monomeric units are small to intermediate-size proteins (approximate molecular weights 3,000 to 18,000), whereas the aggregates vary up to one to two million. By using polyacrylamide disc electrophoresis at alkaline pH in the presence of high molarities of urea, it has been established that the protein constituents of bovine fetal enamel matrix contain at least 20 electrophoretic components. Protein purification techniques have allowed isolation of some of the proteins from developing bovine enamel. Amino acid analyses of the monomeric units thus far isolated show a consistent pattern, *i.e.*, all are rich in proline, glutamic acid, histidine, and methionine, and contain no half-cystine.

The proteins of both developing and mature bovine enamel have been shown to contain relatively large amounts of phosphate which appears to be covalently linked to the amino acid residue, serine. Seyer and Glimcher have prepared four highly purified organic phosphorous-containing polypeptides from the organic matrix of developing bovine enamel. Two of the four peptides constitute 15 to 20% of the neutral pH-soluble proteins and have been studied in detail. One polypeptide is characterized by its high content of leucine while the other contained relatively large amounts of tyrosine. The molecular weight of both polypeptides was estimated to be 6,000. A possible role of protein-bound serine phosphate in initiating nuclea-tion of the inorganic crystals of enamel has been proposed.

PROTEIN MATRIX OF DENTINE AND CEMENTUM

The decalcified matrix of human and bovine dentine is composed essen-tially of collagen. Dentinal protein possesses the distinctive wide-angle x-ray

Table 2–2. Amino Acid Composition of Some Collagens

Amino Acid	Dentine		Cementum	Tendon
	Human[1]	Bovine[2]	Bovine[3]	Bovine[4]
	RESIDUES OF AMINO ACIDS/1000 RESIDUES			
3-Hydroxyproline	—		1	2
4-Hydroxyproline	99	99	105	90
Aspartic acid	46	50	50	47
Theonine	17	17	19	17
Serine	33	38	39	34
Proline	116	118	124	120
Glutamic acid	74	71	80	74
Glycine	329	326	307	331
Alanine	112	125	115	112
Valine	25	21	21	23
Half-cystine	0	0	<0.5	0
Methionine	5	4	3	5
Isoleucine	9	11	12	12
Leucine	24	25	27	27
Tyrosine	6	4	3	5
Phenylalanine	16	12	14	14
Hydroxylysine	10	9	11	9
Lysine	22	19	25	22
Histidine	5	5		5
Arginine	52	47	51	51

[1] From Piez, K. A.: Amino Acid Composition of Some Calcified Proteins, Science, *134*, 841, 1961.

[2] From Veis, A. and Schleuter, R. J.: The Macromolecular Organization of Dentine Matrix Collagen, Biochemistry, *3*, 1650, 1964.

[3] From Glimcher, M. J., Friberg, U. A., and Levine, P. T.: The Identification and Characterization of a Calcified Layer of Coronal Cementum in Erupted Bovine Teeth, J. Ultrastruct. Res., *10*, 76, 1964.

[4] From Lidsky, M. D., Sharp, J. T., and Rudee, M. L.: Isolation, Chemical Composi-tion, and Demonstration of Collagen with an Unusual Hydroxylysine : Hydroxyproline Ratio, Arch. Biochem., *121*, 496, 1967.

diffraction pattern and amino acid composition of collagen (Table 2–2). No significant difference in amino acid composition of dentine is observed as the tooth matures.

Decalcified bovine dentinal matrix contains, in association with collagen, a phosphoprotein component which is presumably covalently linked to collagen via a hydroxylysine-glycosidic linkage. A similar soluble phosphoprotein has been isolated from EDTA extracts of unerupted bovine dentine. The phosphoprotein is present at approximately 0.024% of the total weight of undecalcified dried teeth. Analysis of the phosphoprotein has shown it to be a conjugated protein with the protein moiety accounting for only approximately 50% of the total. Aspartic acid, serine, and serine phosphate account for approximately 75% of the protein moiety. Another striking feature of the protein is the presence of hydroxylysine at concentrations estimated at 10 per 1000 residues. The function of the phosphoprotein has not been established. However, it has been suggested that the matrix-bound and soluble phosphoproteins may serve the dual roles of locating the deposition of mineral on the collagen matrix and of inhibiting the calcification of the predentine.

Collagen also constitutes the major portion of the demineralized organic matrix of cementum (Table 2–2). Glimcher has presented evidence indicating the existence of a layer of cementum covering the crown of the erupted bovine tooth. The coronal cemental layer has both the x-ray diffraction pattern and amino acid composition of collagen and is continuous with cementum surrounding the root of the tooth.

COLLAGEN

Collagen is the major protein of the extracellular connective tissues and functions as a structural protein serving principally as the prime mechanical support of tissues. The amount of collagen varies from one species to another and from tissue to tissue within the same species. Collagen comprises as much as one-third of the total protein in the vertebrate body and in certain invertebrates, such as representative sponges and echinoderms, collagen may account for an even larger proportion of the total protein of the organism. Collagen content of normal human dentine has been estimated to be 18% by dry weight.

Physicochemical Properties

From the standpoint of protein structure, collagen is a unique molecule. Its most distinctive feature, the wide-angle x-ray diffraction pattern obtained in the solid state, is accepted as a fundamental defining criterion for collagen. The x-ray pattern represents a unique polypeptide configuration consistent with a structure of three chains arranged linearly in a helix (Fig. 2–1). When viewed with the electron microscope, collagen from mesenchymal tissue is

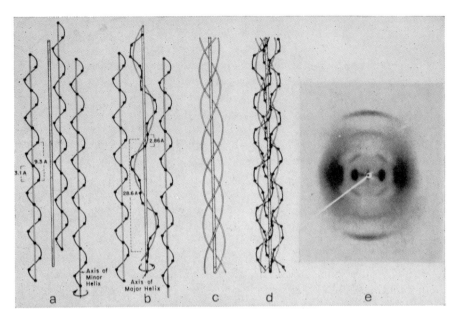

Fig. 2–1. Diagram of the coiled-coil structure of the collagen macromolecule with its wide-angle x-ray diffraction pattern. (*a*) Each of the three polypeptide chains is wound around its own axis in a left-handed threefold screw fashion. Axes are parallel. The screw repeat for polyglycine is 9.3 Å and the amino acid residues (black dots) are 3.1 Å apart. (*b*) In the center, deformation of the axis of one polypeptide chain in order to coil the chain around the axis of the major helix. The amino acid residues are 2.86 Å apart and the screw repeat of the major helix is 28.6 Å. (*c*) and (*d*). Deformation of the axis of the three chains to give the right-handed major helix. (*e*) Wide-angle x-ray diffraction pattern. (Adapted from Rich and Crick, The molecular structure of collagen. J. Mol. Biol., *3*, 433, 1961.

composed of fibrils having a repeated pattern of cross striations, termed the 640 Å (700 Å in the hydrated form) repeating period (Fig. 2–2).

Chemically, collagen possesses some characteristic features. One-third of the amino acid residues are glycine, while the amino acids proline and hydroxyproline account for about 20 to 25% of the total. Half-cystine residues notably are not found in most vertebrate collagens but have been found in invertebrate collagens. Collagens are further characterized by the presence of hydroxylysine and the low content of tyrosine and phenylalanine.

Structure

In the native state, most collagen is insoluble. However, native soluble collagen can be obtained *in vitro* under certain conditions. Soft-tissue collagen from young, rapidly growing animals can be extracted with either cold neutral salt solution, dilute acetic acid, or citrate buffer, yielding a solution of the monomer or fundamental unit of collagen. Radioisotope-labeling

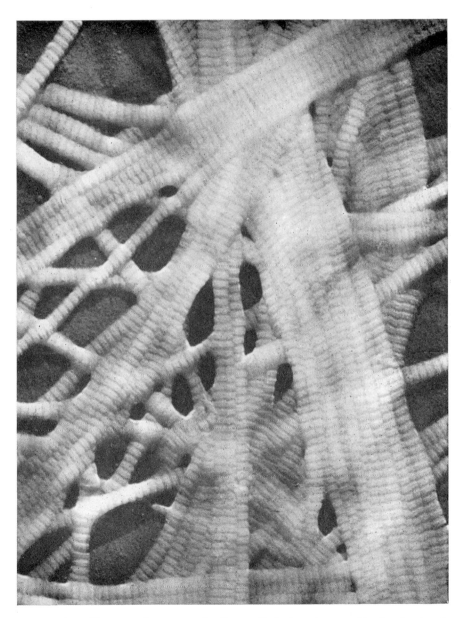

FIG. 2–2A. Electron micrograph of collagen fibrils from human skin showing bands spaced about 700 Å apart. 42,000 ×. (From Gross, J.: Collagen. Sci. Amer., *204*, 120–128, 1961.)

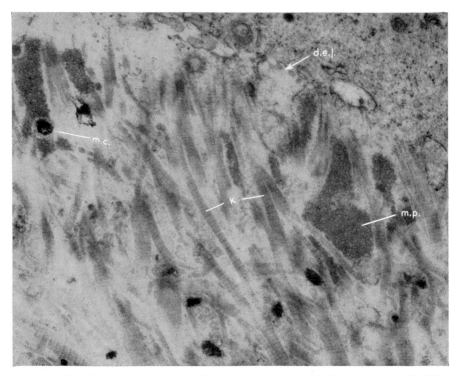

Fig. 2–2B. Electron micrograph illustrating the collagen fibrils in dentine. ×36,000. (From Bevelander, G., and Nakahara, H.: Formation and mineralization of dentine. Anat. Rec., *156*, 303, 1966.)

studies have indicated that neutral salt extracts of soluble collagen represent the most recently synthesized extracellular collagen. Presumably, the collagen is still soluble because it has not yet formed cross-linkages with adjacent collagen molecules.

The solubilized collagen molecule is highly asymmetric, being 2,800 Å long × 14 Å wide, and has a molecular weight of about 300,000.

A collagen monomer consists of three polypeptide chains, each chain being twisted into a left-handed helix. The three helices in turn form a right-handed super or major helix (Fig. 2–1). The triple helical structure is possible only because of the high incidence (one-third) of glycine. The pitch of the helix is determined by the frequent proline and hydroxyproline residues which do not permit the more common helical arrangements.

Denaturation of collagen results in the appearance of three molecular components, termed α-, β-, and γ-components. When a solution of native collagen is denatured by heating or by the action of urea, thiocyanate, or guanidine, the three components can be detected by ultracentrifugation, ion exchange chromatography, or gel electrophoresis (Fig. 2–3). The molecular weight of the α-component is considered to represent any single

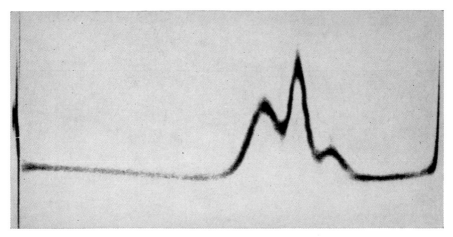

FIG. 2–3. Sedimentation velocity pattern of denatured dogfish skin collagen showing boundaries resulting from single (α), double (β) and triple chain(γ) components in order of increasing sedimentation rate (left to right). (From The Characterization of Collagen from the Skin of the Dogfish Shark, Squalus Acanthias, J. Biol. Chem., *239*, 3336, 1964 by Lewis, M. S. and Piez, K. A. Reproduced by courtesy of The American Society of Biological Chemists, Inc.)

chain of which there are three in the collagen molecule. By chromatographic means, the components from the major portion of vertebrate collagen, including dentine and cementum, are separable into two distinct units, designated α_1 and α_2, which have approximately the same molecular weight (100,000) and are present in a ratio of 2:1; that is, the chain composition is $[\alpha_1]_2 \alpha_2$.

Recently, collagens with alpha chains with amino acid compositions different from α_1 and α_2 have been described. Arbitrarily, these alpha chains have been designated α_1 in conjunction with a Roman numeral designating their sequence of discovery. Previously described alpha chains with amino acid compositions different from α_1 have retained their original nomenclature, *e.g.*, α_2 and α_3. Thus, the first described and predominant collagen type contains $\alpha_1(I)$ and α_2 type chains and has a chain composition of $[\alpha_1(I)]_2\alpha_2$.

A minor but significant portion of vertebrate collagens have chain compositions different from $[\alpha_1(I)]_2\alpha_2$ (Table 2–3). For example, cartilage collagen is comprised almost entirely of molecules containing three identical chains with respect to amino acid composition and sequence. These chains are designated $\alpha_1(II)$ and the molecular chain composition is designated $[\alpha_1(II)]_3$. Other vertebrate tissues containing genetically distinct α-chains and collagen molecules with three identical chains are skin and basement membrane. In addition to collagens with three identical chains, the collagen monomer of codfish skin contains three nonidentical α-chains and consists of chain composition $[\alpha_1, \alpha_2, \alpha_3]$.

Table 2–3. Tissue Distribution and Molecular Form of Known Types of Collagen α-Chains

Chain	Molecular Form	Distribution
$\alpha_1(I)$ and α_2	$[\alpha_1(I)]_2\,\alpha_2$	Bone Dentine Tendon Dermis
$\alpha_1(II)$	$[\alpha_1(II)]_3$	Cartilages
$\alpha_1(III)$	$[\alpha_1(III)]_3$	Young dermis Cardiovascular system
$\alpha_1(IV)$	$[\alpha_1(IV)]_3$	Several basement membranes

From Miller, E. J., and Matukas, V. J.: Biosynthesis of Collagen, Fed. Proc., *33*, 1199, 1974.

The β-components have a molecular weight of 200,000 and an amino acid composition indicating they are dimers consisting of two α-chains. These are formed by covalent cross-links between the α-chains.

Gamma-components have the same amino acid composition as that of unfractionated tropocollagen and probably represent many possible combinations of trimers of covalently linked α-chains.

Primary Structure of α-*Chains.* Significant advances have been made in elucidating the primary structure of α-chains. The use of carboxymethyl-cellulose chromatography for separation of collagen α-chains and classic techniques in protein chemistry have led to the determination of the complete amino acid sequence of an $\alpha_1(I)$ chain (more than 1000 amino acid residues). From this work, the collagen α-chain may be defined as a linear sequence of amino acids, linked only by α-amino, α-carboxyl peptide bonds. The α-chains are characterized by glycine at every third position for more than 95% of their length.

Amino- and carboxy-terminal ends of collagen α-chains do not contain the repetitive glycine structure. Therefore, short sequences (16 or 17 residues) called telopeptides, which differ in structure from the rest of the collagen molecule in that they are probably devoid of the polyproline kind of helical structure, are present at the terminal ends of the α-chains. The N-terminal telopeptide region of the α-chains contains the specific lysine and hydroxylysine residues that eventually take part in intramolecular cross-link formation. Also, the N-terminal region contains part of the immunogenic determinants of the collagen molecule.

Carbohydrate Content

Highly purified collagens contain a small amount of carbohydrate, identified as hexoses, covalently bound to the collagen polypeptide chains through the hydroxyl groups of hydroxylysine. Some hydroxylysine residues in vertebrate collagen are glycosidically linked to one molecule of galactose, whereas others are glycosidically linked to the disaccharide unit 2-O-α-D-glucopyranosyl-D-galactose (Fig. 2–4). The monosaccharide and disaccharide units are covalently bound through O-glycosidic linkages to the δ-carbon of hydroxylysine.

The number of carbohydrate groups in an α-chain is correlated with the number of hydroxylysine residues in the chain. α_1(I)- and α_2-chains, which possess the smallest amount of hydroxylysine, contain one to two carbohydrate units per chain; α_1(II)-chains contain an intermediate amount of hydroxylysine and have approximately 10 carbohydrate units per chain; and α_1(IV)-chains have much higher quantities of hydroxylysine and contain over 30 carbohydrate groups.

Patterns of carbohydrate content of the same collagen type may vary among tissues. For example, when the carbohydrate content in collagen from adult human skin is compared with human bone, the same proportion (about 30%) of the hydroxylysine is glycosylated in both, but the ratio of glucosylgalactosylhydroxylysine to galactosylhydroxylysine in bone (0.5) is different from that in skin (2.0). The physiological significance of different patterns of collagen glycosylation in mineralized and soft tissues is not understood.

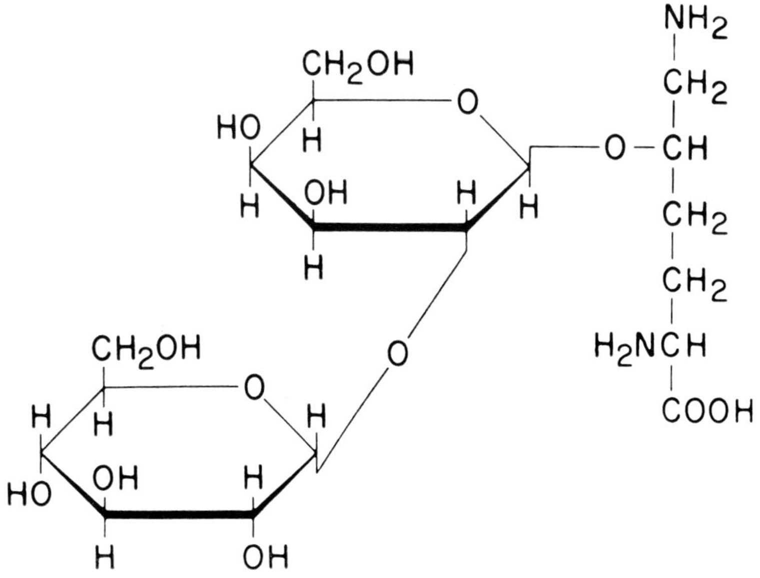

FIG. 2–4. 2-0-α-D-glucopyranosyl-0-β-D-galactopyranosylhydroxylysine.

Cross-links

In general, stability and solubility properties of proteins can be imparted by several molecular forces, such as hydrogen bonds, hydrophobic bonds, electrostatic bonds, or covalent bonds. Available information indicates that stability and solubility properties of collagen are, for the most part, imparted by a system of covalent bonds called cross-links. The cross-linking system consists of covalent bonds between alpha chains and includes both intramolecular and intermolecular cross-links. The cross-links are derived from protein-bound lysine and hydroxylysine and their aldehyde derivatives, allysine and hydroxyallysine. Cross-linking may be conceived as forming between chains through an aldol condensation reaction between allysyl or hydroxyallysyl residues or as Schiff bases arising from lysine or hydroxylysine and their aldehyde derivatives (Fig. 2–5).

Several types of cross-links have been isolated from collagens derived from various tissues. Depending on the participating residues, the initial condensation product, and the subsequent chemical modifications, collagens may contain any of a variety of cross-links. A major type of cross-link in highly insoluble collagens of calcified structures, such as bone, dentine and cartilage, has been identified as dehydrodihydroxylysinonorleucine and its derivatives (Fig. 2–6). Evidence suggesting that dehydrodihydroxylysinonorleucine is present in tissues in the reduced form (dihydroxylysinonorleucine) or as the keto-amine derivative has been presented. Such stabilized forms of

A. LYSINE TO ALLYSINE CONVERSION

$$P-CH_2-CH_2-CH_2-CH_2-NH_2 \longrightarrow P-CH_2-CH_2-CH_2-CHO$$

Lysine　　　　　　　　　　　　　　　　Allysine

B. ALDOL CONDENSATION

$$P-CH_2-CH_2-CH_2-CHO + OHC-CH_2-CH_2-CH_2-P'$$
$$\downarrow$$
$$P-CH_2-CH_2-C = CH-CH_2-CH_2-CH_2-P'$$
$$|$$
$$CHO$$

Aldol Condensation Product

C. SCHIFF BASE FORMATION

$$P-CH_2-CH_2-CH_2-CH_2-NH_2 + OHC-CH_2-CH_2-CH_2-P'$$
$$\downarrow$$
$$P-CH_2-CH_2-CH_2-CH_2-N = CH-CH_2-CH_2-CH_2-P'$$

Dehydrolysinonorleucine

FIG. 2–5. Represenative reactions of collagen cross-link formation. P represents the polypeptide portion of a collagen α-chain. Hydroxylysine may replace lysine in the reactions shown.

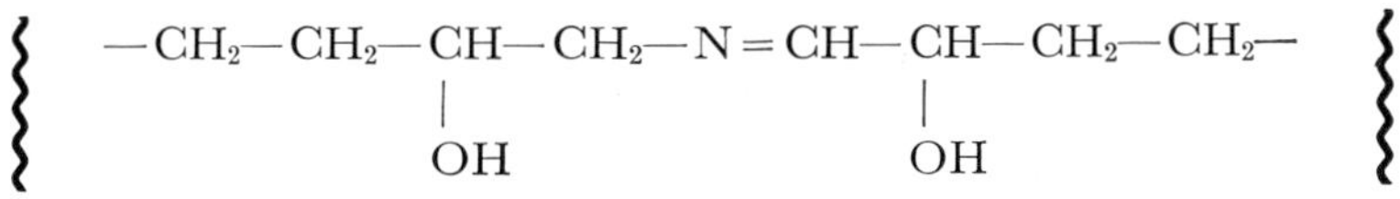

$$\Big\{ \;-CH_2-CH_2-CH-CH_2-N=CH-CH-CH_2-CH_2- \;\Big\}$$
$$\qquad\qquad\qquad\quad | \qquad\qquad\qquad\qquad\quad |$$
$$\qquad\qquad\qquad\quad OH \qquad\qquad\qquad\qquad OH$$

FIG. 2–6. Dehydrodihydroxylysinonorleucine is a proposed intermolecular cross-link of dentine collagen. Its structure is consistent with its derivation from one residue of hydroxylysine and one residue of hydroxyallysine.

dehydrodihydroxylysinonorleucine have been suggested to be the residues responsible for the insolubility of collagen from mineralized tissues.

Cystine disulfide bridges participate in cross-linking in many proteins. The absence of half-cystine residues in collagens with chain compositions $[\alpha_1(I)]_2\alpha_2$ and $[\alpha_1(II)]_3$ excludes cystine disulfide bridges from participation in cross-linking in these collagens. However, half-cystine residues have been identified in $[\alpha_1(III)]_3$ collagen and disulfide bridges may serve as cross-links in this type of collagen.

BIOSYNTHESIS OF COLLAGEN

Biologic mechanisms for the biosynthesis of collagen α-chains are similar to mechanisms leading to the biosynthesis of other protein polypeptide chains. In general, polypeptides are synthesized by components residing in the microsomal and soluble fractions of the cell. Polypeptides are assembled on aggregates of ribosomes (polyribosome or polysome) through the interaction of (1) messenger ribonucleic acid (mRNA), (2) soluble or transfer RNA (tRNA), (3) soluble enzymes required for the formation of amino acyl-tRNA complexes and for the transfer of these complexes to mRNA on the polysome, (4) energy source (adenosine triphosphate generating system), (5) Mg^{++}, and (6) guanosine triphosphate (Fig. 2–7).

Experimental evidence from *in vitro* collagen-synthesizing systems indicates that collagen α-chain polypeptides are assembled by the activation of intracellular free amino acids, then coupled with specific transfer RNAs, and subsequently incorporated into peptide linkages in an order directed by messenger RNA for collagen. Pulse labeling experiments have demonstrated that the α-chains are assembled throughout their length by sequential addition of individual amino acids. The chick embryo polysome fraction that is capable of completing and releasing nascent α-chains is the size expected for a monocistronic message.

Procollagen

Similar to the biosynthesis of many other proteins, the α-chains of collagen are initially synthesized as larger precursor molecules which are subsequently modified by proteolysis to the functional protein. The biosynthetic precursor of collagen, procollagen, has been identified and studied in some detail.

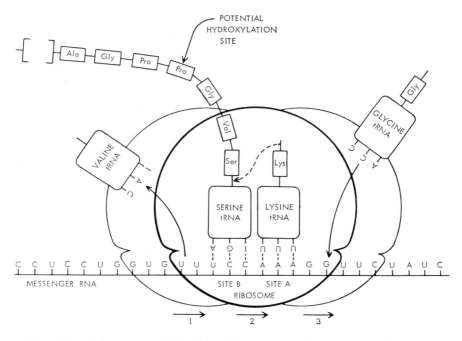

Fɪɢ. 2–7. Collagen is synthesized by ribosomes according to coded instructions of messenger ribonucleic acid (mRNA). The code letters of mRNA are four bases: adenine (A), guanine (G), cytosine (C), and uracil (U). A sequence of three bases, called a codon, is required to specify each amino acid, except hydroxyproline and hydroxylysine. Each amino acid (again, except hydroxyproline and hydroxylysine) is carried to the ribosome by a particular form of RNA called transfer RNA (tRNA) which carries an anticodon (three bases) that forms a temporary bond with one of the codons in mRNA. The ribosome is shown moving along the chain of mRNA. Two binding sites for tRNA appear to exist on the ribosome: one site (A) for a newly arrived tRNA molecule and another (B) for holding the growing polypeptide chain. Hydroxylation of proline and lysine occurs after these amino acids are incorporated into the growing polypeptide chain.

Denaturation of procollagen yields pro-α-chains with a molecular weight greater than α-chains by approximately 15 to 20%. Evidence for an NH₂-terminal location for at least a major part of the additional amino acid residues in procollagen was obtained by electron microscopic studies. Amino acid analysis of the pro-α₁-chain of chick bone collagen indicated that the additional sequence unique to the precursor lacked the one-third glycine and high imino acid content characteristic of collagen. Instead, the sequence, when compared with collagen, was rich in aspartic acid, glutamic acid, and serine, contained a higher content of tyrosine and histidine, and contained cystine.

After the synthesis of procollagen, functional collagen is formed by several steps: (1) hydroxylation of proline and lysine, (2) helix formation, (3) gly-

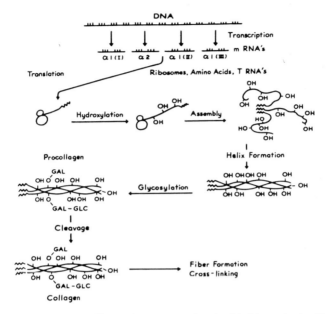

FIG. 2–8. Schematic diagram illustrating the steps involved in biosynthesis of functional collagen. (From Miller, E. J., and Matukas, V. J.: Biosynthesis of Collagen, Fed. Proc., *33*, 1198, 1974.)

cosylation, (4) transport and secretion, (5) procollagen–collagen conversion, (6) fiber formation, and (7) cross-linking (Fig. 2–8).

Hydroxylation of Proline and Lysine

Both proline and lysine are incorporated into growing collagen α-chains but hydroxyproline and hydroxylysine are not. Therefore, hydroxylation of these residues must occur after their incorporation into α-chains. Hydroxylation of peptide-bound proline is catalyzed by peptidyl proline hydroxylase. Peptidyl proline hydroxylase requires as cofactors molecular oxygen, ferrous iron, α-ketoglutarate, and ascorbic acid. Purified peptidyl proline hydroxylase is devoid of lysyl hydroxylase activity. Another enzyme, peptidyl lysine hydroxylase, hydroxylates certain lysyl residues which are, for the most part, those located in the third position of the collagen triplet. Peptidyl lysine hydroxylase requires the same cofactors as peptidyl proline hydroxylase.

Some progress has been made in understanding the nature of the peptidyl proline hydroxylase substrate. The best evidence indicates that the major part of hydroxyproline synthesis is accomplished prior to release of polypeptides from ribosomes. In the growing chains, prolyl residues preceding glycyl residues constitute the potential substrate for the hydroxylating enzyme. The minimal length of ribose-bound polypeptide required for the initiation of hydroxylation has not been established. However, studies with synthetic polypeptides of the form $(Pro-Pro-Gly)_n$ as substrate for peptidyl proline hydroxylase have shown that the effectiveness of the substrate increases as n increases from 5 to 20. For the series $(Pro-Pro-Gly)_n$ the maximal velocity of the hydroxylation reaction remains constant but the Km with respect to the substrate concentration decreases about two orders of magnitude as n increases from 5 to 20. Evidence that suggests that the hydroxylation reactions are terminated as the procollagen assumes the triple helical conformation has been presented.

Ascorbic acid has been considered as a reducing reagent in the hydroxylating reactions. It has been suggested that the requirement of ascorbic acid as a cofactor represents a partial explanation of connective tissue defects observed in the scorbutic animal. However, cell-free studies using partially purified peptidyl proline hydroxylase and substrates such as protocollagen (unhydroxylated collagen) have demonstrated that a number of reducing agents including tetrahydropteridine, tetrahydrofolate, and dithiothreitol are capable of stimulating hydroxylation. Recently, evidence has been presented indicating that ascorbic acid may stimulate an activating system for the conversion of an inactive precursor form of peptidyl proline hydroxylase to an active enzyme.

Helix Formation

Whether helix formation takes place as the chains are synthesized or after release from the polysomes is not known. Results of recent studies have shown that unhydroxylated collagen is not sufficiently stable to maintain triple-helical conformation at 37° C. Therefore, it would be reasonable to assume that helix formation occurs following hydroxylation. The additional amino-terminal sequence of procollagen α-chains has been postulated to play a key role in alignment of the chains for helix formation. Current evidence suggests that after the procollagen molecule is synthesized, interchain disulfide bonds are formed and that such bonds may function to assure alignment and stabilize the precursor structure.

Glycosylation

Another intracellular event in the completion of functional collagen molecules is glycosylation of the protein. Carbohydrate groups incorporated into vertebrate collagens are disaccharide and monosaccharide moieties (glucosylgalactose and galactose) covalently bound through O-glycosidic linkages to the δ-carbon of hydroxylysine. Two different enzymes participating in the glycosylation of collagen have been described. One enzyme, a galactosyltransferase, catalyzes the formation of peptide-bound galactosylhydroxylysine. Another enzyme, a glucosyltransferase, transfers a glucosyl residue to the peptide-bound galactosylhydroxylysine substrate. Apparently the major determinant for the number of carbohydrate groups attached to a given chain is the number of available hydroxylysine residues and not transferase specificity. Since galactosyl and glucosyltransferases are membrane-bound enzymes, glycosylation must occur after hydroxylation and prior to secretion of the molecule from the cell.

Transport and Secretion

After completion of the intracellular events contributing to collagen formation, the molecule is secreted from the cell into the interstitial space. Three modes of transport and secretion are currently proposed. One proposal suggests that after synthesis on ribosomes of the endoplasmic reticulum, collagen is transported within the endoplasmic reticulum to the Golgi region where secretory vacuoles are formed. The collagen-containing vacuoles subsequently move to the cell surface, fuse with the cell membrane, and discharge their contents. A variation of the first proposal suggests that collagen-containing vesicles are derived from the endoplasmic reticulum and move directly to the plasma membrane. It has also been suggested that collagen synthesized in the endoplasmic reticulum moves directly into the cell cytoplasm and to the plasma membrane where direct passage of the molecule into the extracellular space occurs.

The exact mechanism of collagen translocation and secretion has not been resolved. However, the known role of the Golgi complex in other transport systems makes the hypothesis for collagen secretion that involves the Golgi region an attractive one. Strong evidence for passage through the Golgi complex in the case of collagen secretion by odontoblasts has been presented in the work of Weinstock and Leblond. Experiments utilizing microtubule inhibitors such as colchicine and vinblastine have shown that collagen secretion is markedly inhibited by these drugs. Therefore, the inference can be made that a microtubular system participates in guiding collagen-filled vacuoles to the cell surface.

Procollagen-Collagen Conversion

Physiologic events leading to the formation of a functional collagen molecule include the enzymatic removal of the amino-terminal extensions of procollagen. The presence of collagen precursors in the medium of cultured fibroblasts demonstrates that procollagen–collagen conversion is not necessary for secretion and suggests that the conversion of procollagen occurs extracellularly. An enzyme called procollagen peptidase, which catalyzes procollagen conversion, has been obtained in extracts of embryonic chick cranial bone as well as bovine skin, aorta, tendon, lung, and cartilage. Both avian and bovine enzymes are neutral proteases which are inhibited by EDTA. Whether the conversion of procollagen to collagen is a single enzymatic step utilizing only procollagen peptidase or a multienzymatic step remains to be established.

Fiber Formation

When procollagen is secreted into the extracellular space, polymerization into microfibrils begins only after procollagen–collagen conversion. Procollagen is incapable of polymerization, and when the NH$_2$-terminus of collagen is degraded by proteolytic enzymes polymerization will not occur. Therefore, it may be inferred that an appropriate sequence at the NH$_2$-terminus formed by the action of procollagen peptidase is necessary for microfibril formation. After initiation, polymerization is thought to occur spontaneously by the direction of specific interactions of the charged side groups of collagen α-chains. The microfibrils then polymerize into collagen fibrils in a definite manner, so that associated microfibrils are in register

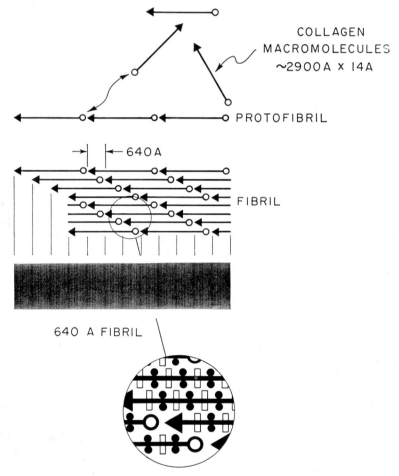

Fig. 2–9. A schematic diagram of the aggregation of tropocollagen to form collagen fibrils. The quarter-stagger array produces the typical 640 Å spacing. (From Glimcher, M. J.: Calcification in Biological Systems, R. F. Sognnaes (Ed.). Washington, D. C., Am. Assoc. Adv. Science, 1960, p. 437.)

with one another, conferring upon the fibril the unique repeating pattern seen by electron microscopy (Fig. 2–9).

Cross-linking

After fibril formation, the collagen fibers are distributed three-dimensionally in particular tissues by a process which has not yet been investigated. In addition to tissue distribution, the collagen fibers undergo maturation, which consists of the formation of covalent chemical bonds between adjacent collagen molecules both within the same microfibril and in adjacent microfibrils within the collagen fibril (Fig. 2–10).

Covalent cross-links between the individual collagen molecules comprising the fiber endow the collagen fiber with characteristics suitable to function as the major structural component of various tissues. There now exists con-

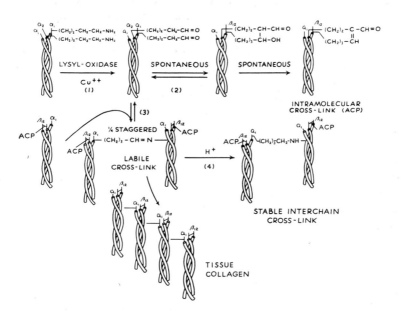

FIG. 2–10. Schematic representation of the steps involved in the formation of cross-links in collagen. (1) The first step of the reaction is the enzymatic oxidation of the ε-amino group of a specific lysyl (or hydroxylysyl) residue to yield α-amino adipic acid-δ-semialdehyde. (2) The second step is the spontaneous aldol condensation to form a β-hydroxyaldehyde. This compound will also dehydrate spontaneously to form the dehydrated "aldol condensation product" (ACP). The ACP represents the intramolecular cross-links in the soluble collagens. (3) Upon proper alignment of collagen fibrils (one-quarter staggering), the residues of α-amino adipic acid-δ-semialdehyde (or hydroxyl derivative) will form a Schiff base with the ε-amino group of a hydroxylysyl (or lysyl) residue, thus forming the "labile" intermolecular cross-link. (4) Available information indicates that the major intermolecular cross-links of mineralized tissue are stabilized after reduction or Amadori rearrangement (oxidation–reduction to the keto-amine derivative). (Adapted from Perez-Tamayo, R., and Rojkind, M.: *Molecular Pathology of Connective Tissues*, New York, Marcel Dekker, Inc., 1973, p. 141.)

vincing evidence that the cross-links are mediated through aldehydes derived from lysyl and hydroxylysyl residues. The initial step in cross-link formation occurs through oxidative deamination of the ε-carbon of specific lysyl and hydroxylysyl residues. The product of the oxidative deamination of lysine is the δ-semialdehyde of α-amino adipic acid (allysine). Oxidative deamination of the ε-amino group of peptidyl-bound lysine is catalyzed by an amine oxidase, designated lysyl oxidase. It may be presumed that the aldehyde derivative of hydroxylysine, δ-hydroxy, α-amino adipic-δ-semi-aldehyde (hydroxyallysine) is also formed by enzymatic oxidative deamination of the ε-amino group of hydroxylysine. Lysyl oxidase appears to be a pyridoxal phosphate and copper-containing enzyme. Lathyrogens, such as β-aminopropionitrile, inhibit lysyl oxidase which indicates that the inhibitory effect of these reagents in cross-link formation is at the step requiring oxidative deamination of lysyl or hydroxylysyl residues.

After the formation of allysyl and hydroxyallysyl residues, intramolecular and intermolecular cross-link formation is thought to follow spontaneously. Available information indicates that the initial intramolecular cross-link of soluble collagen is derived by aldol condensation. In intermolecular cross-links, Schiff base formation is apparently the predominating mechanism. However, intermolecular cross-linking by aldol condensation has not been ruled out. In many soft tissue collagens the initial intermolecular cross-link formed appears to be derived from one residue each of lysine and hydroxylysine, whereas in bone, dentine, and cartilage collagens the predominant cross-link (dehydrodihydroxylysinonorleucine) is derived from two residues of hydroxylysine. As the collagen fibril matures, further chemical modifications, such as reduction or oxidation–reduction (Amadori rearrangement), of the cross-link may occur.

Finally, the mechanisms regulating the biochemical events leading to the biosynthesis of functional collagen remain to be established.

SELECTED REFERENCES

BALAZS, E. A.: Chemistry and Molecular Biology of the Intercellular Matrix. Vol. I, Collagen, Basal Laminae, Elastin. New York, Academic Press, 1970.

BARNES, M. J.: Biochemistry of Collagens form Mineralized Tissues. Hard Tissue Growth, Repair and Remineralization. CIBA Foundation Symposium. Amsterdam, Elsevier-Associated Scientific Publisher, 1973, pp. 247–261.

BORNSTEIN, P.: The biosynthesis of collagen, Ann. Rev. Biochem., *43*, 567–603, 1974.

EASTOE, J. E.: The amino acid composition of proteins from the oral tissues—II, Arch. Oral Biol., *8*, 633–652, 1963.

EGGERT, M. F., ALLEN, G. A., and BURGESS, R. C.: Amelogenins. Purification and partial characterization of proteins from developing bovine enamel, Biochem. J., *131*, 471–484, 1973.

GALLOP, P. M., BLUMENFELD, O. O., and SEIFTER, S.: Structure and metabolism of connective tissue proteins, Ann. Rev. Biochem., *41*, 617–672, 1972.

GLIMCHER, M. J.: Studies of the Proteins of Embryonic and Mature Dental Enamel; The "Enamelins." Chemistry and Physiology of Enamel. University of Michigan Symposium, 1971, pp. 2–4.

GLIMCHER, M. J., BONAR, L. C., and DANIEL, E. J.: The molecular structure of the protein matrix of bovine dental enamel, J. Mol. Biol., 3, 541–546, 1961.

GLIMCHER, M. J., FRIBERG, U. A., and LEVINE, P. T.: The isolation and amino acid composition of the enamel proteins of erupted bovine teeth, Biochem. J., 93, 202–210, 1964.

————: The identification and characterization of a calcified layer of coronal cementum in erupted bovine teeth, J. Ultrastuct. Res., 10, 76–88, 1964.

GLIMCHER, M. J., LEVINE, P. T., and MECHANIC, G. L.: Studies on the source of hydroxyproline in bovine enamel, Biochim. Biophys. Acta, 136, 36–44, 1967.

GROSS, J.: Studies on the formation of collagen, J. Exp. Med., 107, 247–263, 1958.

————: Collagen, Scientific American, 204, 120–128, 1961.

KUBOKI, Y., and MECHANIC, G. L.: The distribution of dihydroxylysinonorleucine in bovine tendon and dentin, Conn. Tiss. Res., 2, 223–230, 1974.

MILLER, E. J., and ROBERTSON, P. B.: The stability of collagen cross-links when derived from hydroxylysyl residues, Biochem. Biophys. Res. Commun., 54, 432–439, 1973.

PIEZ, K. A.: Crosslinking of collagen, birth defects, Original Articles Series, 2, 5–9, 1966. (Published by the National Foundation-March of Dimes, N.Y.)

PIEZ, K. A., EIGNER, E. A., and LEWIS, M. S.: The chromatographic separation and amino acid composition of the subunits of several collagens, Biochemistry, 2, 58–66, 1963.

RASMUSSEN, H., and BORDIER, P.: The Physiological and Cellular Basis of Metabolic Bone Disease. Baltimore, The Williams & Wilkins Co., 1974.

UNDENFRIEND, S.: Formation of hydroxyproline in collagen, Science, 152, 1335–1340, 1966.

VEIS, A. and SCHLEUTER, R. J.: The macromolecular organization of dentine matrix collagen, Biochemistry, 3, 1650–1657, 1964.

WEINSTOCK, M., and LEBLOND, C. P.: Formation of collagen, Fed. Proc., 33, 1205–1218, 1974.

Chapter 3

Carbohydrate Components of Teeth

NICOLA DI FERRANTE, M.D., Ph.D.

A completely developed tooth represents a very specialized type of tissue, since it consists of three different calcified structures. Dentine is the most abundant and innermost one, limiting the pulp cavity and protecting its delicate content of blood vessels and nerve endings. Dentine itself is protected by enamel at the level of the exposed portion of the tooth and by cementum over the dental roots. The amount of minerals in the three tissues is quite different, varying from approximately 50% by weight in cementum to 75% in dentine and 98% in enamel. In view of the elevated inorganic content, the role that the minute amounts of organic components play in the sequence of biochemical events leading to mineralization must indeed be remarkable, and suggests a careful study of the identity, localization, and function of the various macromolecular components. Whereas other chapters of this book address themselves to protein components, this chapter describes the macromolecular carbohydrate components (glycans) of teeth.

Although our interest is more specifically focused on the structural aspects of human dental tissues, many of the studies to be reported have been performed on species other than human. The results obtained reflect minimal species-specific differences, and are particularly useful because they indicate the entity and type of changes occurring in connection with general physiological events such as development, eruption, and mineralization of the tooth.

The glycans found in connective tissue may be either nutritional or structural. Glycogen is the nutritional homoglycan (that is, a polysaccharide made from one kind of sugar), which is found intracellularly and consists of α-D-glucose linked by α (1$\rightarrow$4) glycosidic bonds to neighboring residues, with occasional α (1$\rightarrow$6) bonds occurring approximately every four α (1$\rightarrow$4). The resulting highly branched structure appears in the cells as discrete particles consisting of aggregates of several molecules reaching a molecular weight of about 10^7. Approximately two-thirds of these particles is water, but several enzymes involved in the synthesis and breakdown of glycogen are also present therein. The function of glycogen is to store, as a polymer of glucose, nutritional compounds provided in amounts exceeding the immediate needs, and to make glucose available to the cell whenever it is needed, either as a source of energy required for synthetic processes or as a building block for the synthesis of other glycans. In view of this specific function, which benefits every single cell of the organism, little mention will be made of the presence of glycogen in the various cells of dental tissues.

The structural glycans include two types of macromolecules, the proteoglycans (PG) and the glycoproteins (Fig. 3–1). They have in common a

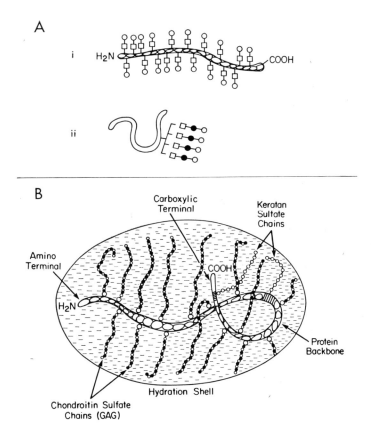

Fig. 3–1. Schematic representation of glycoproteins and proteoglycans. Ai, A segment of a glycoprotein such as those secreted by the salivary glands, showing abundance of oligosaccharide chains. □, N-acetylgalactosamine; ○, N-acetylneuraminic acid. Aii, Segment of a glycoprotein containing a minor number of more complicated oligosaccharide chains. □, N-acetylglucosamine; ●, galactose; ○, N-acetylneuraminic acid. B, Cartilage proteoglycan showing the peptide backbone with chondroitin sulfate and keratan sulfate chains. The exact location of the latter ones is not known. The complex has a strong negative charge when not saturated by counter ions and has a discrete amount of water of hydration, not available to other macromolecules.

single peptide chain serving as a backbone to which several glycan structures of various length are attached through covalent bonds. The two types are not sharply separated, but usually may be differentiated on the basis of their physicochemical properties, which depend to a large extent on the following structural characteristics of their carbohydrate components.

The glycoproteins have one or several short, often branched carbohydrate chains (oligosaccharides) consisting of various monosaccharides linked in a non-ordered sequence (heteropolysaccharides) rather specific for each glycoprotein, and accounting for less than 1 to more than 80% of the weight of the molecule. When the commonly occurring monosaccharides are D-galactose, D-mannose, D-glucose, L-fucose, D-xylose, N-acetyl-D-glucosamine, N-acetyl-D-galactosamine, the carbohydrate chains have a neutral charge. Frequently, however, sialic acid residues or its various derivatives are present at the free terminal of the chain, conferring on it a strong negative charge; hexuronic acid and sulfate are normally absent (Fig. 3-1Ai, Aii).

Gross analyses of glycoproteins of connective tissue reveal that the polypeptide is usually the major component of the molecule, so that the protein/carbohydrate ratio is frequently in favor of the former. Thus, their overall properties are not very different from those of pure proteins, with a somewhat increased affinity for aqueous solvents and resistance to proteolysis and denaturing conditions.

The proteoglycans may be considered as specialized members of the glycoprotein family, since they have numerous long, linear heteropolysaccharide chains, called glycosaminoglycans (GAG) or acid mucopolysaccharides (Fig. 3-1B). They consist of alternating sequences of monosaccharides, whose structure, type of linkage, and sulfate content account for several types of repeating units. Hexuronic acid (D-glucuronic and/or L-iduronic) and aminosugars (D-glucosamine or D-galactosamine) are the main components of these repeating units, whereas sialic acid and fucose may be present only in rare and specific instances. Because of the presence of hexuronic acids and sulfate groups, the GAG have a high density of negative charges. These, combined with a protein/carbohydrate ratio heavily in favor of the latter, impart to the proteoglycans physicochemical properties quite different from those of pure proteins and most glycoproteins.

Several types of linkage may be found between the glycan chains and the respective polypeptide backbones. In the proteoglycans, a link between the reducing group (carbon 1) of xylose and the hydroxyl group of serine or threonine is frequent, whereas in glycoproteins, an N-acetylaminosugar may be found in place of xylose. These bonds are particularly sensitive to alkali, a finding of considerable importance either for the extraction of glycans or for their fixation *in situ* prior to staining. Another common type of linkage found in glycoproteins or proteoglycans occurs between the reducing group of an N-acetylaminosugar and the amide group of asparagine, this type being resistant to alkaline hydrolysis.

A third type of linkage, commonly found in a variety of collagens, basement membranes, lens capsules of the eye, and some components of the complement system, is formed between the reducing group of D-galactose and the hydroxyl group of hydroxylysine present in a peptide chain. Frequently, a D-glucose residue is attached through an α-glycosidic linkage to the carbon 2 of the galactose residue.

Keratan sulfate is a GAG having molecular parameters, structure, and properties that place it between proteoglycans and glycoproteins. It is usually linked to a protein backbone (in the skeleton, probably the same one to which chondroitin-6-sulfate is attached, see Fig. 3-1B) either through an N-acetylgalactosamine-hydroxyaminoacid, alkali-labile linkage (as in skeletal keratan sulfate) or through an N-acetylaminosugar-asparaginamido, alkali-resistant linkage (as in corneal keratan sulfate). Its chains are rather short, contain D-galactose (instead of D-glucuronic acid) and N-acetyl-D-glucosamine, are branched and, although sulfated, also contain appreciable amounts of sialic acid, fucose, and mannose.

The glycans of teeth have been studied with histochemical and analytical procedures. Both approaches have specific advantages and inherent limitations.

The histochemical methods consist of staining a properly fixed tissue section with various dyes specific for different types of natural compounds. As the properties of these macromolecules approach those of pure glycans and deviate from those of proteins, the problems that the histochemist encounters increase considerably, since glycans are chemically more inert and more difficult to fix in an insoluble form. Thus, aldehyde fixatives (which usually form derivatives of free amino groups present in proteins) are ineffective, and organic solvents (which usually denature proteins and make them insoluble) leave the glycans *in situ* but do not prevent their subsequent solution in aqueous reagents which might be used at a later stage. Heavy metals, which usually fix proteins efficiently, have little effect on glycans, especially those charged negatively. Thus, quite frequently tissue glycans are poorly visualized or altogether absent because of losses occurring prior to their staining. Cationic compounds (positively charged), which may be either colorless or colored (dyes), are capable of forming ionic linkages with negatively charged glycans (polyanions), rendering them insoluble and fixing them *in situ*, provided they penetrate the section of the tissue being studied.

The considerable progress made by histochemistry in the last decades reflects an improved knowledge of the chemical structure of the substrates to be visualized.

The proteoglycans and the glycoproteins containing sialic acid have a strong negative charge at physiological pH (Fig. 3–1); these charges may be balanced with positively charged counter ions, which not only may contribute to their fixation but, when colored, impart a definite coloration to the substrate. Some of these counter ions may be electron dense and suitable for electron microscopy (ruthenium red). When the little specificity involved in electrostatic reactions (that is, reactions occurring between positively and negatively charged compounds) is considered, additional procedures must be followed in order to establish a certain amount of specificity for each given condition.

Thus, advantage may be taken of the different dissociation constants of the acid groups of glycans or other biopolymers by reacting them with increasing concentrations of neutral electrolytes (NaCl or $MgCl_2$, critical electrolyte concentration). These techniques may neutralize the carboxylic groups present in proteins or the phosphate groups of nucleic acid, leaving dissociated and, therefore, negatively charged, only the sulfate-containing compounds. Specific hydrolases may also be used to treat one of two adjacent sections prior to staining both of them. Under optimal condition of fixation and with the use of highly specific enzymes, any difference in the amount of stainable material between the two sections could be ascribed to the removal of a specific substrate. The availability of newly discovered specific bacterial glycosidases and glycosulfatases and their use in conjunction with bacterial or testicular hyaluronidase make the identification of various GAG in tissue sections easier and more reliable. Moreover, ingenious chemical manipulations of the tissue sections have made periodate oxidation suitable for the differentiation of neutral glycans from specific types of GAG.

In spite of all this progress, the histochemical methods remain essentially qualitative, and they are subject to great variability because of differences in purity of various batches of dye, minor variations in the technique employed, and the subjective interpretation of the investigator. Moreover, they still suffer from a limited specificity, as they usually fail to differentiate among compounds belonging to the same class and are frequently hindered by steric factors, which do not allow the various reagents to reach, fix, and stain their substrates. These steric factors may also prevent the action of various enzymes specific for substrates possibly present in the histochemical sections. The latter limitation is particularly evident in mineralized tissues where specific staining may take place only after demineralization. Unfortunately, during demineralization, organic components, especially when scarce, may easily be removed along with the inorganic ones.

Despite these limitations, the histochemical methods offer the paramount advantage of showing the relationship among the different compounds in a given section and frequently reveal zonal, tissual, temporal, or species heterogeneities which may be of physiopathological relevance.

The analytical methods consist of suitable extraction procedures, followed by purification and separation steps dictated by the chemical specificity of the compounds to be isolated. The final products, analyzed with highly specific chemical or enzymatic tests, provide a quantitative measurement of the various tissue components which were extracted and carried through the procedure.

The analytical methods usually involve large-scale preparative procedures to obtain sufficient amounts of material for analyses; only seldom is a quantitative recovery of the various compounds originally present in the tissue achieved. Thus, frequently the results represent an average of the molecular species retained through the various procedural steps but not necessarily of those originally present in the tissue. The analytical methods involve homogenization of the original material, and this unavoidably leads to a disruption of the structural relationship among the various tissue components, as well as to a disappearance of any structural or functional heterogeneity of the sample.

These considerations indicate that histochemical and analytical methods are complementary rather than exclusive of one another. Therefore, it is with a great deal of expectation that the biologist looks upon some recently refined methods utilizing adjacent sections of the same specimen for histochemistry and microanalytical determinations, thus providing an excellent correlation between chemical and morphological structure of a given tissue.

CARBOHYDRATE COMPONENTS

Tooth Germs

The presence of glycosaminoglycans (GAG, acid mucopolysaccharides), glycogen, and other carbohydrate-containing macromolecules in human tooth germs has been demonstrated with histochemical methods by several authors. Fullmer and Alpher and Matthiessen have studied in detail complete series of human teeth at various stages of differentiation and development. In their studies the glycogen content was low at the bud stage, higher at the cap stage, and lower again at the bell stage, when intercellular substance started to accumulate. The onset of enamel formation (amelogenesis) occurred after the appearance of GAG in the dentine and at the dentino-enamel junction; in connection with it there was a decrease of glycogen content, and eventually its complete disappearance in the functioning ameloblasts, suggesting its utilization for the onset of protein synthesis.

The dental papilla, predentine, dentine, and newly formed enamel gave a positive periodic acid-Schiff reaction (PAS), suggesting the presence of glycoproteins.

The GAG were identified in the epithelial components of the tooth germ and, along with the surrounding vessels, have been considered to determine the development of the enamel reticulum. However, the GAG were not demonstrable in the formed enamel, whereas they could be seen not only in the dental papilla, but also in the predentine and dentine.

Histochemical staining methods used in conjunction with incubation of the sections with hyaluronidase suggested that the GAG of human tooth germs are mainly chondroitin-4-sulfate (CS4) and chondroitin-6-sulfate (CS6). The same methods performed at various pH values indicated that hyaluronate (HA) is also present in the papilla.

A biochemical study of human tooth germs was performed recently by Matthiessen and Gelin. The material extracted with and without papain digestion was precipitated with cetyl pyridinium chloride (CPC) and analyzed. On the basis of glucosamine or galactosamine content and sensitivity of the material isolated to testicular hyaluronidase, the presence of HA in an amount roughly double that of CS4 and/or CS6 has been confirmed. Moreover, the results indicate that only half of the CS was protein bound, while the HA seems to be free of protein.

Comparison of the data obtained with the histochemical and biochemical analyses of tooth germs clearly indicates the excellent agreement that may be achieved with the two different approaches, each one possessing specific features capable of providing valuable data for a meaningful correlation between structure and function.

Periodontal Ligament

Studies of the biochemical composition of the periodontal ligament are important because of the ligament's major functions in supporting the teeth during mastication and in maintaining the cementum and alveolar bone in optimal condition.

Bovine molar teeth were isolated with the periodontal ligament still attached, split to remove the dental pulp, defatted, and varnished with silicone except over the periodontal membrane.

In order to dissolve the constituents of the ligament, the teeth so prepared were digested with papain. The digest was deproteinized with trichloracetic acid, and the GAG present in the supernatant were fractionated (1) by precipitation with CPC at various salt concentrations, (2) by precipitation with ethanol, and (3) by column chromatography on an anion exchange supporting medium.

Eventually the various fractions were analyzed, subjected to electrophoresis on cellulose acetate strips, and tested for sensitivity to testicular hyaluronidase. The results obtained confirmed previous histochemical findings and demonstrated the presence of CS4 and CS6, dermatan sulfate (DS), heparan sulfate (HS), and hyaluronate (HA). The amount of CS (4 and/or 6) was roughly twice that of HA, and the sum of CS4 and CS6 was much higher than the amount of DS, to give a composite pattern of GAG not different from that described by Meyer and associates for tendon and heart valves.

Dental Pulp

Histochemically, the extracellular matrix of human dental pulp is characterized by the presence of glycoproteins, GAG, and proteins containing appreciable amounts of ε-amino groups (collagen). The structure of the glycoproteins is not known. Some seem to contain sialic acid as suggested by a decrease of specific staining after treatment with sialidase. As indicated by the study of the chemical and immunological properties of glycoproteins of various organs or tissues, it is possible that some glycoproteins of dental pulp possess a specific structure different from that of similar compounds occurring elsewhere. The basement membrane of the blood vessels of the dental pulp is particularly rich in glycoproteins.

The macromolecules of the dental pulp have amphoteric properties. At a physiological pH, the carboxyl groups of collagen, the glycoproteins, and the GAG confer a negative charge to the extracellular matrix. This has been considered to be responsible for the binding not only of specific dyes, but also of cations of physiological importance.

The extracellular matrix of the dental pulp consists of two fractions, one readily soluble in water and saline solution and the other insoluble and resistant to extraction with neutral or acidic buffers. These two phases are considered to be in equilibrium, and their relative amounts vary in physiological and pathological conditions. Some of these changes occur with age; for instance, the collagen increases and replaces the ground substance, the matrix itself becomes more resistant to proteolytic enzymes and less soluble, and its water content decreases. These changes suggest that in old dental pulp, as in old connective tissue present elsewhere in the body, there is an increase of cross-linked collagen at the expense of glycoproteins and GAG. These changes may be responsible for modification in the distribution of electrolytes and for the high incidence of calcification in aged dental pulp.

In recent years, Linde has been responsible for several biochemical investigations concerning the carbohydrate macromolecules of dental pulp. In one of his first investigations, he studied the GAG of dental pulp from unerupted and erupted permanent mandibular pig teeth. The material was dehydrated, defatted, and digested with papain. The GAG present in the digest were precipitated with CPC and fractionated on a cellulose column as CPC complexes. The various fractions were analyzed electrophoretically for aminosugar type and content, and by infrared spectrophotometry.

The results indicated that the amount of HA present in the pulp increases considerably (from 10 to 25% of total GAG) during development, whereas that of HS remains almost constant and those of CS (4 or 6) and DS decrease considerably (from 81 and 6% to 67 and 2%, respectively).

Some of these GAG (HS and probably DS) may represent contributions from the blood vessels of the pulp, whereas others may be specific constituents of the tissue. The latter are considered responsible for interaction with collagen fibers and water molecules to form an elastic compartment capable of compensating the high pressures that develop in the dental cavity during mastication. These pressures have been reported to be the highest ones in the body, and an elastic tissue would act as an incompressible cushion, protecting the blood vessels, nerve endings, and the odontoblast layer.

The increase of HA during development would be eminently suited for this purpose, and the decrease of CS could be related to the process of impending calcification. The role of GAG and proteoglycans in the process of

3

calcification has been discussed for a long time, and opposite theories have been proposed. In recent years the theory of the possibility that proteoglycans might act as inhibitors of calcification (see section on calcification) has gradually gained acceptance, since it has been demonstrated that these macromolecules bind calcium ions and prevent the precipitation of metastable calcium phosphate. Therefore, calcification would be initiated after the disappearance of proteoglycans and GAG, probably by the activation of specific degradative enzymes.

In agreement with this hypothesis, Linde has demonstrated the presence of relatively high proportions of CS (75% of the total GAG) in the pulp of continuously growing rat incisors. Moreover, he has found that the turnover of these GAG is faster than that measured for the same compounds in other tissues, such as cartilage and skin, confirming that a modification of their metabolism may be connected with the development and growth of the tooth.

It is likely, then, that changes in the GAG composition of the dental pulp might be related intimately to the various phases of tooth development and that the presence of infecting microorganisms capable of causing their premature degradation could severely interfere with the physiological sequence of events.

Cementum, Dentine, Enamel, and Their Cells

Histochemically, the cytoplasm of cementoblasts and cementocytes is usually basophilic. Cementum itself, when demineralized, reacts strongly with periodic acid-Schiff's reagent (PAS) and with Hale's colloidal iron reagent. It is also metachromatic, especially around lacunae, cementocytes, Sharpey's fibers, and the interlamellar regions. The cytoplasm of odontoblasts is intensively stained with PAS; since the stainable component is not removed by a previous treatment with diastase, it is not glycogen.

Demineralized dentine stains readily with PAS, while nondemineralized dentine fails to do so. Sections of demineralized dentine from normal, fully formed but unerupted teeth stain strongly with alcian blue and show metachromasia (to indicate the presence of GAG), whereas predentine does not stain. In nondemineralized sections, however, predentine stains metachromatically but dentine remains unstained. Sections of formalin-fixed, demineralized dentine from infants are intensely metachromatic; with increasing age, the metachromasia is replaced by a moderate basophilia which, in turn, decreases gradually with further aging.

Engle, Wislocki, and Sognnaes have demonstrated that glycogen is present in large amounts in the oral epithelium, dental lamina, outer enamel epithelium, and stellate reticulum of fetal teeth. Perceptible reactions for glycogen were also recorded in the stratum intermedium, ameloblasts, odontoblasts, and dental papillae of a human fetus 130 mm long. Although histochemical methods failed to show glycogen in adult teeth, Egyedi claims to have demonstrated chemically its presence in the insoluble portion of the organic matrix of enamel and, to a lesser extent, in dentine. The presence of carbohydrate-protein complexes in the dentine and enamel matrices of rat teeth and of glycoprotein granules in the cytoplasm of odontoblasts and ameloblasts has been reported. PAS-positive material has been described as occurring in the interstitial matrix of nondecalcified ground sections of dentine from human and monkey teeth, but these findings have not been confirmed. The periphery of dentinal tubules has a substance that is not only metachromatic, but also strongly basophilic at pH 2 to 3. This material surrounds the odontoblastic processes.

The calcifying enamel in the regions between the rods and the cross striation of the prisms is strongly metachromatic.

In summary, various histochemical contributions suggest that glycogen is present in osteogenic and odontogenic cells before the onset of calcification, and carbohydrate-protein complexes are present within the cytoplasm of active osteoblasts, cementoblasts, odontoblasts, and ameloblasts and in the ground substance surrounding them. The ground substance of the stellate reticulum of the enamel organ and the interprismatic regions of calcifying enamel prisms seem to be rich in GAG, as indicated by metachromasia and basophilia. The same reactions for GAG are evident in the ground substance of the dental papilla, in the peripheral regions of the dentinal tubules, in the ground substance of the dental sac, and around the Sharpey's fibers of cementum.

Various attempts have been made to extract and characterize the carbohydrate-containing components of teeth. In 1950, Pincus extracted a GAG from dentine which, on the basis of qualitative tests, was considered akin to chondroitin sulfate. Defatted human dentine powder was extracted with calcium chloride, and the extract was deproteinized with a chloroform-amyl alcohol mixture. The final product, obtained by precipitation with ethanol and glacial acetic acid, when analyzed revealed an excess of nitrogen and low hexosamine and hexuronic acid values. This led Pincus to believe that chondroitin sulfate existed in dentine as a protein complex. It is also conceivable, however, that the material isolated was contaminated by protein not covalently linked to chondroitin sulfate.

In 1952 Hess and Lee extracted powdered dentine from normal human molars with a solution of potassium chloride-potassium carbonate, according to the method of Einbinder and Schubert. Concurrently, they extracted dry bovine tracheal cartilage with the same method to obtain a reference sample of chondroitin sulfate and dry dentine powder with the method previously used by Pincus. The percentage of chondroitin sulfate extracted from dentine with Einbinder and Schubert's and Pincus' methods was 0.64 and 0.75, respectively. The analytical data of the two products, however, were quite different, as the one prepared with the Pincus method was associated with a discrete amount of protein (Table 3-1).

In 1965, Clark, Smith, and Davidson measured the total amount and distribution of aminosugars in enamel and dentine-cementum and isolated

Table 3–1. Glycosaminoglycans Extracted from Dentine

Sample source	Aminosugars %	Hexuronic acid %	Nitrogen %
Bovine tracheae	28.07	29.20	2.13
Dentine (Einbinder & Schubert)	27.78	25.08	2.63
Dentine (Pincus)	15.3	14	
Theory for $C_{14}H_{19}NSO_4.4H_2O$	29.49	31.96	2.31

(From Hess, W. C. and Lee, C.: The isolation of chondroitin sulfuric acid from dentin. J. Dent. Res., *31*, 793–797, 1952.)

various GAG present in the same material. Whole human teeth were cleaned, dried, crushed, and ground. The fine powder was treated with a mixture of 91% bromoform and 9% acetone, of specific gravity 2.7, to separate enamel from dentine-cementum. Dried aliquots of the two fractions were decalcified with 5% EDTA, deproteinized, dialyzed, and concentrated. The solutions were precipitated with CPC, and the precipitates were solubilized with increasing concentrations of sodium chloride (0.4 M, 1.20 M, and 2.1 M). After removing the CPC the dialyzed solutions were analyzed for hexuronic acids and for total aminosugars. It was found that the dentine-cementum and enamel fractions of human teeth contain, respectively, 0.08 and 0.03% total aminosugars. Of these amounts glucosamine represents 42 and 47% of the total, respectively, in dentine-cementum and enamel, and galactosamine represents 43 and 54%. Dentine-cementum also contained a third compound (accounting for 15% of total hexosamine) which reacted with the Elson-Morgan reagent but behaved differently from glucosamine and galactosamine on column chromatography. A similar component, hitherto unidentified in its structure, has been described in sheep wool, human hair, and epidermis. The GAG isolated from dentine-cementum were HA, CS4, and CS6, the latter ones being differentiated by infrared spectroscopy, paper chromatography, and optical rotation. The ratio between sulfated and nonsulfated GAG in dentine-cementum was 20:1. The same GAG were isolated from enamel, the ratio between the sulfated and nonsulfated ones being 10:1.

If one assumes that the extraction and recovery of the GAG were quantitative, the GAG accounted for 45% of the total aminosugars present in dentine-cementum and for 9% of those present in enamel, the balance probably being represented by glycoproteins which were degraded by the proteolytic enzymes to products eliminated during dialysis. In this connection, it is pertinent to mention that sialic acid, a component of many glycoproteins, has been isolated from dentine.

In 1972, Engfeldt and Hjerpe studied the GAG of dentine and predentine, with particular emphasis on their qualitative and quantitative modifications in connection with their possible role during mineralization. Because low amounts of predentine may be recovered from normal teeth, these authors obtained it from teeth of rachitic young dogs, in which the zone of predentine is considerably widened and provides more material for dissection.

The dentine and predentine were obtained by microdissection, and the defatted and dried materials were digested with papain. The GAG precipitated with CPC were first analyzed by infrared spectrophotometry and then fractionated by chromatographic microtechniques; the specific aminosugars present in each chromatographic fraction were then identified.

The results indicated that, when calculated on the basis of organic dry weight, the amount of GAG in predentine is significantly larger than that in dentine.

Only galactosamine-containing GAG could be demonstrated, and their chromatographic behavior identified them as CS4 and CS6, the former more abundant in dentine, the latter, in predentine.

In agreement with the theories that claim that a loss of GAG occurs prior to mineralization, the total amount of GAG was found to be lower in the mineralized tissue. Moreover, Urist and co-workers and Buddecke and Drzenick have demonstrated that CS6, which is more abundant in predentine, has a higher Ca-binding capacity than CS4, which is more abundant in dentine. Thus, a decrease in the CS6/CS4 ratio from predentine to dentine would represent a decrease of Ca-binding capacity of GAG, with consequent availability of calcium for the precipitation of hydroxyapatite crystals.

The sulfated and nonsulfated GAG of enamel and dentine seem to be involved in the initiation and progression of dental caries. The softening of dentine in carious teeth has been ascribed, at least in part, to loss of HA and CS due to the action of streptococcal enzymes similar to hyaluronidase. This sequence of events is supported by the demonstration that streptococci isolated from human carious teeth are capable of growing on media whose only source of carbon is hyaluronic acid or chondroitin sulfate. Moreover, the dentino-enamel junction and peritubular dentine have small quantities of fibers relatively rich in GAG. These findings may constitute one of the reasons why the dentino-enamel junction is the site where dentine caries begins (after caries destruction of enamel is completed) and why streptococci penetrate the tubules and produce a soft, leathery carious dentine in the peritubular regions rather than in the highly fibrillar intertubular regions.

METABOLISM OF GLYCOPROTEINS AND PROTEOGLYCANS

Biosynthesis

The biosynthesis of glycoproteins and proteoglycans requires specific enzymic mechanisms responsible for the attachment of carbohydrate units to the peptide chain being synthesized or already synthesized. The structure of the carbohydrate chains in these compounds requires for their assembly mechanisms completely different from those responsible for peptide synthesis, since each single monosaccharide can be linked to the preceding one through a variety of glycosidic linkages.

Several studies performed with tissue slices, organ perfusion, or intact systems have shown that the sugars are attached to a "precursor" bound to the membranes of the endoplasmic reticulum. Any interference with the continuous synthesis of the precursor (as caused by puromycin) is soon followed by an impairment of the synthesis of the carbohydrate chains, the internally located monosaccharides being more affected than the peripheral ones.

Thus, it is believed that one sugar at a time becomes attached to the peptide precursor, starting from the inner ones and progressing away from the peptide backbone. This process is catalyzed by a series of glycosyltransferases that transfer an activated sugar from its nucleotide carrier to the macromolecular acceptor. The specificity of this enzymic system, which also resides on the endoplasmic reticulum, is dictated by the specificity of each transferase for the base and the sugar moiety of the sugar nucleotide and for various characteristics of the acceptor, such as size of the peptide chain, sequence of amino acids in the vicinity of the glycopeptide bond to be formed, and nature and configuration of the terminal sugar to which the new sugar is to be attached.

The various enzymes probably work in sequence on the peptide already released from the ribosomes and migrating along the endoplasmic reticulum; the product of one enzymic reaction becomes the substrate for the next one. For example, the disaccharides linked to hydroxylysine present in collagens and basement membranes are synthesized by a mechanism consisting of two enzymes: the first transfers D-galactose from uridine diphosphate (UDP)-galactose to the hydroxyl group of hydroxylysine only when the latter is in a high molecular weight peptide chain and its ε-amino group is unsubstituted; the second enzyme transfers D-glucose from UDP-glucose to the already linked galactose (but not to any differently linked galactose or free galactose) to form an α (1→2) glycosidic linkage.

The biosynthesis of the linkage region of the proteoglycans seems to take place in the rough endoplasmic reticulum, and involves a xylosyltransferase that transfers xylose from UDP-xylose to the hydroxyl group of a serine residue which is part of the peptide acceptor (Fig. 3–2). After this enzymatic reaction, two different galactosyl transferases are required: one transfers D-galactose from UDP-galactose to xylose (β [1→4] linkage), and the other transfers the second galactose to the first one (β [1→3] linkage). Thereafter, a special transferase attaches D-glucuronic acid from UDP-glucuronic acid to the last galactose (β [1→3] linkage).

In the synthesis of glycans, D-glucose is the precursor of the various monosaccharides. Since these reactions of interconversion are described in

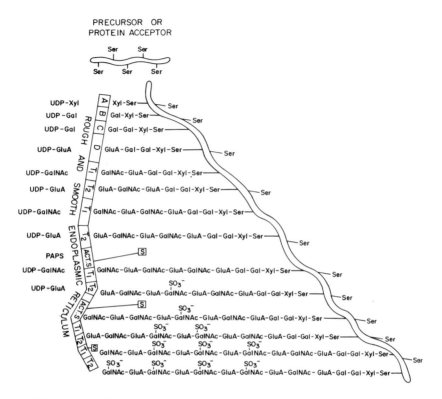

A   UDP-XYLOSYL TRANSFERASE
B and C   UDP-GALACTOSYL TRANSFERASES
D   UDP-GLUCURONIC ACID TRANSFERASE
T_1 and T_2 POLYMERIZING TRANSFERASES or DIFFERENT CENTERS of SAME ENZYME
S   PAPS, or ACTIVE SULFATE

Fig. 3–2.   Biosynthesis of proteoglycans. A series of glycosyl transferases, located in the endoplasmic reticulum, transfer various sugars, derived from their nucleotide diphosphate precursors, to the serine residue of a peptide acceptor. Sulfation of the growing glycan chains is performed by transferases and by active sulfate.

detail in books of general biochemistry, I shall mention only the reactions leading to the formation of aminosugars, hexuronic acids, and xylose, mainly because these sequences and their end products participate in the mechanism of regulation of glycan synthesis (Fig. 3–3).

In the hemolytic streptococcus, glucosamine is synthesized from fructose-6-phosphate (F-6-P) and the amide group of glutamine. This irreversible reaction has a great functional importance because at its level acts one of the most efficient control mechanisms for the synthesis of glycans. In some tissues, the synthesis of glucosamine requires not glutamine but ammonia, as indicated by the following reaction:

$$NH_3 + \text{fructose-6-phosphate} \rightleftharpoons \text{glucosamine-6-phosphate} + H_2O.$$

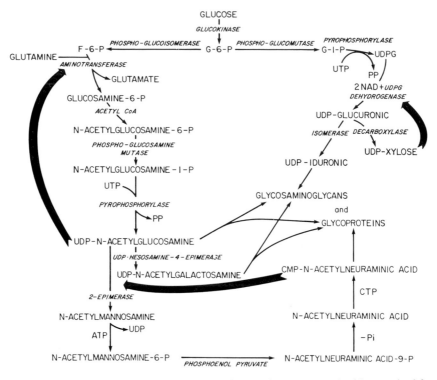

Fig. 3–3. The biosynthesis and activation of the various monosaccharides required for the synthesis of glycosaminoglycans and glycoproteins. Large arrows indicate feedback inhibition of key enzymic reactions of the biosynthetic pathway.

Acetylation of the glucosamine-6-phosphate by coenzyme A and an appropriate enzyme pulls the reversible reaction to the right. As soon as N-acetylglucosamine-6-phosphate is transformed by a mutase to N-acetylglucosamine-1-phosphate, the latter reacts with uridine triphosphate (UTP) to produce uridine diphospho-N-acetylglucosamine (UDP-NAcGlu) and pyrophosphate.

Glucuronic acid is produced from oxidation of uridine diphosphoglucose (UDPG) by a specific dehydrogenase with the coenzyme, nicotinamide-adenosine dinucleotide (NAD). The uridine diphosphoglucuronic acid (UDPGA) thus formed is ready for interaction with the specific transferase in order to participate in the synthesis of the glycan. Two specific transferases, or one with two active centers, located in the smooth endoplasmic reticulum, transfer alternatively N-acetyl-D-hexosamine and D-glucuronic acid to the growing glycan, establishing glycosidic bonds typical of the various GAG (Fig. 3–4). In this process, the nucleotide uridine diphosphate is set free. Some GAG (like chondroitin sulfate) contain N-acetylgalactosamine and sulfate ester groups. A UDP-hexosamine-4-epimerase transforms UDP-N-acetylglucosamine to UDP-N-acetylgalactosamine while the synthe-

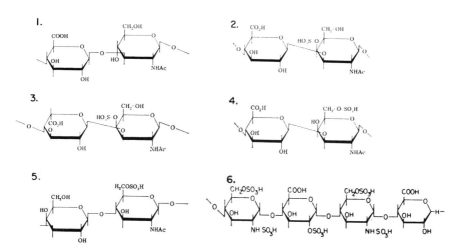

Fig. 3–4. The structure of repeating units of various GAG: (1) hyaluronic acid; (2) chondroitin-4-sulfate; (3) dermatan sulfate; (4) chondroitin-6-sulfate; (5) keratan sulfate; (6) heparin.

sis of the sulfate esters (and that of the sulfoamido groups of heparin and heparan sulfate) requires the presence of "active sulfate" or adenosine-3'-phosphate-5'-phosphosulfate or PAPS. This nucleotide is formed in two steps by enzymes widely distributed in various organs (Fig. 3–5). First, adenosine-5'-phosphosulfate is formed by a sulfurylase which eliminates pyrophosphate from ATP and substitutes it with sulfate. Then, a phosphokinase transfers the terminal phosphate of another ATP to position 3' of adenosine-5'-phosphosulfate thus producing the "active sulfate." A series of specific sulfotransferases transfers the sulfate groups of "active sulfate" to various substrates like phenolic compounds, steroids, and GAG. Whether sulfation occurs in the smooth endoplasmic reticulum or in the Golgi apparatus is not established. Moreover, it is not quite clear whether the synthesis of sulfate esters takes place at the oligosaccharide level or after the glycosidic chain has been formed. Some investigators believe that the sulfate esters are introduced after completion of the polymer. The transfer of ester sulfates to the last residue of N-acetylgalactosamine present in the growing polymer would prevent the additional incorporation of glucuronic acid, thus ending the synthetic process (Fig. 3–2).

Another epimerization reaction accounts for the presence of L-iduronic acid in dermatan sulfate and heparin; this epimerase acts on UDP-D-glucuronic acid, transforming it to UDP-L-iduronic acid. Whether such epimerization of hexuronic acids might occur during or after the polymer has been synthesized is not clear as yet (Fig. 3–3).

Decarboxylation of UDP-D-glucuronic acid to UDP-D-xylose requires NAD and provides the precursor for the xylose needed for the synthesis of the linkage region.

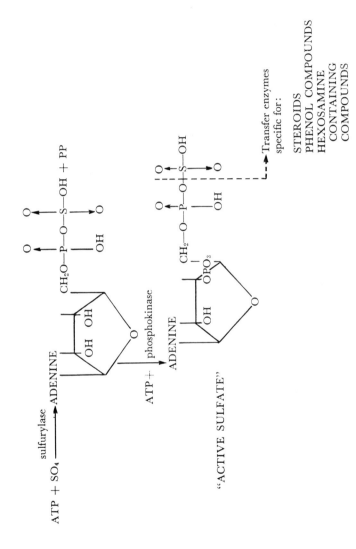

Fig. 3–5.   Synthesis of "active sulfate."

Besides the stimulating or inhibiting effect of hormones, vitamins, and drugs on the synthesis of GAG, particularly interesting is the regulatory activity performed by some intermediates of the synthetic process itself (feedback inhibition). For instance, UDP-xylose inhibits the dehydrogenase that produces UDP-glucuronic acid from UDP-glucose (Fig. 3–2). Thus, when the utilization of UDP-xylose is slow, its accumulation produces a secondary accumulation of UDP-glucose. This, in turn, may cause specific enzymes to direct glucose-1-phosphate toward different metabolic pathways (toward the glycolytic pathway, for instance, after glucose-1-phosphate has been transformed to glucose-6-phosphate). Similarly, when UDP-N-acetylglucosamine accumulates, the aminotransferase responsible for transferring the amino group of glutamine to fructose-6-phosphate becomes specifically inhibited, causing a decreased production of the nucleotide temporarily not utilized and a shunt of fructose-6-phosphate toward different pathways (Fig. 3–3).

Similarly, the accumulation of cytidine monophosphate-N-acetylneuraminic acid (CMP-N-acetylneuraminic acid), which is the activated form of neuraminic acid and participates in the synthesis of glycoproteins, inhibits the epimerization of UDP-N-acetylglucosamine to N-acetylmannosamine, thus decreasing its own synthesis (Fig. 3–3).

The glycoproteins and proteoglycans are products mainly destined to be exported from the cell; since from the moment of their synthesis, they are always kept segregated from the cytoplasm by the membranes of the reticulum and of the Golgi apparatus. While inside these structures, they are the substrates of the various post-ribosomal enzymic modifications (transfer of additional monosaccharides, sulfation, and the like), and eventually are packaged in vesicles originating from the Golgi region in order either to be transported to the cell surface and outside of it, or to remain inside the cell within special vesicles. These are identified as primary lysosomes, recognizable because their glycoprotein content consists mainly of hydrolases capable of degrading a variety of structural macromolecules.

Degradation

The study of several inborn errors of metabolism has provided a great deal of information on the normal mechanisms of glycan degradation. Individuals affected by these diseases inherit the inability to synthesize (or the inability to synthesize correctly) a certain enzyme that participates in the degradation of a specific macromolecule.

Because of this degradative block, all the subsequent enzymes cannot function and the macromolecule accumulates in a progressive manner, with deleterious effects on the cellular economy. It is evident that a great number of degradative enzymes are lysosomal glycoproteins possessing hydrolytic activities with a rather acidic pH optimum. They possess a particular specificity for the terminal residue that has to be cleaved and for the bond that it forms with the preceding residue. However, the nature of the macromolecule to which the monosaccharide to be removed is attached does not dictate the specificity of the degradative hydrolases, and this fact explains why the absence of a single lysosomal hydrolase may result in the accumulation of two different macromolecules. The macromolecules to be digested include proteoglycans, glycoproteins, lipids, gangliosides, cerebrosides, glycogen; by pinocytosis they are brought inside the cell, included in vesicles that merge with primary lysosomes to form the secondary lysosomes or digestive vacuoles. Therein, the various degradative enzymes and their substrates come in contact.

Various lysosomal proteases, called cathepsins, are capable of digesting the peptide backbone of glycoproteins and proteoglycans, and an almost endless list of acidic glycosidases, capable of cleaving every one of the glycosidic linkages found in naturally occurring macromolecules, has been compiled and is being continuously updated. These enzymes remove the terminal monosaccharides, and therefore they must operate in a sequential manner until all the glycan is degraded. The monosaccharides released may be used as a source of energy or may be reutilized for new synthetic processes. A variety of lysosomal sulfatases capable of removing sulfate from the various sulfate esters or sulfoamido groups present in different GAG also have been described. Absence or faulty function of any degradative enzyme results in an arrest of the process with formation of a "dense body," which is a residual lysosome containing undigested material.

Structure and Function

The glycosaminoglycans are high molecular weight heteropolysaccharides containing aminosugars. Previously referred to as acid mucopolysaccharides, they may be conveniently represented by a "repeating unit," which is repeated many times to produce chains of different length. Eight different GAG have been isolated and characterized on the basis of (1) the structure of the repeating unit, (2) optical rotation, (3) solubility in alcoholic solutions, and (4) enzymic degradation. The acidic character of these compounds is due to the presence of three different functional groups: carboxylic ($-COOH$), ester sulfate ($-O-SO_3H$), and sulfoamide ($-N-SO_3H$). Figure 3–4 shows the repeating units of several GAG and Table 3–2 summarizes some of their properties.

Hyaluronic acid is a linear polysaccharide composed of equimolar amounts of D-glucuronic acid and D-N-acetyl-glucosamine, linked by alternating β (1→3) and β (1→4) glycosidic linkages (Fig. 3–4, 1). It has been isolated from various sources such as vitreous humor, umbilical cord, rooster comb, embryonic pig skin, human serum, Rous sarcoma, synovial fluid, brain and spinal cord, platelets, electric organ of the eel, and several bacteria. It is rapidly depolymerized by bacterial, testicular, and leech hyaluronidase, the latter being specific for this substrate.

Table 3–2. Properties of Isolated Glycosaminoglycans

	Hyaluronic Acid	Chondroitin	Chondroitin-4-Sulfate	Dermatan Sulfate	Chondroitin-6-Sulfate	Keratan Sulfate	Heparin	Heparan Sulfate
Optical rotation [α]D	−70°, −80°	−21°	−28°, −32°	−55°, −63°	−16°, −22°	−13°, +5°	+44°	+39°, +50°
Ethanol concentration precipitating Ca salts			30–40%	18–25%	40–50%			
Sensitivity to hyaluronidase: testicular	++	++	+	+, −	+	−	−	−
bacterial	++	−	−	−	−	−	−	−
leech		−	−	−	−	−	−	−
chondroitinase AC		++	++	−	++	−	−	−
ABC		++	++	+	++	−	−	−
heparinase							+	+
chondrosulfatase* 4			+	+	−			
6			−	−	+			
Aminosugar	acetylglucosamine	acetylgalactosamine	acetylgalactosamine	acetylgalactosamine	acetylgalactosamine	acetylglucosamine	glucosamine-N-sulfate	acetylglucosamine and glucosamine-N-sulfate
Hexuronic acid	glucuronic	glucuronic	glucuronic	iduronic	glucuronic	absent	glucuronic	glucuronic
Anionic groups	carboxylic	carboxylic	carboxylic + sulfate esters	carboxylic + sulfate esters	carboxylic + sulfate esters	sulfate esters	carboxylic, sulfate esters, and amides	carboxylic, sulfate esters, and amides
S%	—	0–2%	6–7%	6–7%	6–7%	6–9%	11–12%	6%
Anticoagulant activity	−	−	−	−	−	−	+	−

* Active on sulfated disaccharides obtained with chondroitinase AC and ABC.

Hyaluronic acid isolated from vitreous humor consists of several fractions of different molecular weight (from 7.7×10^4 to 1.5×10^6). These fractions contain a small protein component which seems to be an integral part of the polymer. It has been demonstrated that oxidation–reduction processes may remove most of the protein moiety and depolymerize the carbohydrate chains. The hyaluronic acid–protein complex of synovial fluid behaves like a semi-rigid coil with a molecular weight of approximately 4×10^6. In solution, these macromolecules resist compression and limit the flow of solvent and the diffusion of other solutes, either small or large. In fact, when in solution hyaluronic acid secludes the volume of solvent necessary for its solubilization, preventing its function as a solvent for other molecules or its free flow in the intercellular space. This effect on the solvent, quite different from that shown by salts or protein in solution, is referred to as "excluded volume." This property of hyaluronic acid in solution explains the absence of plasma proteins in normal synovial fluid and their presence in those pathological fluids in which the degree of polymerization of hyaluronic acid may be reduced. Moreover, the recent demonstration that in the joints the hyaline cartilage is covered by a thin layer of hyaluronic acid seems to support the theory that water layers may be interposed between the articular surfaces, serving as a lubricating and shock-absorbing device.

Chondroitin-4-sulfate and chondroitin-6-sulfate (previously referred to as chondroitin sulfate A and C) are quite similar linear polymers found in various connective tissue areas and mainly in cartilage, bone, cornea, vascular walls, chordoma, and chondrosarcoma.

Composed of equimolar amounts of D-glucuronic acid and D-N-acetyl-galactosamine, linked by alternating β $(1\rightarrow3)$ and β $(1\rightarrow4)$ glycosidic linkages (Fig. 3–4, 2 and 4), chondroitin-4-sulfate and chondroitin-6-sulfate are both depolymerized by testicular hyaluronidase and by chondroitinase AC, but they are resistant to bacterial hyaluronidase. They differ in optical rotation (Table 3-2) and in the position of the sulfate groups located in position 4 of the acetylgalactosamine in chondroitin-4-sulfate and in position 6 in chondroitin-6-sulfate (Fig. 3–4). This structural difference may be demonstrated with colorimetric determinations, with infrared analyses, or with the use of specific chondrosulfatases.

Dermatan sulfate (previously identified as chondroitin sulfate B) is similar to CS4 but has large amounts of L-iduronic acid and smaller amounts of D-glucuronic acid in addition to D-N-acetylgalactosamine, sulfated in position 4. On occasion, sulfate ester groups are found in position 2 or 3 of the iduronic acid residues. Because of the presence of L-iduronic acid, the glycosidic linkages between this monosaccharide and the following amino-sugar are α $(1\rightarrow3)$ and are cleaved by a specific lysosomal enzyme α-L-iduronidase. Dermatan sulfate, found mainly in skin, tendon, lung parenchyma, and aortic tissue, is depolymerized by chondroitinase ABC (Table 3–2).

Heparin is synthesized in the mast cells as a proteoglycan whose protein moiety is cleaved and the carbohydrate chain reduced in length before it is exported extracellularly. It is composed of roughly equimolar amounts of N-sulfoamido-D-glucosamine and D-glucuronic acid, linked by α (1→4) glycosidic linkages. The presence of L-iduronic acid and N-acetyl-D-glucosamine in this GAG has been demonstrated. The sulfate ester groups are in position 6 of the aminosugar. Heparan sulfate, which is found mainly in vascular structures, is similar to heparin since approximately half the amino groups of the D-glucosamine residues is acetylated and half sulfated; the sulfate esters on D-glucosamine are also in position 6. The glucosidic linkage between D-glucosamine and D-glucuronic acid is α (1→4), but the one between D-glucuronic acid and the aminosugar is now believed to be β (1→4). Keratan sulfate (KS), found in skeletal tissues and in cornea, is the only GAG without hexuronic acid. It is composed of D-galactose and N-acetyl-D-glucosamine, linked by alternating β (1→4) and β (1→3) glycosidic linkages, the sulfate esters being in position 6 of the aminosugar and frequently also of the galactose.

The different types of chondroitin sulfate, and in particular, dermatan sulfate present in a given tissue may stimulate or inhibit the formation or growth of the collagen fibers, thus influencing the types of fibers eventually appearing in the tissue. All the glycosaminoglycans occur naturally in the form of protein complexes (proteoglycans), and although there have been doubts about hyaluronic acid, even this GAG seems to have a small co-valently linked protein moiety. Although the proteoglycans of cartilage matrix have been more extensively studied because of their availability, the conclusions reached may apply to those present in other tissues. They consist of a protein backbone to which are covalently attached 50 to 60 chains of chondroitin sulfate through the linkage region, consisting of xylose and galactose described previously. The molecular weight of each GAG chain is approximately 2.5×10^4 and that of the whole complex is about 1.5×10^6 (Fig. 3–1B). The physical and biological properties of the proteoglycans are different from those of the respective GAG, represented by CS4, CS6, and some KS. Whether the latter is attached to the same protein backbone of the CS chains has been argued for a long time, but it seems quite certain that KS and CS6 have the same protein moiety.

When in solution, the stiffness of the glycosidic chains and the repulsion of the numerous anionic groups cause the proteoglycans to spread and to occupy a vast domain, thus subtracting a large volume of solvent for the transit of other solutes. For this reason, cartilage and other tissues rich in proteoglycans have a large water content which is incompressible. Because the proteoglycans hold the water in the tissue and do not allow it to be forced out, the whole tissue acquires a certain resistance to compression. This high affinity for water is a property of large molecular weight complexes (proteoglycans and their aggregates; hyaluronic acid) and is related to their tendency to occupy a large domain in solution. Because the water held by the proteoglycans is not available as a solvent for other macromolecules, its volume has been defined as "excluded volume." The effects of this phenomenon, which limits the free flow of water or the solution of other macromolecules, are greatly increased by the formation of supramolecular aggregates among various proteoglycan units. Recent investigations indicate that minute amounts of HA might serve as a nucleus for the aggregation of the proteoglycans. The presence of collagen fibrils alongside the proteoglycans confers some rigidity to what otherwise would be a highly viscous solution. The final organization of the tissue has been compared to a "rather rigid sponge," which may be compressed to some extent and may lose some water, but regains normal shape and water content when the pressure is released.

The interaction between collagen and proteoglycans has been studied extensively with physical methods. For instance, when cartilage proteoglycans were mixed with a solution of collagen, centrifugation yielded a pellet containing the proteoglycans enmeshed in a net of collagen. The pellets retained water and had a rubber-like consistency. When CS replaced the proteoglycans, or when these were treated with proteolytic enzymes, the physical properties of the pellets could not be reproduced.

The proteoglycans play a role of paramount importance in calcification. Small amounts of these complexes added to an aqueous suspension of metastable calcium phosphate prevent the sedimentation of the salt upon centrifugation. However, if the proteoglycan is treated with proteolytic enzymes or with testicular hyaluronidase, its degradation allows the immediate sedimentation of the calcium salt as if it were in aqueous suspension. The calcium phosphate present in the plasma and in the extracellular fluid is in supersaturated, metastable solution, and the presence of proteoglycans in tissues may represent one of the factors preventing its precipitation. It is relevant to mention that proteases capable of degrading the protein part of the complex have been described in cartilage, and this may account for the reduction in the amount of this protein immediately prior to the onset of calcification.

The role of proteoglycans in calcification should be considered along with that of collagen, elastin, and matrix vesicles. The latter are extracellular membranous vesicles, 1000 Å in diameter, first recognized with the electron microscope in epiphyseal cartilage but present also in dentine and calcifying aorta. They are different from lysosomes and contain alkaline phosphatase, adenosine triphosphatase, and pyrophosphatase. It was postulated and eventually demonstrated that, because of their enzymic content, these vesicles might initiate calcification (1) by increasing the concentration of inorganic phosphate through hydrolysis of appropriate substrates; (2) by hydrolyzing ATP and utilizing its energy for the active transport of Ca ions inside the vesicle for the formation of hydroxyapatite; and (3) by hydrolyzing pyrophosphate, which is considered an inhibitor of calcification.

When physiological conditions are maintained, the first hydroxyapatite-like crystals appear within the vesicles. Once released outside of the membrane, they might find a "support" or template on the collagen fibers, which would thus contribute to the accretion and growth of the initial crystals.

The role of the proteoglycans and elastin may be one of calcium storage, so as to make it available to the matrix vesicles only at the appropriate time. Although proteoglycans bind calcium efficiently, they release it when the protein moiety is cleaved or degraded, an event that, with various techniques, has been demonstrated to occur prior to calcification. This affinity of proteoglycans for calcium ions may compete with the affinity that elastin and collagen have for the same ions.

Urry has postulated that the high glycine content of collagen and elastin causes and stabilizes a left-handed β-helical turn, which provides binding sites for cations by coordination with the neutral acyl oxygens of the peptide bonds. Once they bind calcium with this mechanism, the proteins become positively charged and attract charge-neutralizing ions, such as phosphate and carbonate, which decrease the space-charge saturation and allow further calcium binding. Although it has been proposed that this repetitive mechanism might itself constitute nuclei for crystallization of hydroxyapatite, it is also possible that it might represent a storage of calcium no longer available to the matrix vesicles, but capable of initiating pathological or ectopic calcifications.

Thus, the proteoglycans of calcifying tissues, by binding calcium, might perform several functions: compete with elastin and collagen for calcium, thus decreasing the possibility of abnormal calcification; store calcium temporarily and release it at the proper time, making it available to the matrix vesicles; and prevent the deposition of metastable calcium phosphate at sites not meant to undergo calcification.

Bernard has studied by electron microscopy the process of dentine and enamel calcification in developing mouse molar tooth buds. When predentine begins to calcify, the first hydroxyapatite crystals are inside or adjacent to cellular "buds," which are derived from the odontoblasts near the dentino-enamel junction. These structures, analogous to the previously mentioned "vesicles," may be filled with amorphous substance, may be granular, or may contain crystals. In the earliest stages of crystal formation, they are still intracellular and limited by an intact membrane. Later, when crystal growth is more abundant, their membrane disappears and the matrix becomes involved in the crystals' further growth. From these initial calcifications, crystals grow more and first become arranged into spheroidal forms and then spread onto and between collagen fibrils. Coalescence of nodules with calcified collagen forms seams of calcified dentine (mantle dentine), characterized by unevenness due to the random arrangement of the collagen. Thereafter, the crystals grow into the predentine, where the oriented collagen fibrils provide a patterned structure for crystal growth.

Prior to complete formation of mantle dentine, the basement lamina underlying the ameloblasts disappears, and the enamel protein is rapidly synthesized in the pre-enamel. The continuity thus established with the already calcified mantle dentine allows the enamel protein to calcify rapidly, the first crystals being clearly derived from the hydroxyapatite of the dentine and showing the same x-ray diffraction pattern. However, because of the special orientation of enamel protein, the hydroxyapatite crystals therein have a particularly elongated shape different from those of dentine.

Thus, the process of dentino-enamel calcification recapitulates the types of calcification seen in other tissues: the calcification of mantle dentine is initiated cellularly and follows a pattern similar to that of cancellous bone and calcified cartilage, whereas that of the dentine surrounding the pulp and of the enamel proceeds in the matrix and is similar to that seen in lamellar bone.

SELECTED REFERENCES

BERNARD, G. W.: Ultrastructural observations of initial calcification in dentine and enamel. J. Ultrastruct. Res., *41*, 1–17, 1972.

BUDDECKE, E., and DRZENICK, R.: Stabilitatskonstanten der calcium komplexe von sauren mucopolysacchariden. Hoppe-Seylers Z. Physiol. Chem., *327*, 49–64, 1962.

CLARK, R. D., SMITH, J. G., JR., and DAVIDSON, E. A.: Hexosamine and acid glycosaminoglycans in human teeth. Biochim. Biophys. Acta, *101*, 267–272, 1965.

ENGFELDT, B., and HJERPE, A.: Glycosaminoglycans of dentine and predentine. Calcif. Tissue Res., *10*, 152–159, 1972.

FULLMER, H. M., and ALPHER, N.: Histochemical polysaccharide reactions in human developing teeth. Lab. Invest., 7, 163–170, 1958.

HESS, W. C., and LEE, C.: The isolation of chondroitin sulfuric acid from dentin. J. Dent. Res., *31*, 793–797, 1952.

LINDE, A.: Glycosaminoglycan turnover and synthesis in the rat incisor pulp. Scand. J. Dent. Res., *81*, 145–154, 1973.

MATTHIESSEN, M. E.: Histochemical studies of the prenatal development of human deciduous teeth. Acta Anat., *55*, 201–223, 1963.

MATTHIESSEN, M. E., and GELIN, G.: Acid glycosaminoglucuronoglycans of human tooth germs. Scand. J. Dent. Res., *81*, 174–176, 1973.

MEYER, K., DAVIDSON, E., LINKER, A., and HOFFMAN, P.: The acid mucopolysaccharides of connective tissues. Biochim. Biophys. Acta, *21*, 506–518, 1956.

TEN CATE, A. R.: Histochemical investigations on the stellate reticulum of human foetal teeth. J. Anat. (Lond.), *91*, 609–610, 1957.

URIST, M. R., SPEER, D. P., IESEN, K. J., and STRATES, B. S.: Calcium binding by chondroitin sulphate. Calcif. Tissue Res., *2*, 253–261, 1968.

URRY, D. W.: Neutral sites for calcium ion binding to elastin and collagen. Proc. Natl. Acad. Sci. USA, *60*, 810–814, 1971.

WISLOCKI, G. B., SINGER, M., and WALDO, C. M.: Some histochemical reactions of mucopolysaccharides, glycogen, lipids and other substances in teeth. Anat. Rec., *101*, 487–505, 1948.

Chapter 4

Lipids in Teeth and Membranes

THOMAS R. DIRKSEN, D.D.S., Ph.D.

JAMES J. VOGEL, Ph.D.

LIPIDS IN SOUND AND CARIOUS DENTIN

Histology

Early experimenters on teeth utilized histochemical methods to demonstrate the lipid components of enamel and dentin. Odontoblastic tubules in fully mineralized teeth readily stain for fat as do the incremental lines of enamel. Sections of carious teeth show additional lipid in enamel as well as in the peritubular matrix of dentin. Although much carious staining is related to the presence of bacteria, some also results from bound lipids which are "unmasked" during partial or total removal of mineral. That such lipid is endogenous in origin was confirmed by Opdyke who detected lipid staining in acid-demineralized sound teeth. The teeth were exposed to sterile agar media containing lactic acid. Over a 20-day period of progressive decalcification, the teeth stained sequentially for calcium, later protein, and finally lipid.

Identification and Quantitation of Lipids

Paper chromatographic methods were used to identify specific classes of lipids in sound and carious dentin. Dirksen reported cholesterol esters, triglycerides, fatty acids, cholesterol, diglycerides, monoglycerides (tentative), and various phospholipids such as phosphatidyl inositol, sphingomyelin, lecithin, phosphatidyl ethanolamine, lysolecithin, and three unidentified phosphatides in sound dentin.

The presence of phosphatidyl serine was confirmed in carious dentin. Since this lipid was not extracted from non-carious material, a possible binding of inorganic salt by lipid was suggested, which prompted lipid analysis of demineralized dentin matrix. Lipid extracts of sound and

EDTA-demineralized dentin were separated and quantitated, the results of which are shown in Table 4–1. Total lipid weights were determined gravimetrically before column separation, and it is obvious that the combined weights of the individual lipid classes do not approximate the total weights. Studies by Prout and Shutt suggest that about 50% of total fatty acids in mineralized tissues exists as free fatty acids, a lipid class not quantitated in the aforementioned study. The finding that lipid extracts of calcified tissues (this includes bone) differ as to type as well as amount, depending upon whether sample material is demineralized or not, has been verified many times.

Shapiro and associates studied lipid extracts of bovine enamel and dentin obtained (1) before demineralization, (2) after demineralization, and (3) with acidified chloroform-methanol. On a dry weight basis, enamel contained some 20 times more phospholipid than dentin (0.06 vs. 0.003%). The major portion of neutral phospholipids was removed before demineralization, whereas the acidic phospholipids were obtained only after demineralization or by the use of acidified solvents. In dentin, 56% of total phospholipid was identified as lecithin with 50% being extracted before EDTA treatment. No phosphatidyl serine, phosphatidyl inositol, or phosphatidic acid was extracted from the tissue until after demineralization. Quite comparable results were obtained with enamel. This again suggests a high degree of association between phospholipids and mineral. Similar observations were made by Odutuga and Prout with human teeth. Enamel and dentin contain 0.51% and 0.33% total lipid, respectively.

Total fatty acids have been extracted from fossil teeth as old as 230,000,000 years. Over 60% of the fatty acids were present as palmitic, stearic, and

Table 4–1. Comparison of the Lipid Content of Sound Dentin Prepared by Two Extraction Procedures

	I†	II‡
Total lipid weight	40.90*	176.60
Cholesterol esters	2.89	4.14
Free cholesterol	3.42	6.53
Triglycerides	1.59	1.61
Diglycerides	0.75	1.15
Monoglycerides	0.45	0.80
Phospholipids	0.45	4.95

* All values based on mg per 100 gm of dried dentin.
† Chloroform-methanol extraction.
‡ EDTA decalcification.

oleic acids. The distribution of fatty acids in freshly extracted human teeth has also been examined. Both enamel and dentin showed similar patterns: palmitic, 19 to 25% of total fatty acids; stearic, 14 to 17%; and oleic, 20 to 21%. In general, this distribution is not unlike that observed for other tissues.

THE SUDANOPHILIC REACTION AT SITES OF CALCIFICATION

Using specific histochemical techniques and the light microscope, Irving has been able to demonstrate a sudanophilic reaction at sites of active calcification. Sudan black B is a frequently utilized stain in lipid studies. The method involves tissue fixation, pyridine or ethanol-benzene extraction, demineralization, gelatin embedding, frozen sectioning, and Sudan black B staining. The junction between predentin and dentin, as well as enamel where it becomes acid soluble, specifically demonstrates a sudanophilic line. A similar reaction is also seen in the epiphyseal zone of long bone where hypertrophic cartilage cells become calcified.

Wuthier microdissected calf epiphyseal plate in an attempt to isolate and identify the lipid (or lipids) that might be responsible for this staining reaction. Again, quantities of acidic phospholipids are extracted only after demineralization, which points to their possible involvement in calcification. Subsequent work with enamel, however, suggests a possible role of hydrophobic proteins as well as lipids in the staining reaction.

Anderson isolated extracellular matrix vesicles from the epiphyseal plate of bone that might also be involved in the sudanophilic reaction. These vesicles, isolated by density centrifugation, contain calcium, a larger percentage of acidic phospholipids than whole cartilage, and enzymes, including pyrophosphatase and alkaline phosphatase. Electron micrographs have shown these vesicles to be the site of initial calcium phosphate deposition. Similar matrix vesicles have been observed in dentin but not in enamel. The involvement of phospholipids in the calcification process should therefore be considered during the initial mineral deposition of either amorphous calcium phosphate or apatite. Once formed, crystal growth can continue by apposition into the surrounding area of cartilage, bone, dentin, or enamel.

FAT-SOLUBLE VITAMINS

When their solubility is considered, vitamins are classified into two major groups. The water-soluble vitamins and derivatives function as coenzymes in various metabolic pathways of the body. The fat-soluble vitamins, however, serve in other capacities, some of which remain to be elucidated. Vitamins A, D, E, and K are found associated with the lipid fraction of foods, and their absorption into the body depends upon the presence of bile for emulsification. The structures of the fat-soluble vitamins are shown in Figure 4–1.

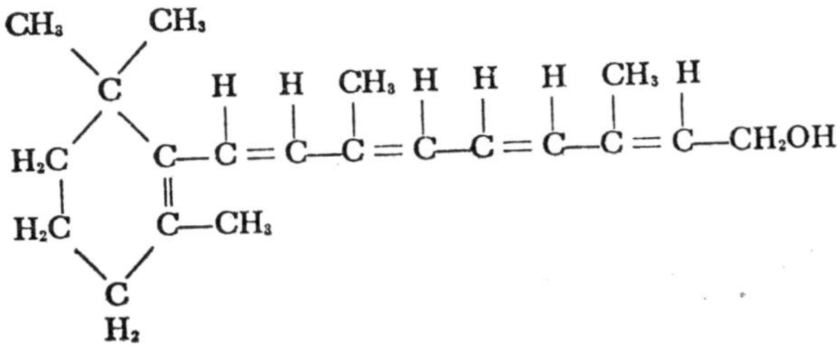

Vitamin A₁

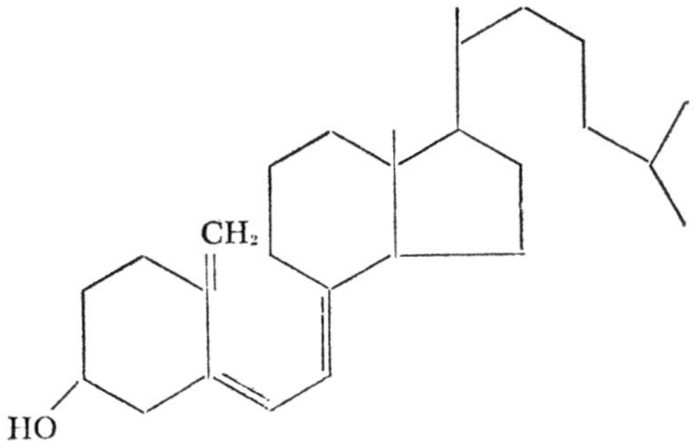

Vitamin D₃

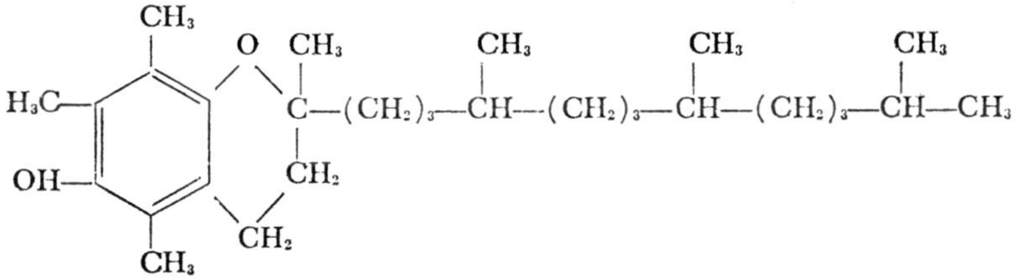

Vitamin E (α-Tocopherol)

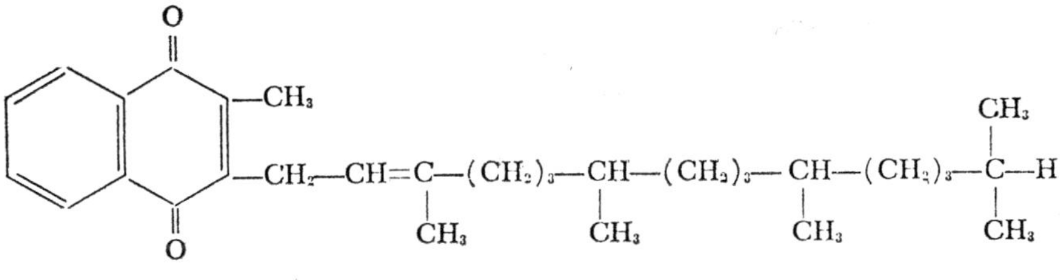

Vitamin K₁

FIG. 4–1.   Structures of the fat-soluble vitamins.

Vitamins E and K

There is a paucity of information available regarding the effects of vitamins E and K upon mineralization of bone and teeth. Vitamin K, the antihemorrhagic factor, is essential for synthesis of the clotting factor, prothrombin. During coagulation, prothrombin is converted to thrombin, which in turn is necessary for conversion of fibrinogen into a fibrin clot.

Vitamin E was isolated when it was found that vitamin E-deficient diets produced sterility in the rat, thus its designation as the antisterility factor. Its metabolic function probably involves the ability to function as an antioxidant, which in turn helps to stabilize biological membranes. In the rat, vitamin E deficiency, in addition to producing sterility, destroys the integrity of the enamel organ. Hypovitaminosis E causes elaboration of chalky white enamel with the enamel organ becoming edematous and disorganized.

Vitamin A

Definitive work on vitamin A occurred when the biochemical mechanisms of vitamin D were established. More than one form of vitamin A exists. Vitamin A_1 is an unsaturated primary alcohol. Other forms include an aldehyde, retinal; an acid, retinoic acid; and esters that are all biologically active. Plant precursors of vitamin A, the carotenes, may be converted to vitamin A during digestion and absorption.

The search for and eventual discovery of vitamin A was initiated when a component of butter was found to be necessary for growth in experimental animals and for the prevention of blindness in children. The presence of vitamin A precursors in the yellow pigments of certain vegetables was also established. In animals, the main stores of vitamin A occur in the liver with minor amounts in kidneys, adrenal glands, and adipose tissue. The large vitamin A content in certain fish oils led to its early confusion with vitamin D.

The important role of vitamin A in the visual cycle and in the prevention of follicular hyperkeratosis is well known. Chronic hypovitaminosis A leads to xerophthalmia, keratomalacia, and permanent blindness. Collection of excess keratin into white foamy patches on the cornea (Bitot's spots) is also characteristic of hypovitaminosis A. Such symptoms are mainly attributed to alterations in epithelial structures during hypovitaminosis A in which epithelial cells degenerate toward a stratified squamous type with increased keratinization.

Effects of vitamin A on calcified tissues have been well documented. Vitamin A deficiency disturbs the pattern of bone resorption and bone formation so that bone becomes unusually thickened. Histological sections show superfluous bone in certain areas with complete or partial failure of bone resorption in other areas. The normal positions of osteoblasts and osteoclasts during growth appear reversed and result in abnormal bone patterns. Compression of various cranial and vertebral nerves from bone growth frequently results in severe nerve damage. Vitamin A is therefore considered to direct the action of both osteoclasts and osteoblasts in the normal growth and remodeling of bone by mechanisms not yet understood.

Excess vitamin A is toxic and symptoms are quick to appear. Eskimos and Arctic explorers have died from eating livers of certain Arctic animals that contained as much as 7,500,000 IU of vitamin A per pound. Severe headache, abdominal pains, excessive sweating, peeling of skin, and death can occur within a short time. Chronic hypervitaminosis A is occasionally seen in food faddists and in children of well-meaning parents. The concept that "if one vitamin pill is good, two are better" is difficult to counter, and toxic symptoms are frequently interpreted by the non-professional as a call for increasing dosage.

In vitro experiments show that vitamin A exerts a direct action upon bone which leads to the appearance of osteoclasts and increased bone resorption. In tissue culture, ^{35}S previously incorporated into cartilage is released when vitamin A is added to culture media and further incorporation of ^{35}S is inhibited. It has been suggested that vitamin A in optimal concentrations helps to stabilize cell membranes. Vitamin A in excess may possibly alter membrane properties that release the enzymes responsible for bone resorption.

Vitamin D

Of the four fat-soluble vitamins, efforts devoted toward elucidating the physiological action of vitamin D have been the most rewarding during the past decade. Symptoms of hypovitaminosis D were experienced by ancient man whose skeletal remains bear evidence of both rickets and osteomalacia. The "cod liver oil" cure was probably known to laymen in the sixteenth century but like so many other important discoveries was not fully appreciated. Originally confused with vitamin A, the uniqueness of vitamin D was established after oxidative destruction of vitamin A in correlated feeding experiments.

Demonstration of the antirachitic effects of ultraviolet light and sunlight on either skin or food caused considerable misunderstanding in the 1920s, until it was established that certain sterols may be photochemically converted to vitamin D. Under ultraviolet irradiation (250 to 305 nm), ergosterol of plants is converted to vitamin D_2 (ergocalciferol). In the malpighian layer of the epidermis, vitamin D_3 or cholecalciferol is synthesized from 7-dehydrocholesterol, a metabolic intermediate during cholesterol synthesis, through the action of sunlight. The increasing prevalence of rickets, concomitant with decreasing skin pigmentation as ancient man migrated from his equatorial origins toward the poles, bears testimony to the beneficial effect of sunlight. Indeed, the adaptive changes of skin coloration to preclude hyper- or hypovitaminosis D are believed to be involved in the evolution of man's skin coloration.

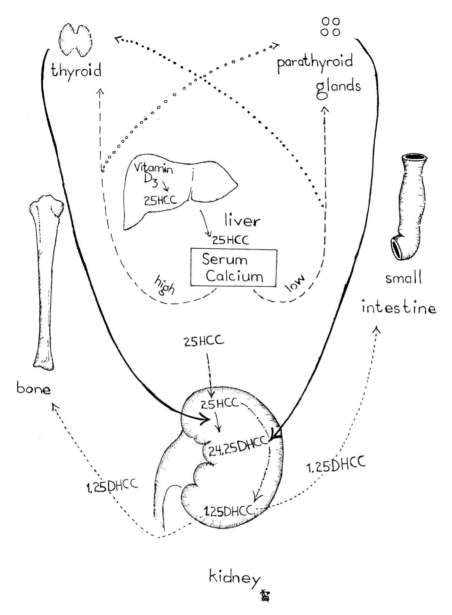

FIG. 4–2. A proposed mechanism for interrelating parathyroid hormone, calcitonin, and vitamin D action. Hypocalcemia releases parathyroid hormone (PTH) into the circulation. PTH is known to stimulate conversion of 25-HCC to 1,25-DHCC in the kidney. This polar metabolite is transported to the intestine where calcium transport increases, and to bone cells where osteoclastic and osteolytic activity is stimulated. Both actions result in increased serum calcium levels, which in turn lowers serum PTH and increases that of calcitonin (CT). CT may in some manner be involved by diverting metabolism of 25-HCC from 1,25-DHCC to the less active 24,25-DHCC. This scheme, although attractive and supported by a variety of observations, must be viewed as a hypothesis until conflicting evidence has been resolved. (Drawing courtesy of Saint-Paul Gaffney, Jr.)

Probably the most critical function of vitamin D is to maintain normal blood serum calcium and phosphorus levels. It is generally considered that vitamin D must be activated before effecting this physiological function. The metabolism of vitamin D is shown in Figure 4–2.

Dietary vitamin D is absorbed from both the ileum and jejunum. The process requires bile and essential fatty acid, and lipid-soluble vitamin deficiencies should be considered if difficulties in fat absorption are prolonged. The absorbed vitamin enters the systemic circulation through the thoracic duct and is apparently transported initially by serum lipoproteins. With time, the transport of vitamin D, as well as its succeeding metabolites, is transferred to a serum alpha globulin with an approximate molecular weight of 50,000 to 60,000.

Initial metabolism of dietary or *in vivo*-synthesized vitamin D_3 occurs in the liver to produce 25-hydroxycholecalciferol (25-HCC). Metabolism of vitamin D_2 is believed to follow a similar pathway. Hepatectomized rats are unable to convert vitamin D_3 to 25-HCC. The 25-hydroxylase system is found in liver endoplasmic reticulum, has a pH optimum of 6.9, and requires molecular oxygen as well as reduced pyridine nucleotide. Although *in vivo* and *in vitro* experiments suggest that the enzyme system is inhibited by 25-HCC, massive vitamin D administration can overwhelm this safeguard, resulting in toxic effects such as soft-tissue mineralization, bone resorption, and kidney stones.

The next important reaction occurs in the kidney where 25-HCC is converted to more polar metabolites: 1,25-dihydroxycholecalciferol (1,25-DHCC), 24,25-dihydroxycholecalciferol (24,25-DHCC), and 1,24,25-tri-hydroxycholecalciferol (1,24,25-THCC) are among the products so far identified. The 1-hydroxylase system is a mixed function oxidase and is found in kidney mitochondria. It is sensitive to various metabolic inhibitors, requires reduced pyridine nucleotide, and utilizes molecular oxygen. The physiological actions of 24,25-DHCC and 1,24,25-THCC are not yet well documented.

It is apparent that 1,25-DHCC is the active form of vitamin D that affects calcium absorption in the intestine and bone resorption by bone cells. 1,25-DHCC is severalfold more active in this regard than its parent compound, 25-HCC or vitamin D_3. Since 1,25-DHCC is produced within the body at a site distant from bone and intestine, it is frequently referred to as a hormone rather than as a vitamin.

The exact mechanisms whereby 1,25-DHCC increases intestinal transport of calcium still remain debatable. The appearance of a calcium-binding protein and a calcium-dependent ATPase some 12 hours following vitamin D administration to rachitic animals suggests the role of protein synthesis in stimulating calcium transport. Another theory holds that the hydroxylated metabolite exerts its action by altering properties of the intestinal membrane during calcium transport. The 1,25-DHCC also has a direct effect upon bone. Addition of 1,25-DHCC to bone cell cultures results in bone resorption with increased calcium levels in the media.

Vitamin D metabolites have occasionally been used to treat vitamin D-resistant rickets and other bone diseases. Patients with metabolic bone disease resulting from liver or kidney disease in which vitamin D metabolism has been limited have benefited from the administration of either 25-HCC or 1,25-DHCC.

LIPIDS IN MEMBRANES

Cellular organization is dependent upon the presence of continuous structures that provide barriers between aqueous phases. These structures, called *membranes*, are characterized by a high lipid content and are impermeable to most water-soluble compounds. Each cell is surrounded by a membrane, and the various organelles of the cell are also bounded by membranes. In fact, an intact cell membrane is an absolutely essential feature of all living cells. In addition to separating cells into discrete compartments, membranes provide a framework for certain specialized metabolic units of the cell.

The calcification processes involve the movement of ions, particularly calcium and phosphate, across membranes, and since the recent discovery that membranous structures are associated with the initiation of calcification, a discussion of membrane structure and function has been included in this chapter.

Composition

Lipids and proteins are the major components of membranes with proteins making up 45 to 60% of the dry weight. An exception is myelin which is about 70% lipid. The bulk of the lipid consists of phospholipid which is

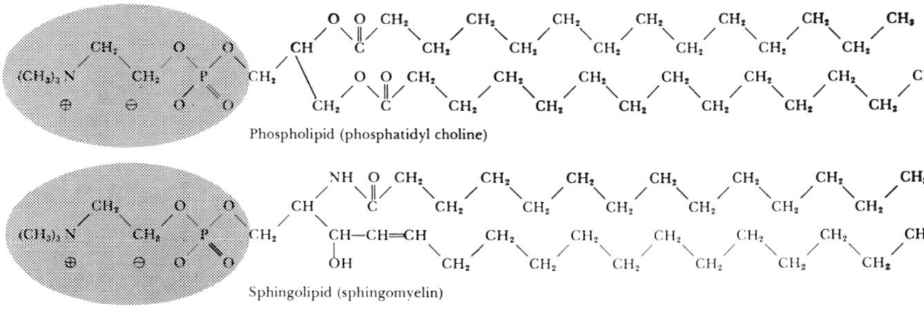

Phospholipid (phosphatidyl choline)

Sphingolipid (sphingomyelin)

Fig. 4–3. General structures of two types of lipids commonly found in membranes. The areas enclosed in the shaded ovals represent the polar head, whereas the unshaded acyl chains are the nonpolar tails. In other phospholipids, the choline residue of the polar head is replaced with ethanolamine, serine, inositol, or inositol phosphates. In other sphingolipids, the choline residue is replaced with oligosaccharides such as galactose. In addition, the acyl chains can vary in length and number of double bonds.

Table 4–2. Relative Composition of Some Membranes

Source of Membrane	mg Phospholipid / mg Protein	Phospholipids (% of total)						
		PC	PE	PS	PI	SPH	CL	PA
Rat liver cells:								
Plasma	0.46	31	20	9	9	19	(4.3)	
Mitochondrial								
(outer)	0.88	49	31	8	5	—	3	—
(inner)	0.30	41	35	3	7	—	21	—
Microsome	0.39	70	21	5	13	5	0.5	—
Bovine epiphyseal cartilage:								
Matrix vesicles	0.25	34	21	13	8	15	3	2.6

Note the similarity between the phospholipid composition of plasma membranes and the matrix vesicles. PC, phosphatidyl choline; PE, phosphatidyl ethanolamine; PS, phosphatidyl serine; PI, phosphatidyl inositol; SPH, sphingomyelin; CL, cardiolipin; PA, phosphatidic acid.

about 20 to 40% of the membrane dry weight. The two most commonly found phospholipids are phosphatidyl choline and phosphatidyl ethanolamine. Another class of lipids found in relatively large amounts in certain membranes is the sphingolipids such as sphingomyelin. The general structures of phospholipids and sphingolipids are shown in Figure 4–3. A characteristic feature of cell plasma membranes is the relatively high level of sphingomyelin. Cardiolipin (diphosphatidyl glycerol) is a unique phospholipid present in the inner mitochondrial membrane. The phospholipid composition can thus be used as a means of characterizing membranes. Some membranes, particularly the plasma membrane of erythrocytes, contain significant amounts of cholesterol. Various glycolipids, peptidoglycans, and glycoproteins are also minor constituents of certain membranes.

A wide variety of proteins are associated with membranes both as structural components and as bound enzymes. For example, more than 25 different proteins have been found to be associated with the erythrocyte plasma membrane. Membrane proteins vary considerably in size, ranging from 10,000 to 200,000 in molecular weight. Structural proteins that are an integral part of the membrane are globular proteins with a high α-helical content. The relative distribution of lipids and proteins in a variety of membranes is summarized in Table 4–2.

Structure

Basically, the phospholipids are the molecules that define membrane structure. These compounds are amphipathic in nature, which means that

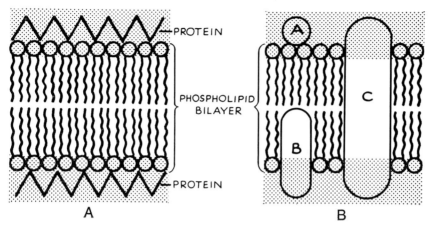

Fɪɢ. 4–4. Diagrams of membrane models. A, Unit membrane of Robertson. B, Lipid-globular protein mosaic model in which A represents hydrophilic proteins, B represents bimodal proteins, and C represents predominantly hydrophobic proteins which are part of the membrane continuum.

they contain both polar and nonpolar regions. The polar end is the base that is covalently bound to glycerol phosphate. The nonpolar region is the fatty acid side chains of the glycerol esters. When phospholipids are placed in water, the fatty acids become sequestered together away from contact with water through *hydrophobic* interactions. The polar ends project into and associate with water through *hydrophilic* interactions. The most stable arrangement for phospholipids in an aqueous environment is as a continuous bilayer made up of a double layer of molecules with the fatty acids projected toward each other (Fig. 4–4).

The lipid bilayer is the essential part of membrane structure proposed by Danielli and Davson in 1935. Robertson expanded this structure into a unit membrane theory in which all membranes consist of bimolecular lipid leaflets with a complete protein coat on each side (Fig. 4–4A). Electron micrographs of membranes show a trilaminar structure 60 to 100 Å in thickness, which is consistent with the bilayer theory. Although it is generally accepted that the phospholipid bilayer is an essential feature of membrane structure, there is still debate as to whether the protein coating is continuous. For example, the inner mitochondrial membrane has been proposed to consist of lipoprotein units in which the protein molecules are an integral part of the structure rather than being a surface coat. More recently, Singer has proposed a lipid-globular–protein mosaic model for membrane structure (Fig. 4–4B). This model implies a basic phospholipid bilayer continuum; however, the protein molecules, rather than forming a surface coating, are dispersed. Some proteins are located on the surface, whereas others penetrate into the hydrophobic core of the membrane. There is evidence that some proteins extend completely through the lipid bilayer and as such would be part of the membrane continuum. Nonpolar proteins have been isolated from membranes and obviously interact with the hydrophobic core. Others are amphipathic, containing both polar and nonpolar regions. The lipid-protein mosaic model is attractive because it incorporates all the possible lipid bilayer-protein interactions, from electrostatic binding on the surface to hydrophobic bonding within the interior of the membrane.

Another feature of membrane structure is that it is asymmetric. Not only are different protein molecules found on opposite sides of the bilayer, but variations in the types of phospholipids also occur. For example, phosphatidyl choline and sphingomyelin are found on the outside of the erythrocyte plasma membrane, whereas phosphatidyl ethanolamine is found on the inside. Glycoproteins occur almost exclusively on the outer surfaces of cell membranes.

Functions

The primary function of membranes is to separate various aqueous phases in biological systems. In the living cell, the plasma membrane is a functional barrier between the cell's interior and its external environment. The membrane also contains the mechanisms by which cells take in and maintain those substances needed for normal metabolism.

Since most polar molecules cannot penetrate the lipid core of the membrane, special mechanisms have been established in order to move these substances across membranes. These mechanisms are known as transport systems and can be either passive or active.

Passive Transport. Passive transport systems facilitate the movement of polar substances down a concentration gradient and require no energy expenditure. One concept of passive transport requires the presence of protein molecules that penetrate the lipid bilayer and provide a hydrophilic core through which ions and molecules can diffuse. The nature of the protein provides specificity as to what type of substance can diffuse through, *i.e.*, size and charge.

Another type of passive transport is through the coupling of the molecule with a carrier substance, most likely protein, that shields the hydrophilic character and allows penetration through the membrane. This type of transport has been called "facilitated diffusion." An example is the entry of glucose into erythrocytes.

Active Transport. Active transport systems are the most important means by which cells acquire adequate concentrations of essential nutrients and regulate their internal ionic environment. Active transport is characterized by a requirement for expenditure of energy, the movement of substances against a concentration gradient, and by being unidirectional. Active transport systems either require ATP for energy or are coupled with a system that uses ATP. A classic example is the (Na^+-K^+) ATPase transport system found in virtually all cell plasma membranes. The primary

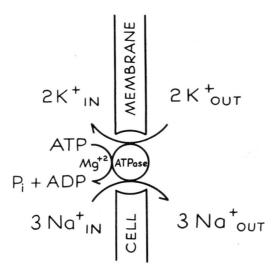

Fig. 4–5. Mechanism of Na⁺-K⁺ ATPase transport. The inside of the cell is on the left. For each molecule of ATP hydrolyzed, 3 Na⁺ ions are transported out and 2 K⁺ ions are transported in. Mg⁺² is required to transfer a PO₄ group from ATP to the enzyme (ATPase).

function of the system is to move K^+ ions into and Na^+ ions out of the cell. The mechanism is summarized in Fig. 4–5. Amino acids and some sugars are actively transported by being coupled to the Na^+-K^+ transport system.

Calcium transport, which is important to the metabolism of calcified tissues, occurs through a similar mechanism requiring ATP and an intermediate phosphorylated transport protein (E).

1. $ATP + E \rightarrow E \sim P + ADP$

2. $E \sim P \rightarrow E + Pi$

$$Ca^{+2}_{out} \qquad Ca^{+2}_{in}$$

Membranes also provide a structural framework for various complexes of metabolic enzymes. For example, the enzymes required in the mitochondria for oxidative phosphorylation and electron transport are membrane bound. Cell movement and adhesion are dependent upon the plasma membrane. Changes in cell shape such as occur during pinocytosis and phagocytosis involve membranes. The glycoproteins comprising antigen-antibody reactions are associated with cell membranes.

SELECTED REFERENCES

Lipids

AVIOLI, L. V., and HADDAD, J. G.: Progress in endocrinology and metabolism. Vitamin D: Current concepts. Metabolism, 22, 507–531, 1973.

BARNICOT, N. A., and DATTA, S. P.: Vitamin A and bone. In *The Biochemistry and Physiology of Bone*, Vol. II. G. H. Bourve (Ed.), New York, Academic Press, Inc., 1972, Chapter 5.

DAS, S. K., and HARRIS, R. S.: Fatty acids in the tooth lipids of 16 animal species. J. Dent. Res., *49*, 119–125, 1970.

DAS, S. K., and HARRIS, R. S.: Lipids and fatty acids in fossil teeth. J. Dent. Res., *49*, 126–130, 1970.

DELUCA, H. F.: Vitamin D: The vitamin and the hormone. Fed. Proc., *33*, 2211–2219, 1974.

DIRKSEN, T. R.: Lipid components of sound and carious dentin. J. Dent. Res., *42*, 128–132, 1963.

DIRKSEN, T. R., and IKELS, K. G.: Quantitative determination of some constituent lipids in human dentin. J. Dent. Res., *43*, 246–251, 1964.

DIRKSEN, T. R., and MARINETTI, G. V.: Lipids of bovine enamel and dentin and human bone. Calcif. Tissue Res., *6*, 1–10, 1970.

IRVING, J. T., and WUTHIER, R. E.: Histochemistry and biochemistry of calcification with special reference to the role of lipids. Clin. Orthop., *56*, 237–260, 1968.

IRVING, J. T.: The patterns of sudanophilia in developing rat molar enamel. Arch. Oral Biol., *18*, 137–140, 1973.

ODUTUGA, A. A., and PROUT, R. E. S.: Lipid analysis of human enamel and dentine. Arch. Oral Biol., *19*, 729–731, 1974.

OPDYKE, D. L. J.: The histochemistry of dental decay. Arch. Oral Biol., 7, 207–219, 1962.

PERESS, N. S., ANDERSON, C. H., and SAJDERA, S. K.: The lipids of matrix vesicles from bovine fetal epiphyseal cartilage. Calcif. Tissue Res., *14*, 275–281, 1974.

PINDBORG, J. J.: The effect of vitamin E deficiency on the rat incisor. J. Dent. Res., *31*, 805–811, 1952.

PROUT, R. E. S., and SHUTT, E. R.: Analysis of fatty acids in human root dentine and enamel. Arch. Oral Biol., *15*, 281–286, 1970.

SHAPIRO, I. M., WUTHIER, R. E., and IRVING, J. T.: A study of the phospholipids of bovine dental tissues. I. Enamel matrix and dentine. Arch. Oral Biol., *11*, 501–512, 1966.

WUTHIER, R. E.: A zonal analysis of inorganic constituents of the epiphysis during endochondral calcification. Calcif. Tissue Res., *4*, 20–38, 1969.

WUTHIER, R. E.: The role of phospholipids in biological calcification. Clin. Orthop., *90*, 191–200, 1973.

Membranes

CAPALDI, R. A.: A dynamic model of cell membranes. Sci. Am., *230*, 26–33, 1974.

ROTHFIELD, L. I. (Ed.): *Structure and Function of Biological Membranes*. New York, Academic Press, 1971.

SINGER, S. J., and NICOLSON, G. L.: The fluid mosaic model of the structure of cell membranes. Science, *175*, 720–731, 1972.

STOECKENIUS, W., and ENGELMAN, D. M.: Current models for the structure of biological membranes (review). J. Cell Biol., *42*, 613–646, 1969.

Chapter 5

Histochemistry of Developing Teeth

J. P. KENNEDY, Ph.D.

The development of human teeth is a complex, dynamic physicochemical process that begins about the sixth or seventh week of intrauterine life. Each tooth develops from a tooth germ which is derived from two embryonic tissues, ectoderm and mesoderm. The tooth germs of either deciduous or permanent teeth undergo similar structural and chemical transformations. Morphodifferentiation of tooth germs specific for premolars is different from that of tooth germs that give rise to incisors. This is a brief discussion of certain histochemical changes in the development of a human tooth from initiation through the formation of hard dental tissues which begins about the twentieth week of intrauterine life.

Human enamel is formed from the epithelial dental organ or enamel organ which is derived from part of the ectodermal epithelium that lines the oral cavity. Dentine and pulp are formed from the dental papilla which is derived from the mesenchyme that condenses and lies partly within the inverted cup-like epithelial dental organ. Mesenchyme is a loosely arranged, unspecialized embryonic tissue that is the source of all connective tissue. Cells, fibers, tissue fluid, and ground substance are the components of connective tissue. The epithelial dental organ and its subjacent dental papilla are invested by a connective tissue follicle, the dental sac. Cementum, peridental ligament, and part of the alveolar bone are derived from the dental sac. Thus, the epithelial dental organ, dental papilla, and the dental sac produce all components of teeth exclusive of the nerve and vascular supply (Table 5–1).

Oral tissues contain several chemical constituents which reflect their epithelial and connective tissue origin and structure. These chemical substances include mucopolysaccharides, glycoproteins, mucins and certain enzymes.

4

Table 5–1. Schema of Tooth Development

ectodermal epithelium	dental lamina	epithelial dental organ	outer dental epithelium stellate reticulum stratum intermedium inner dental epithelium (ameloblasts)	enamel Nasmyth's membrane Hertwig's epithelial sheath
mesoderm		dental papilla	odontoblasts Korff's fibers blood vessels	dentine pulp
		dental sac	osteoblasts fibroblasts cementoblasts	alveolus peridental membrane cementum

HISTOGENESIS

The derivation and development of dental tissues may be considered in the physiological and histogenetic phases of (1) initiation, (2) proliferation, (3) histodifferentiation and morphodifferentiation, and (4) apposition. The life cycle of a tooth is depicted in Figure 5–1. Variability in prenatal tooth development should be acknowledged in a discussion of histogenetic and histochemical dental events even when there is reference to conventional stages of tooth development. First trimester male human fetuses are dentally advanced in comparison to their female counterparts.

Continuity and interrelationships in the histogenesis of dental tissues have been described in general, but much additional critical study is needed before a precise and coherent understanding is possible. Even with information obtained from studies using techniques such as historadiography, autoradiography, electron microscopy, special histochemical procedures, and others, the histogenesis and histochemistry of dental tissues remain controversial and inadequately known. Methods of histology and cytology are described by Bloom and Fawcett, histochemistry by Pearse and instrumental or physical techniques by Newman in their respective publications. A simple and fundamental account of the developing tooth germ follows.

Initiation or the beginning of tooth development is a brief but significant process that occurs in human embryos of about 11 mm in length. Initiation

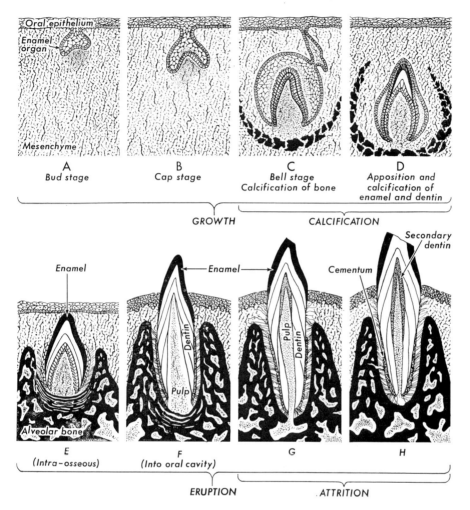

Fig. 5–1. Diagram of the life cycle of a human deciduous incisor. (Bloom, W., and Fawcett, D. W.: *A Textbook of Histology*, 10th ed. Philadelphia, W. B. Saunders Co., 1975.)

is clearly indicated by the appearance of the dental lamina, a local thickening of the ectodermal epithelium which outlines the future dental arches. Mitotic cells of epithelium and mesenchyme are present. Glycogen is evident in the cytoplasm. By subsequent ingrowth the dental lamina presents a continuous band-like ridge into the mesenchyme. At points indicative of specific deciduous teeth, small epithelial buds appear from the dental lamina. These bud-like structures with pertinent underlying mesenchyme are the developing tooth germs.

Proliferation or cell multiplication and growth continue at a rapid but unequal rate until the epithelial tooth germ caps a condensing mass of

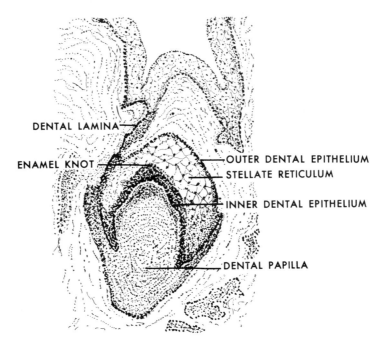

DENTAL LAMINA

ENAMEL KNOT

OUTER DENTAL EPITHELIUM

STELLATE RETICULUM

INNER DENTAL EPITHELIUM

DENTAL PAPILLA

FIG. 5–2. Intermediate stage of epithelial dental organ.
(Redrawn and modified from Bevelander.)

mesenchyme, the dental papilla. The cap-like epithelial tooth germ continues to proliferate and begins to histodifferentiate into a bell-shaped structure, the epithelial dental organ, which partially encloses the dental papilla. At this early stage of development the epithelial dental organ consists of an outer dental epithelium separated from the inner dental epithelium by a fluid-filled cellular network, the stellate reticulum (Fig. 5–2). Metachromatic properties of the stellate reticulum ground substance suggest the presence of acid mucopolysaccharides. At a later stage an additional layer is seen between the stellate reticulum and the inner dental epithelium. It is the stratum intermedium which may be derived from some of the subjacent cells of the inner dental epithelium. The cuboidal cells of the stratum intermedium may be pertinent to the formation of the future epithelial attachment of the cervix of the tooth to the oral mucosa. The cuboidal cells of the outer dental epithelium are arranged radially; the low columnar cells of the inner dental epithelium appear regular and increase in height to form the ameloblasts.

Functions of the stellate reticulum and the stratum intermedium are problematical. It is doubtful that they serve solely as a cushion to be replaced by hard tissue. The presence and similar commencement of enzymatic activity in the stellate reticulum and the stratum intermedium suggest a

Table 5–2. Enzyme Activity of Certain Cells Associated
with Developing Teeth

	Alkaline Phospha- tase*	Acid Phospha- tase*	Amino Pepti- dase†	Cyto- chrome Oxi- dase†	Succinic Dehydro- genase†
Stellate reticulum	++	0	+	+	+
Stratum inter- medium	++	0	+	+	+
Ameloblasts (molar)	0	0	0	0 or +	0
Odontoblasts	+ or ++	0	+	+	+

0 = no staining; + = less active; ++ = more active.
* Frozen-dried paraffin-embedded tissues
† Fresh-frozen tissues
(After Sicher, H., and Bhaskar, S. N. (Eds.): *Orban's Oral Histology and Embryology*, 7th ed. St. Louis, C. V. Mosby Co., 1972.)

metabolic function. Dehydrogenase activity in these two layers has been reported (Table 5–2).

After the disintegration of the epithelial remnant that connected the epithelial dental organ to the oral epithelium, the tooth germ is completely invested by the dental sac. Within the dental sac a small epithelial strand projects from the lingual surface of the epithelial dental organ. It is the dental lamina or successional lamina of the permanent tooth. Molars that are not preceded by deciduous teeth develop from the extension of the dental lamina posterior to the position of the second deciduous molar.

The epithelial dental organ is important in the formation of human enamel. It also influences the elaboration of dentine and the shape of the tooth root through the formation of Hertwig's epithelial sheath. Hertwig's sheath consists of the inner and outer dental epithelium that extends inward about the apical region of the tooth apparently to function as a diaphragm during root formation. Nasmyth's membrane or cuticle covers the enamel of the erupting tooth. It is derived from the stratum intermedium. The cuticle is resistant to certain acids and may be protective.

HISTOCHEMISTRY

Histochemical properties of the developing dental papilla may be summarized before discussing the elaboration of dentine and enamel. The ground substance of the dental papilla contains an acid mucopolysaccharide as inferred by metachromasia with toluidine blue. Cells of the dental

the premise that the odontoblasts function in the formation of protocollagen which, when extracellular, forms some collagen fibrils of the dentine.

It is generally believed that collagen or reticular fibers form the fibrous part of the dentinal matrix. The genesis of these fibers is controversial, but a dual origin is not unreasonable. Small width, randomly arranged fibers that are located near the odontoblast process apparently result from odontoblast activity. The larger fibers of Korff probably originate from the pulp. Interestingly, regardless of their size all show staining and structural characteristics indicative of collagen.

Numerous histochemical investigations, mostly of rodent teeth, report the presence of various and diverse compounds in the developing odontoblastic layer and subjacent pulp. These compounds include glycogen, mucopolysaccharides, acid polysaccharides, alkaline phosphatase, acid phosphatase, 5 nucleic acid, lipid (sudanophilic droplets), sulfhydryl and disulfide groups and ascorbic acid. The odontoblasts show dehydrogenase activity which may be related to citric acid and pentose cycles. Histochemical techniques have indicated the presence of succinic, malic, isocitric, glutamic, lactic, β-hydroxybutyrate, α-glycerophosphate, glucose-6-phosphate and 6-phosphogluconate dehydrogenases and DPN and TPN diaphorases in the teeth of 5-day-old rats. In general, enzymatic activity precedes the microscopic evidence of dentine and enamel; activity of dehydrogenases is seemingly related to the differentiation and function of the odontoblasts. This inventory of compounds in developing teeth, particularly in the odontoblastic layer and pulp, indicates a metabolic role of these tissues in dentinogenesis.

Predentinal apposition always precedes the formation of dentine. Predentine appears near the developing occlusal surface of the tooth just before the formation of enamel. Concomitant with the deposition of predentine, changes are evident in the odontoblasts. The once columnar odontoblasts recede pulpward leaving cytoplasmic processes that course within small canals, the dentinal tubules, toward and sometimes slightly beyond the dentino-enamel junction. Thus, the formation of dentine consists first in the elaboration of a zone of predentine which contains fibers, a mucopolysaccharide ground substance and the vital odontoblast processes or Tomes' dentinal fibrils, which do not calcify.

At thicknesses of about 10 to 20 microns mineralization of predentin begins, nearest the dentino-enamel junction. Dense granules of approximately 100 Å containing an acid mucopolysaccharide appear and may represent the first part of the matrix to undergo mineralization. Subsequently, small mineral crystals appear on the periodic 640 Å bands of the collagen fibers. These fibers appear to be coated with an acid mucopolysaccharide similar to that of the interfibrillar matrix. Development and coalescence mainly through crystal growth lead to the homogeneous mineralized matrix with mature apatite crystals.

Mineralization is usually at first intertubular and mineralization of this matrix is followed by the formation of peritubular dentine within the dentinal tubules. Peritubular dentine stains intensely and metachromatically with toluidine and methyl blue at pH 2.6 and 3.6 respectively. It stains deeply with alcian blue at pH 2.6. This indicates a high acid mucopolysaccharide content of peritubular dentine. Symons believes that the content of other polysaccharide is apparently low because of the failure to stain with the PAS method. It should be made clear that peritubular zone first begins to appear in the mineralized dentine within the dentinal tubule.

According to Bevelander and Nakahara the functional odontoblast elaborates an acid mucopolysaccharide which is probably chondroitin sulfate and is transported to the sites of mineralization. However, the mechanism that initiates crystal formation in the dentinal matrix is not fully understood (see Chapter 6). The acid mucopolysaccharide may serve to transport mineral from the cell to the dentinal matrix. Sulfated mucopolysaccharides may attract or bind positively charged metals such as calcium.

The process of predentine formation and its mineralization is repeated as long as dentine formation continues. As previously indicated, mineralization occurs first at the future dentino-enamel junction in the developing tooth and later at the dentine-predentine border after the first increment of dentine is formed. Thus, dentine formation is by apposition of incremental zones. Estimates of the rate of daily dentine deposition in mammalian teeth, exclusive of the continuously growing teeth of rodents, range from about 2 to 16 microns.

AMELOGENESIS

Amelogenesis may be considered as occurring in two conspicuous phases: (1) organic matrix formation and (2) maturation of enamel. After the initial formation of dentine, cells of the inner dental epithelium begin the formation of enamel and are referred to as ameloblasts. The formation of enamel and dentine is depicted in Figure 5–4.

On the basis of functional and cytological differences, two kinds of ameloblasts may be recognized. They are the tall ameloblasts which are synthesizing and secretory cells engaged in the initial elaboration of the enamel matrix, and the short or post-secretory ameloblasts which function in the maturation of enamel through the removal of organic material and possibly water from the enamel.

The tall ameloblasts are associated with a stratum intermedium in which enzymatic activity is seemingly intense. The close association of the stratum intermedium with blood vessels and its high alkaline phosphatase content suggest that this layer may serve as a barrier involved in the selective transport of certain material to the proximal or basal part of the ameloblasts, which is nearest the stratum intermedium. The precise role of alkaline phosphatase is not known, but it can be associated with biological transport mechanisms. It has also been suggested that the stratum intermedium func-

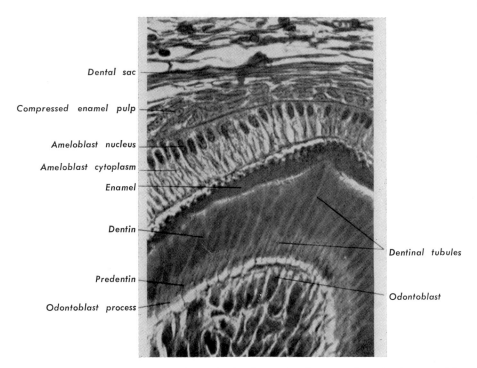

Dental sac

Compressed enamel pulp

Ameloblast nucleus

Ameloblast cytoplasm

Enamel

Dentin

Predentin

Odontoblast process

Dentinal tubules

Odontoblast

Fig. 5–4. Formation of enamel and dentine in the developing incisor of a 5-month-old human fetus. Mallory-azan stain. (Bloom, W., and Fawcett, D. W.: *A Textbook of Histology*, 10th ed. Philadelphia, W. B. Saunders Co., 1975.)

tions as a barrier and that alkaline phosphatase splits inhibitory organophosphates.

There is evidence that the formation of enamel involves an extracellular secretion rather than an intracellular transformation. Consideration of the enamel matrix as keratin or keratin-like is unjustified according to Reith and Butcher. Protein formation is intracellular, that is, the product of the proteinizing cell is retained. Nevertheless, protein has been considered an important structure in the formation of the enamel matrix. This conclusion has been supported by similarities in the staining properties of developing enamel and certain amino acids. It seems clear that enamel contains a protein with SH groups which stain intensely red with Mallory's trichrome stain. However, the sulfhydryl reaction is not specific for keratin and conclusions of the specific identity of this protein matrix must be made with caution. Other techniques suggest that the protein matrix has a cross-beta configuration in which polypeptide chains course transversely to the axis of the fibrils.

Tall secretory ameloblasts contain highly organized cisternae of granular endoplasmic reticulum. The demonstration of a plasma membrane between the cytoplasm of the secretory ameloblasts and the apparent product of these cells supports the premise that enamel is an extracellular product. This interpretation is at variance with the traditional view that the enamel matrix is a transformation of the apical cytoplasm or Tomes' process and that enamel prisms are essentially an intracellular elongation of the ameloblasts.

It is believed that the ameloblasts elaborate enamel matrix which calcifies extracellularly. Calcification begins at the periphery of each prism. During maturation organic material and fluid are removed and calcium salts enter the developing enamel apparently by means of the epithelial dental organ. Inorganic crystallization begins after the initial deposition of the organic enamel matrix. Apatite crystal growth continues and subsequently mature apatite crystals appear. In mature enamel the organic material is almost entirely replaced by a calcified matrix.

CEMENTOGENESIS

Cementogenesis consists of the formation of an uncalcified layer of cementoid tissue and its subsequent transformation into calcified cementum. The process is suggestive of the formation of dentine and bone.

Dentine formation in the root is influenced by Hertwig's epithelial sheath which for a time separates dentine of the root from the surrounding dental sac. As the epithelial sheath degenerates, cells from the inner zone of the dental sac are observed near the root surface. These cells differentiate into cuboidal cells, the cementoblasts, which elaborate cementoid tissue. The formation of cementum is always preceded by the deposition of a thin layer of cementoid tissue.

The argyrophilic fibers of the dental sac apparently serve as a source of collagen for the formation of the collagen fibrils of the cementoid substance. Mucopolysaccharides from the connective tissue are transformed into the cementoid ground substance. Calcification involves a depolymerization of the ground substance, the incorporation of calcium phosphate and the deposition of apatite crystals along the collagen fibrils.

Fibers of the peridental ligament course into cementum and into alveolar bone where they are known as Sharpey's fibers. Cementum, peridental ligament, and alveolar bone form the suspensorium for a tooth. Interestingly, cells of the peripheral zone of the dental sac differentiate into osteoblasts of the periosteum of the alveolus. Cementum may be classified as cellular or acellular, but there is no functional difference.

SELECTED REFERENCES

BLOOM, WILLIAM and FAWCETT, DON W.: *A Textbook of Histology*, 10th ed., Philadelphia, W. B. Saunders Co., 1975.

BEVELANDER, GERRIT: *Outline of Histology*, 7th ed., St. Louis, The C. V. Mosby Co., 1971.

BEVELANDER, GERRIT and NAKAHARA, HIROSHI: The formation and mineralization of dentine, Anat. Record, *156*(3): 303–323, 1966.

BEVELANDER, G., and RAMALEY, J. A.: *Essentials of Histology*, 7th ed., St. Louis, The C. V. Mosby Co., 1974.

GARN, S. M., and BURDI, A. R.: Prenatal ordering and postnatal sequence in dental development, J. Dent. Res., (Suppl.) *6*, 1407–1414, 1971.

KRAUS, B. S. and JORDAN, R. E.: *The Human Dentition Before Birth*, Philadelphia, Lea & Febiger, 1965.

NEWMAN, DAVID N. (ed.): *Instrumental Methods of Experimental Biology*, New York, The Macmillan Co., 1964.

PEARSE, A. G. E.: *Histochemistry—Theoretical and Applied*, 3rd ed., Boston, Little, Brown & Co., 1968.

REITH, EDWARD J. and BUTCHER, EARL O.: Microanatomy and Histochemistry of Amelogenesis, p. 371–397. In A. E. W. Miles (ed.), *Structural and Chemical Organization of Teeth*. New York, Academic Press, Inc., 1967.

SICHER, HARRY (ed.): *Orban's Oral Histology and Embryology*, 7th ed., St. Louis, The C. V. Mosby Co., 1972.

SISCA, R. F., and PROVENZA, D. V.: Initial dentin formation in human deciduous teeth, an electron microscope study, Calcif. Tissue Res., *9*, 1–16, 1972.

SYMONS, N. B. B.: The Microanatomy and Histochemistry of Dentinogenesis, p. 285–324. In A. E. W. Miles (ed.), *Structural and Chemical Organization of Teeth*. New York, Academic Press, Inc., 1967.

Chapter 6

Mineralization of Bones and Teeth

JAMES J. VOGEL, Ph.D.

Certain biological tissues undergo a mineralization process commonly referred to as *calcification*. This process can be defined as a sequence of events whereby specific cells form an organic matrix within which insoluble calcium salts are deposited. The calcium salts can be either carbonates or phosphates depending upon the type of tissue and the environment. In mammalian calcified tissues (bones and teeth) the major calcium salt is a phosphate that is similar in composition to the mineral *hydroxyapatite*, $Ca_{10}(PO_4)_6(OH)_2$. Calcification is a dynamic process with the formation and maintenance of the mineralized matrix controlled by cellular activity. In this chapter, the sources of constituents, theories on the mechanism of initial calcification, the roles of cells, and the maturation of calcified tissues will be discussed.

SOURCE OF CONSTITUENTS OF CALCIFIED TISSUES

The organic components of the calcified tissues are essentially of cellular origin. In addition to cellular constituents, they include a fibrous protein matrix, proteinpolysaccharide ground substances, and lipids. The nature and biosynthesis of the organic components are discussed in separate chapters.

The inorganic constituents must come from external sources, and in mammalian tissues, the source is from the blood pool which is maintained through dietary intake and metabolic turnover. A dynamic equilibrium exists between blood and tissue fluids for some of the inorganic ions. Since calcium and inorganic phosphate are the major constituents of calcified tissues, it is important to understand the interrelations between serum and calcified tissues for these ions.

At physiological pH, calcium and phosphate exist primarily as Ca^{2+} and HPO_4^{2-} ions. The normal concentration of calcium in serum is from 4.5 to 5.5 mEq/L. Approximately 40% of the total calcium is bound by protein and is nondiffusible through a semipermeable membrane. About 45% is ionic calcium and the remaining 15%, although diffusible, is complexed with small anions such as citrate. Approximately 80% of the total serum phosphate exists as HPO_4^{2-} which would amount to a concentration of 1.5 mEq/L. Unlike calcium, little inorganic phosphate is bound to protein.

The relationship between Ca^{2+} and HPO_4^{2-} ions in serum and those in the mineral phase of bone depends upon (1) how ions in serum gain access to the bone tissue fluids and (2) the solubility properties of bone mineral. Generally, serum ions are readily accessible to the fluids surrounding bone mineral as evidenced by the rapid isotopic exchange that occurs when a radioisotope tracer such as ^{45}Ca is used. This means that bone has an adequate blood supply. On the other hand, the net ionic composition of bone tissue fluids is different from that of serum, indicating that a membrane-like barrier is present. Some investigators are of the opinion that the various cell layers in bone provide such a membrane. Thus, although ionic exchange can occur under equilibrium conditions, cellular influences can have a marked effect on the net concentrations of ions. Bone mineral is now believed to consist of two distinct calcium phosphates: an amorphous phase and a crystalline apatite phase. The amorphous phase is deposited first and serves as a precursor for apatite formation. Thus, newly formed bone has a higher concentration of amorphous phase than older bone. Mature bone consists of about 70% apatite and 30% amorphous phase. The presence of two mineral phases has complicated equilibrium studies on Ca^{2+} and HPO_4^{2-} between serum and bone. Since hydroxyapatite is the least soluble salt,

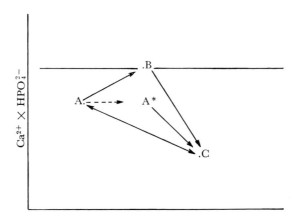

Fig. 6–1. The metastable state of $Ca^{2+} \times HPO_4^{2-}$ is at point A and the solid (hydroxyapatite) state at point C. In order for hydroxyapatite to form, either the ionic product must be increased to point B at which spontaneous precipitation would occur or a catalyst must be introduced which would lower the energy required in forming apatite crystals. This is illustrated by the broken line, the catalyzed intermediate state A* and the line to C. Once hydroxyapatite is formed it is in physical and chemical equilibrium with the ion product of the fluid phase indicated by the double arrow between A and C. The nature of the catalyst will be discussed later in mechanism of calcification.

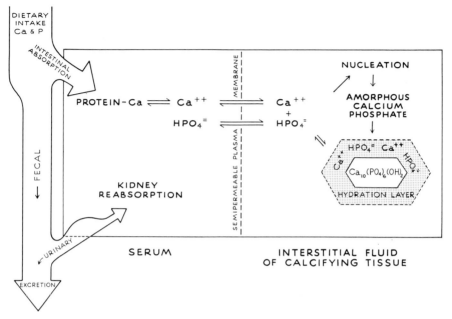

FIG. 6–2.   Routes of calcium and phosphorus in
body fluids and calcified tissues.

most studies have been based upon its solubility.   The $[Ca^{2+} \cdot HPO_4^{2-}]$
product in serum exceeds the experimentally determined solubility product
for hydroxyapatite.   However, the product in serum is not large enough to
result in a spontaneous precipitation of apatite.   Under these conditions the
concentration of Ca^{2+} and HPO_4^{2-} in serum is in a metastable state (Fig.
6 1).   Various factors can influence metastability including the presence of
certain macromolecules and other ions.   The influence of some of these will
be discussed later in this chapter.   Figure 6–2 is a diagram illustrating the
general relationships of Ca^{2+} and HPO_4^{2-} among body fluids and bone
mineral.

The concentrations of Ca^{2+} and HPO_4^{2-} in serum are regulated by a
homeostatic mechanism in which bone, the kidneys, and the intestines all
play important roles.   Three hormones are involved: parathyrin (parathyroid hormone) (PTH), calcitonin (CT), and an active metabolite of vitamin D, 1,25-dihydroxycholecalciferol $[1,25\text{-}(OH)_2D_3]$.   These hormones all
affect target cells in specific ways which either add or remove ions from serum.

Parathyrin (Parathyroid hormone)

The net effect of PTH is to increase the serum calcium concentration.   The
hormone does this by activating the synthesis of the cell messenger, cyclic
AMP, in bone and kidney cells.   In bone, resorption is increased via activa-

tion of both osteocytic and osteoclastic activity while collagen biosynthesis by bone-forming osteoblasts is inhibited. In this way bone calcium is mobilized and transferred to the serum. In order to compensate for the excess phosphate released when bone mineral is dissolved, PTH enhances the renal excretion of inorganic phosphate. The level of calcium in serum regulates the excretion of PTH by the parathyroid glands. A rise in serum Ca inhibits secretion and a fall in serum Ca stimulates secretion.

Calcitonin

Calcitonin (CT) has an effect opposite to that of PTH in that it lowers the level of serum calcium to normal. Its main effect is to inhibit bone resorption which reduces the transfer of Ca^{2+} from bone to serum. The precise mode of action of CT is not fully understood, although its action is also thought to be mediated via cyclic AMP. Higher than normal levels of calcium in serum stimulate the secretion of CT by the thyroid glands. Unlike PTH, calcitonin enhances the renal excretion of both Ca^{2+} and HPO_4^{2-}.

Vitamin D

Before vitamin D can function in the body it must be converted to the active metabolite via two hydroxylation steps. First an OH group is added to the 25 position in the liver and then to the 1 position in the kidney. Newer knowledge indicates that $1,25\text{-}(OH)_2D_3$ functions as a hormone. Its net effect is to maintain adequate concentrations of Ca^{2+} and HPO_4^{2-} in serum and extracellular fluids so that normal bone formation can occur. Its mechanism of action is to program target cells to synthesize a calcium-transporting protein. In the intestine this results in an increase in calcium absorption. The resorption of bone is enhanced by vitamin D but only when PTH is also present. Vitamin D also causes an increase in the serum phosphate concentration by increasing the intestinal absorption, the renal resorption, and the soft tissue mobilization of phosphate. It is the effects on phosphate metabolism that are believed to be the primary effect of vitamin D in preventing or curing rickets.

Other inorganic ions commonly present in calcified tissues include sodium, potassium, magnesium, chloride, fluoride, and carbonate, as well as trace amounts of iron, copper, manganese, and zinc. The bulk of these ions is present in the tissue fluids or located in the hydration layer surrounding the apatite crystals. Bone can serve as a reservoir for many of these ions, particularly magnesium. Certain amounts of Cl^-, F^- and CO_3^{2-} can also be incorporated into the lattice of the crystals. Specific ions have been found to influence the formation and stability of hydroxyapatite. For example, fluoride enhances apatite formation and results in the formation of larger and less-soluble crystals. The incorporation of carbonate into the lattice causes crystals to be more soluble. Magnesium, if present in high enough concentration, stabilizes the amorphous calcium phosphate or retards its conversion to apatite. Whether Mg has a physiological role in this respect is not known; however, the Mg/Ca ratio of bone parallels the amorphous calcium phosphate to apatite ratio with age to some degree. Another function of bone mineral is to remove toxic or harmful ions such as lead and radiostrontium from the body fluids.

MECHANISM OF CALCIFICATION

It is generally accepted that some initial mechanism is required in order for specific tissues to calcify. A great deal of research has been directed toward attempting to understand this initial mechanism responsible for the formation of bones and teeth. The heterogeneous nature of the calcified tissues has complicated these attempts, and as a result, numerous theories on the mechanism of calcification have been proposed.

Since body fluids are metastable with respect to hydroxyapatite, the initiation of calcification can be accomplished in two ways: (1) by a process of *homogeneous nucleation*, whereby the concentrations of calcium and phosphate are increased locally to the point at which spontaneous precipitation of apatite can occur, or (2) by a process of *heterogeneous nucleation*, whereby a catalyst that, in lowering the activation energy, can allow apatite to form from a metastable concentration of calcium and phosphate is present. The various theories on the mechanism of calcification involve either of these two types of nucleation.

One of the earliest theories was that the deposition of calcium phosphate in living animals was initiated by specific protein-metal binding reactions. Later, this concept was expanded to include as a repetitive process calcium binding by protein, complexing of phosphate with the bound calcium, and subsequent release of an insoluble salt. The protein would then bind more calcium to repeat the process. When Robison observed in 1923 that the enzyme alkaline phosphatase was highly active in areas of bone undergoing calcification, the interest shifted from specific ion binding to some means of increasing the ion concentrations to the point of spontaneous precipitation. Robison proposed that alkaline phosphatase split organic phosphate esters and released sufficient quantities of inorganic phosphate to result in precipitation of apatite. After finding that the tissue did not contain enough phosphate esters, he proposed that a secondary booster mechanism was required but never defined it. Some years later, Gutman and Yu, upon demonstrating that glycolysis was active in calcifying tissues, suggested that the breakdown of glycogen could serve as a booster mechanism. The sugar phosphates formed during glycolysis could provide substrates for alkaline phosphatase. Because of its simplicity, the combination of glycolysis and alkaline phosphatase activity was cited for many years as being the initial mechanism for calcification. The theory has some drawbacks, however; it is difficult to explain why other tissues high in alkaline phosphatase, such as intestinal mucosa, do not calcify. Finally, careful histochemical studies indicated that both glycolysis and alkaline phosphatase are associated with cellular activity, whereas calcification occurs in the matrix outside the cells.

When biochemical studies showed that cellular activity could not provide a sufficient quantity of ions to induce spontaneous precipitation of apatite, attention turned to studies on heterogeneous nucleation. The concept of nucleation catalysis was introduced primarily from work in Neuman's laboratory during the 1950s. The catalyst was proposed to be an organic entity that promoted calcification by either epitaxy or a seeding mechanism. Epitaxy implies the presence of a template upon which apatite crystals can form. The seeding mechanism involves the formation of ionic clusters that act as nuclei for crystal formation. Although nucleation catalysis is the theory most widely accepted today, the exact nature of the catalyst has not been totally defined. The various constituents of calcifying tissues that have been implicated are:

Collagen

Collagen has been the constituent most extensively studied in relation to the initiation of calcification. Electron microscopic studies have demonstrated a close morphological relationship between collagen fibers and apatite crystals (Fig. 6-3). Also, reconstituted collagen fibrils will induce apatite formation when placed in a metastable calcium phosphate solution.

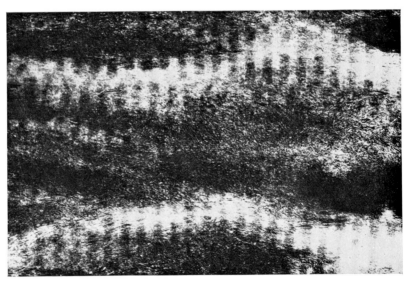

FIG. 6–3. An electron micrograph of an undecalcified, unstained section of embryonic chick bone, showing the ordered disposition of the dense mineral phase along the axial direction of the collagen fibrils. The vertical lines are the collagen banding and the dark, short horizontal lines are apatite crystals. × 110,000. (From Glimcher, M. J. and Krane, S. M.: The organization and structure of bone, and the mechanism of calcification. In *Treatise on Collagen*, Vol. 2B. B. S. Gould (Ed.), New York, Academic Press, 1968, Chapter 2, p. 110.)

Only native fibrils with a ∼700 Å banding pattern are able to function as a catalyst. When polymerized in this native form, the fibrils contain so-called "hole zones" and the initial calcification occurs within these spaces. Although the exact nature of catalysis by the hole zones is not known, Glimcher has provided substantial evidence that covalently bound phosphate is required. Serine residues in the collagen polypeptide chain are phosphorylated by a protein phosphokinase requiring ATP.

$$\text{protein-serine-OH} \rightarrow \text{protein-serine-OPO}_3{}^{2-}$$
$$\text{ATP} \curvearrowright \text{ADP}$$

The bound phosphate groups provide the proper steric sites to bind calcium and initiate calcification. Other investigators have argued that carboxyl groups provide the nucleating sites. The nucleating ability of collagen is not unique, since a variety of other proteins can also induce apatite formation. Among these are the protein of enamel, elastin, and lipoproteins from certain bacteria. In addition, native collagen is found in tissues that do not normally calcify. The difference in ability to calcify, however, could be due to the presence of inhibitory substances.

Mucopolysaccharides

Mucopolysaccharides are now more appropriately referred to as protein-polysaccharides or glycosaminoglycans. The rapid synthesis of glycosamino-glycans occurs in calcifying tissues during mineralization. When chondroitin sulfate was found to be a major constituent, it was suggested that it bound and localized calcium so that nucleation could occur. A demonstration that sulfate-blocking groups inhibited calcification *in vitro* supported such a concept. It is now known that, although cells are rapidly synthesizing glycos-aminoglycans, these compounds are broken down just prior to the time the matrix begins to calcify. It is more likely that, because of their strong calcium-binding capacity, these compounds act as inhibitors of calcification and must be removed before mineralization can occur. The association of certain glycosaminoglycans with collagen thus could govern its ability to calcify.

Lipids

The importance of lipids in calcification was recognized during the early 1960s when Irving observed that the onset of mineral deposition in bones and teeth was preceded by the presence of a lipid substance. Careful biochemical studies by Wuthier showed that acidic phospholipids were the most important component of this lipid substance. Acidic phospholipids, in particular phosphatidyl serine, bind calcium and can stabilize amorphous calcium phosphate. Phospholipid fractions from a number of sources, including calcifying bacteria, can induce apatite nucleation when suspended in metastable calcium phosphate solutions. Furthermore, collagen matrices derived from bone or dentin will not recalcify after acidic phospholipids have been completely removed. A possible role for phospholipids *in vivo* is as a calcium-binding component of membrane-bound structures, vesicles, found to occur in calcifying tissues. A proposed role for these vesicles will be discussed later in this chapter. Synthetic membranes prepared with acidic phospholipids and basic proteins can induce apatite nucleation *in vitro*. Whether similar membrane-induced calcification occurs naturally in calcified tissues has not been established.

Enzymes

Various enzymes that have been proposed to be involved in the calcification mechanism are present in bones and teeth. The roles of alkaline phosphatase and a protein phosphokinase have already been discussed. Another proposed function of alkaline phosphatase has been to remove inhibitory substances from the tissues. Recently, inorganic pyrophosphate was found to act as an inhibitor of calcification. The alkaline phosphatase in bone also has inorganic pyrophosphatase activity and the following mechanism has been proposed (Fig. 6–4). It involves inhibition of calcification by pyrophosphate ions and removal of the inhibition by the pyrophosphatase activity.

Cells

Recent studies have shown that cells elaborating the fibrous protein matrix in bones and teeth also initiate the mineralization process. First of all, these cells have the ability to store large quantities of calcium phosphate in their mitochondria and do so at the time the matrix is being calcified. Second, the cells bud off membrane-bound vesicles that either contain mineral or can accumulate it while in the matrix. These *matrix vesicles* have been postulated to provide the loci for initial calcification, since the earliest apatite crystals that can be seen by electron microscopy occur

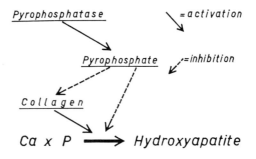

FIG. 6–4.   Possible role of pyrophosphatase in calcification.

within them. The vesicles have both alkaline phosphatase and ATPase enzyme activities which might be involved in the accumulation of mineral. Alkaline phosphatase would provide PO_4^{3-} ions by hydrolyzing phosphate esters and the ATPase activity would provide energy for a Ca^{2+} transport system within the vesicle membrane. Another function of the matrix vesicles might be to merely transport mineral from the cells to the calcification sites within the collagen fibrils. In either case, the transfer of calcium phosphate into the matrix would be under cellular control.

CURRENT CONCEPTS ABOUT INITIATION OF CALCIFICATION

There is ample experimental evidence for both matrix vesicle-induced calcification and apatite nucleation within the hole zones of native collagen fibrils. The relative importance of each process in the formation of calcified tissues remains to be determined. It might be that vesicular calcification represents a form of functional mineralization and that of collagen calcification, a structural form. Another question to be answered is whether both processes occur by a similar basic mechanism.

A multistep process has been proposed for collagen calcification: (1) initial calcium binding by either $R-PO_4^{2-}$ or COO^- groups on the collagen molecule; (2) the formation of a $CaHPO_4$ phase; (3) loss of H^+ to yield an amorphous $Ca_3(PO_4)_2$ phase, and (4) conversion of the amorphous calcium phosphate to crystalline apatite. In going through a series of less structured intermediate phases less energy would be required. A similar process could occur in the matrix vesicles with the initial Ca^{2+} binding by acidic phospholipids present in the membrane. Even though the vesicles can actively accumulate Ca^{2+} via an ATPase transport system, nucleation catalyzed by phospholipids would be more favorable energetically than the spontaneous precipitation of apatite.

Figure 6–5 is a diagram summarizing the calcification processes. The first zone (A) is a layer of cells separated from calcifying matrix by a nonmineralized, proteinpolysaccharide-rich zone (B). Matrix vesicles migrate through this zone and accumulate at the calcification front (C). The phospholipid in the vesicle membranes is largely responsible for the sudanophilia seen histochemically at C. At this point the vesicles appear to disintegrate and release mineral for the calcification of the collagen fibers. Some acidic phospholipids from vesicle membranes are incorporated along with mineral and can only be removed after the bone or dentin is decalcified. The calcification processes occurring at the calcification front have not been completely resolved. It is not known whether the disintegration of the vesicles is due to lytic enzymes or to the accumulation of mineral. Also, the mode of transition of mineral from vesicles to collagen fibers is not understood. Zone D represents the calcification of the collagen fibers. A more detailed description of collagen biosynthesis and fiber formation is given in Chapter 2.

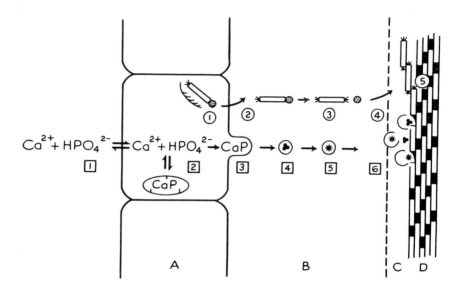

Fig. 6–5. Diagram of cell mediated calcification. The cells can be chondrocytes, osteoblasts, or odontoblasts. The various zones represent: A, cell layer; B, protein-polysaccharide-rich precalcified matrix; C, calcification front; and D, calcified collagen fibers.

The upper sequence summarizes collagen fiber formation: (1) intracellular biosynthesis of procollagen, (2) secretion of procollagen, (3) enzymatic hydrolysis of procollagen to give collagen molecules, (4) polymerization of collagen molecules into fibers, and (5) maturation of fibers.

The lower sequence summarizes proposed steps in calcification: (1) uptake of Ca^{2+} and HPO_4^{2-} ions by cells, (2) storage of ions as CaP in mitochondria, (3) budding of calcifying matrix vesicles from cell membrane, (4) migration of vesicles through zone B with further accumulation of ions and formation of amorphous calcium phosphate (ACP), (5) conversion of ACP to apatite, and (6) clustering of vesicles at the calcification front where they are broken down and release mineral for collagen fiber calcification. Both ACP and apatite are seen within vesicles as well as in the mineralizing region around collagen fibrils. It is possible that the ACP → apatite conversion begins in the vesicles and reaches completion at the calcification front.

DEVELOPMENT AND MATURATION OF CALCIFIED TISSUES

The mechanism of calcification describes the earliest events of the total mineralization process. Once calcification is initiated, the tissue eventually becomes completely mineralized within a framework defined by the organic matrix. As the tissue matures there is an initial loss of some organic material, mainly non-collagenous protein, but the greatest change occurs with the loss of water and the accumulation of mineral. Maturation of the mineral phase includes the conversion of amorphous calcium phosphate to apatite and growth of apatite crystals. The complete process of calcification varies with each type of tissue.

Calcification of Bone

The cells responsible for bone formation are the *osteoblasts* (see Chapter 8). A zone of nonmineralized matrix, called *osteoid*, separates the cells from the calcified bone. The osteoid is a proteinpolysaccharide-rich region where collagen molecules are polymerizing into fibers. In addition, it contains the matrix vesicles that eventually accumulate at the calcification front and disintegrate to release mineral. This sets the stage for the rapid calcification of the collagen fibers.

The first visible mineral deposition within the fibers occurs in the "hole zones." A series of dot-like nuclei form chains parallel to the fiber axis and eventually fuse into needle-like apatite crystals. At first, the mineral fills only the hole zones, which are approximately 15 Å wide and 400 Å long. The deposition of mineral in these hole zones accentuates the $\sim$700 Å banding pattern of native collagen. This stage of mineralization is rapid and accounts for more than 50% of the total bone mineral. Because of the way the collagen microfibrils are packed, channels, which can presumably contain mineral and thus establish a mineral continuum along the entire collagen fiber bundle, exist between them. The combination of mineral in the hole zones and interconnecting channels accounts for about 90% of the total mineral content of bone. The majority of the apatite crystals are oriented with their long axes parallel to the long axes of the collagen fibers. In mature bone, apatite crystals are hexagonal rods 50 Å thick and from 100 to 300 Å in length.

Two general types of bone occur in vertebrates. One is endochondral bone formed upon a calcified cartilage template. As the cartilage is resorbed a dense woven bone is laid down followed by well-structured lamellar bone. In the long bones, such as the femur, lamellar bone is laid down as concentric circular sheets which form a cylinder called a haversian system. Each haversian system contains its own central blood vessel, and the long axis of the cylinder runs parallel to the long axis of the bone shaft. The other type of bone, membranous, is deposited first as a seam of woven bone followed by lamellar bone. Membranous bone functions primarily as a protective covering over vital organs; for example, the bone of the skull is membranous.

Calcification of Cementum and Dentin

The process of mineralization of cementum is virtually the same as that of bone. The cells responsible are called cementoblasts and lie between the edge of the periodontal membrane and a thin layer of uncalcified precementum.

The cells responsible for dentin formation are the odontoblasts, which start the process by elaborating a layer of noncalcified predentin along the basal lamina at the dentino-enamel junction (DEJ). The cells secrete a collagenous matrix, and matrix vesicles bud off the cell membrane to initiate calcification. Like bone, the vesicles calcify and coalesce to form islands of mineral which eventually envelop the collagen fibers. This first highly calcified matrix is called mantle dentin and forms a seam along the basal lamina. The basal lamina disappears after the seam is formed. The layer of odontoblasts then recedes from the mantle dentin, elaborating a more structured calcified matrix called peritubular dentin. The cells are continually separated from calcified dentin by a layer of predentin. In mature dentin the calcified matrix is permeated by a system of parallel tubules from the DEJ to the pulp chamber. These tubules contain odontoblastic processes which extend from cells lining the pulpal cavity all the way to the DEJ. The tubules consist of cylinders of densely mineralized peritubular matrix. An intertubular matrix of less densely calcified collagen fills the space between the cylinders of peritubular dentin. The apatite crystals are oriented along the collagen fibers and are smaller than the crystals found in enamel.

Calcification of Enamel

Enamel calcification does not begin until the basal lamina at the DEJ disappears. The ameloblasts then start elaborating a gel-like protein matrix, and the first apatite crystals appear to grow epitaxially from dentin crystals. Large enamel crystals continue to grow into long ribbons as the ameloblasts recede from the DEJ. The crystals are organized into basic structural units called prisms, which radiate from the DEJ toward the outer surface of the enamel. The prisms have a keyhole-shaped cross section and each prism is possibly the result of a single ameloblast. The apatite crystals in enamel are hexagonal rods approximately 330 Å wide and 300 to 500 Å long. Because the individual crystals are so closely aligned, composites appear to be single crystals, which have been reported to be as long as 5000 Å when seen by the electron microscope. The long axes of the crystals are oriented in the same direction as the axis of the prism. A prismless layer of apatite crystals is present at the outer surface of enamel.

Unlike bone and dentin, enamel does not contain detectable amorphous calcium phosphate and matrix vesicles have not been observed. Thus, the ameloblasts are most likely secreting ions that are being incorporated directly into rapidly forming apatite crystals.

SELECTED REFERENCES

BACHRA, B. N.: Some molecular aspects of tissue calcification, Clin. Orthop., *51*, 199–222, 1967.

IRVING, J. T.: *Calcium and Phosphorus Metabolism*, New York, Academic Press, 1973.

McLEAN, F. C., and URIST, M. R.: *Bone, Dynamics of Calcification*, Chicago, University of Chicago Press, 1961.

MINER, R. W. (Ed.): Recent advances in the study of the structure, composition and growth of mineralized tissues, Ann. N.Y. Acad. Sci., *60*, 543–806, 1955.

RASMUSSEN, H., and BORDIER, P.: *The Physiological and Cellular Basis of Metabolic Bone Disease*, Baltimore, Williams & Wilkins Co., 1974.

SOGNNAES, R. F. (Ed.): *Calcification in Biological Systems*, Washington, D.C., American Association for the Advancement of Science, Pub. #64, 1960.

URIST, M. R.: Origins of current ideas about calcification, Clin. Orthop., *44*, 13–39, 1966.

ZIPKIN, I. (Ed.): *Biological Mineralization*, New York, John Wiley & Sons, 1973.

Chapter 7

Physicochemical Properties of Enamel and Dentine

STUART ZIMMERMAN, Ph.D.

Enamel and dentine, the two primary calcified tissues of the tooth, have certain common features, but differ in other important respects. Therefore in the following discussion many of the physicochemical properties of the mineral phase will be discussed under enamel with exceptions noted where they are applicable to dentine.

ENAMEL CRYSTALLINE STRUCTURE

Unit Cell

The structural organization of the enamel has been extensively studied principally by means of ordinary microscopy, polarization microscopy, infrared spectrophotometry, x-ray diffraction, electron diffraction, and electron microscopy. Since the dimensions of crystallites comprising the enamel mineral phase are considerably smaller than the resolving power of the optical microscope, the latter three techniques have been the most informative. Only indirect evidence of the submicroscopic structure of enamel can be obtained by the optical techniques.

Early chemical analyses indicated that the mineral matter of enamel was a calcium phosphate salt. X-ray diffraction investigations confirmed that the mineral phase belongs to a class of compounds known as apatites. Specifically, hydroxyapatite is the particular apatite present in the enamel. More correctly it should be described as a carbonate apatite. The role of carbonate in enamel will be discussed later. Apatites are characterized by the preservation of a specific crystalline configuration, even under the influence of substitution of some of their chemical constituents. Pure hydroxyapatite can be stoichiometrically represented as $Ca_{10}(PO_4)_6(OH)_2$. However, magnesium, strontium, radium, and hydronium ions can substitute in the calcium position; fluoride can substitute in the hydroxyl position resulting in fluorapatite; and carbonate can substitute somewhere within the crystalline lattice. Naturally occurring geological apatites include francolite, dahllite (both carbonate-containing apatites), and the aforementioned fluorapatite. The crystal can be regarded as built-up of small units of parallel-epiped shape, the "unit cells." Repetition of unit cells in the direction of the threie axes represents the entire crystal. The crystalline unit cell is shown in Fgure 7–1.

The dimensions of the unit cell and the positions of ions within the cell have been determined by the employment of several experimental techniques, principally x-ray diffraction analysis. A discussion of the methodology can be found in Trautz's article. The lengths of the unit cell (horizontal) axes are $a_1 = a_2 = 9.42$ Å, while the (vertical) c-axes are 6.88 Å. The spatial arrangement of ions composing the cell has been described by Trautz as: "The hexagonal unit cell, which is the smallest space unit of the structure containing all the crystallographic symmetry elements of the whole crystal, is a parallelepipedon whose edges are formed by the two horizontal 'a' axes, enclosing an angle of 120°, and by the vertical 'c' axes at right angles to the 'a' axcs. The unit cell contains 10 Ca^{2+}, 6 PO_4^{3-}, and 2 OH^- ions. The

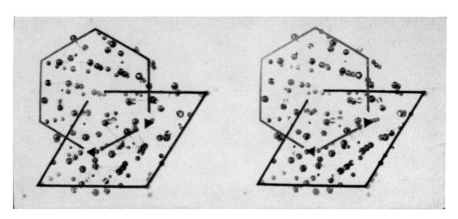

Fig. 7–1. Stereopicture of a model of apatite structure viewed parallel to the hexagonal axis down upon the basal plane. The hexagonal unit cell is outlined by the taped rhombus. (The unit cell contains 10 Ca, 6 PO₄ (tetrahedra), 2 OH on the c-axes at the corners of the rhombus.) The depth of the unit cell extends from the first to the third OH. The taped hexagon indicates the hexagonal symmetry around the c-axis. The PO₄ tetrahedra have one vertical and one horizontal edge and two vertical and two tilted faces. Two symmetry planes perpendicular to the c-axes pass through the horizontal edges of the PO₄ tetrahedra, and through the OH and the Ca ions not lying on the threefold rotation axes.

With a little practice one may succeed, without the use of a stereoscope, in seeing the stereoscopic picture in space. Place the well-illuminated pictures symmetrically before you. Align your eyes parallel by viewing "through the pictures" an imaginary distant spot. While the eyes accommodate to the closer distance of the pictures (25 to 30 cm) the two pictures fuse into a single three-dimensional view. A piece of cardboard placed vertically between the two pictures may be of help at the beginning. (This model was built by Dr. Edward Klein using data of Beevers and Mac-Intyre, 1946.) (Miles, A. E. W.: *Structural and Chemical Organization of Teeth*, New York, Academic Press, 1967.)

phosphate oxygens are arranged in tetrahedral groups enclosing the phosphorus and are tied more strongly to it than to the Ca^{2+} ions, which are interspersed between the PO_4^{3-} groups as such are built into the crystal. The two OH^- ions sit on the hexagonal 'c' axes, each surrounded by three Ca^{2+} ions at the same level. The other four Ca^{2+} occupy positions on the two vertical triagonal axes which pass through the cell at one third and two thirds along the long cell diagonal." The symbolic representation for the apatite is $P6_3/M$. The P denotes a primitive cell, *i.e.* there is one unique arrangement of atoms consistent with the symmetry of the cell. The 6_3 denotes the c axis is a sixfold screw axis. "This means that after rotating the structure about c through $2\pi/6 = 60°$, and simultaneously shifting along the c axes through c $\times$ 3/6, *i.e.* c/2, the appearance of the structure will be identical to what it was originally."

Crystallite Size and Shape

The crystallites in enamel are considerably longer (up to a factor of 10) than those occurring in either bone, dentine, or cementum. Many naturally occurring apatite crystals grow in the form of hexagonal prisms. Developing

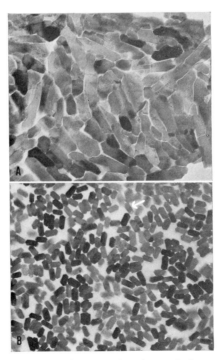

Fig. 7–2. Electron micrograph of cross sectioned crystals from mature human (A) and immature rodent incisor enamel (B). A central dark line (arrow) can be seen in some crystals in both types of enamel. $\times$ 75,000. (Nylen, M. V.: Recent electron microscopic and allied investigations into the normal structure of human enamel, Int. Dent. J., *17*, 719–733, 1967.)

enamel crystallites take the form of either rods or platelets, there being some disagreement about the magnitude of the crystallite width. Crystals ranging in length from 1200 to 2100 Å and width from 150 to 250 Å have been reported (Fig. 7–2).

Investigations of the crystallite shape in developing dentine by stereoscopic techniques provide a view of individual crystals at different angles. Crystals that gave a narrow dense profile in one orientation presented broad, less dense profiles after being tilted about their long axes. A needle-like structure would not behave in this manner, thus it was concluded that dentinal crystals are plate-like structures. As the enamel matures, the crystallites become more densely packed. Two arrangements of the crystallites in mature enamel are suggested in the electron microscopic study of Johansen. In the first pattern (Fig. 7–3) the crystallites are oriented parallel to each other and appear as straight regular crystals. The second pattern contains an irregular arrangement of crystallites of quite variable morphology (Fig. 7–4).

Quite a few of the crystallites deviate from parallelism to some extent with certain divergences reaching the maximum of 90°. Those crystallites found in the irregular arrangement also vary widely in width and shape. Both extensions and indentations are seen in Figure 7–4. Many crystallites in this structural arrangement are formed such that the boundary of one crystallite is in complementary apposition to its neighbors. It has been

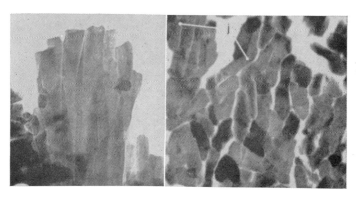

FIG. 7–3.   FIG. 7–4.

FIG. 7–3. Crystallites of sound enamel in parallel and presumably natural arrangement. Homogenate preparation. (× approx. 91,300.)

FIG. 7–4. Section of sound enamel illustrating irregular arrangement and varying morphology of crystallites. Both parallel and diverging crystallites can be seen. Individual crystallites show great variation in size and shape and junctions between terminal ends can be seen (j). Note the structural arrangement whereby the boundary of one crystallite is in complementary apposition with those of adjacent crystallites. (× approx. 113,400.) (Johansen, E.: Comparison of the Ultrastructure and Chemical Composition of Sound and Carious Enamel from Human Permanent Teeth. In *Tooth Enamel*, M. V. Stack and R. W. Fearnhead (Eds.), Bristol, John Wright & Sons, 1965, pp. 177–181).

reasoned that the lateral enlargement of the crystallites during maturation would bring the originally sparsely spaced crystallites into approximation, with their final shape dependent upon the relative rate and direction of growth along with the remaining spatial configuration between adjacent crystallites.

Within the crystallites, the apatite unit cells are oriented with their c-axes almost parallel with the crystallite long axis, the maximum divergence encountered is about 2°. There is considerably more variation in the angle made between the long axis of the enamel crystallite and the long axis of the enamel prism. This will be discussed further when the microanatomy of the enamel is presented.

The minute size of the apatite crystallites plays a decisive role in determining its variable chemical composition. Since the enamel crystallites are only a few unit cells thick, a large fraction of the atoms are located at or near the surface.

Chemical Substituents and the Ca/P Ratio

The large fraction of crystalline ionic sites at or near the crystal surface permits frequent homoionic exchange, *i.e.* exchange of like ions within the crystal lattice, as well as heteroionic exchange. As mentioned earlier, lead, magnesium, manganese, strontium, and hydronium can substitute for the calcium in hydroxyapatite. Arsenate or vanadate can substitute for phosphate and fluoride or chloride can substitute in the hydroxyl position. In addition, ions can be adsorbed to the crystal surface by electrostatic attraction or retained in the strongly bound hydration layer associated with the crystal.

Under all these substitutions, the apatite crystals maintain essentially the same structural configuration. When the substituents do not appreciably change the size of the unit cell, *e.g.* fluorine resulting in fluorapatite, the two isomorphous apatites, such as fluor- and hydroxyapatite, can mix in any proportion and form a continuous series of solid solutions. A dissimilarity of more than 10% in the cell dimensions of the two isomorphous crystals will limit the extent of substitution.

The chemical composition of the enamel mineral reflects the composition of the serum and calcifying fluid environment at the time of calcification. In this way, for example, ^{90}Sr removed from atmospheric fallout will be incorporated into teeth and bones following a period of nuclear testing. Whereas there is rapid exchange in developing enamel, as calcification progresses, ions both natural and foreign become "diffusion locked" due to the restricted intracrystalline space and electrostatic charge repulsion. The fluoride content of human enamel likewise increases with the fluoride content of the drinking water of a given area.

Pure synthetic hydroxyapatite has a Ca/P ratio of 1.67 on a molar basis or 2.15 on a weight basis. In actual analyses of dental enamel, Ca/P ratios of from 1.92 to 2.17 (by weight) have been reported in the literature. In nearly all cases, the ratio is below 2.15. Several explanations have been offered for this phenomenon. Adsorption of phosphate on the crystallites or the substitution of sodium, magnesium, or other ions has been proposed as a contributing factor. Specifically, a substitution of hydronium ion, H_3O^+, for 2 calcium ions has been suggested. More recently, the idea of a reduced Ca/P ratio arising from a defect in the crystalline structure has been postulated. One explanation offered is that calcium ions are missing in certain positions in the lattice. These calcium-deficient apatites appear to be metastable with respect to hydroxyapatite towards which they slowly change by acquiring calcium ions from solution.

Carbonate. Carbonate, among the apatite substituents, has been the subject of many studies and deserves separate mention. The apatite present in dental enamel is not a pure hydroxyapatite, but rather a carbonate apatite with a carbonate content of 2 to 3%. For nearly 30 years there has been a controversy about the location of the carbonate in enamel, dentine, and bone.

One school of thought (Carlstrom, 1955) has maintained that the small fraction of carbonate present in the enamel existed in the form of a non-crystalline phase, adsorbed to the surface of hydroxyapatite crystallites. This carbonate phase, an amorphous calcium carbonate, would not be detectable by x-ray diffraction analysis as the non-crystalline material would not give rise to any lines in the diffractogram.

Another group of workers claims that the carbonate is actually incorporated in the apatite lattice. Most recent investigations support this point of view. There still exists some discussion as to the exact sites in the lattice that are occupied by the carbonate. The aforementioned investigations have analyzed naturally occurring carbonate apatites such as dahllite and francolite along with a series of synthetic carbonate apatites whose carbonate content varied from 0.4 to 22.5%. Crystallographic analysis of these carbonate apatites reveals that with increasing carbonate there is a decrease in the a-axis dimension relative to hydroxyapatite. Also, chemical analyses show that a PO_4 decrease corresponds with a carbonate increase in these series. This evidence led them to propose a substitution of carbonate for phosphate in the lattice.

Other researchers employing infrared absorption spectroscopy report that only a fraction of the carbonate in the enamel is substituted within the lattice and that fraction appears in the hydroxyl position. Thus, while most recent investigators agree that carbonate appears to be substituting within the lattice rather than existing in an amorphous phase, there is still some disagreement as to the actual position of the carbonate.

The presence and location of carbonate in dental enamel may relate directly to the risk of carious attacks. Carbonate has been shown to be leached preferentially from early carious lesions. Further, carbonate content and susceptibility of teeth to dental caries have been correlated. Carbonate apatites have an increased acid solubility which most probably explains the increased caries susceptibility of high carbonate-containing teeth.

Fluoride. Numerous clinical studies have shown that the addition of 1 ppm fluoride to public drinking water or the treatment of teeth with topically applied fluoride solution has been effective in reducing the occurrence of dental caries. Because of this caries-inhibiting effect, fluoride has been studied quite extensively.

Two modes of fluoride interaction with hydroxyapatite dependent on the fluoride concentration are known. With high fluoride concentrations, around 5 to 10%, there is a surface reaction of the hydroxyapatite to form calcium fluoride, CaF_2. This reaction occurs to a certain extent as a result of topical application of sodium fluoride or stannous fluoride. The reaction may be represented by the equation:

$$Ca_{10}(PO_4)_6(OH)_2 + 20\ F^- \rightarrow 10\ CaF_2 + 6\ PO_4 + 2\ OH^-.$$

Calcium fluoride forms a precipitate because of its low solubility product ($K_{sp}3 \times 10^{-11}$). Its formation is associated with the dissolution of the apatite. While calcium fluoride has been found on powdered enamel and on intact enamel surfaces *in vitro* after topical fluoride treatment, there is uncertainty over the fate of calcium fluoride in the mouth. One possibility is that it may dissolve and provide fluoride for the formation of fluorapatite, although the kinetics of this reaction make it a very unlikely possibility.

When fluoride solution at a 1 ppm concentration is applied to hydroxyapatite, fluorapatite is formed by the reaction expressed in the following equation:

$$Ca_{10}(PO_4)_6(OH)_2 + 2\ F^- \rightarrow Ca_{10}(PO_4)_6F_2 + 2\ OH^-$$

Initially, fluoride is deposited in low concentrations, around 30 to 50 ppm, during the formation of the apatite crystals in the calcification phase of enamel development. After calcification is complete, more fluoride is taken up by the external enamel. Before eruption there is an increased uptake from tissue fluids; after eruption, the surface enamel continues to take up fluoride from the oral environment.

Fluoride increases the crystallinity of apatite, whereas bicarbonate reduces it. Octa-calcium phosphate instead of apatite forms when precipitation occurs from a solution of calcite and sodium phosphate under high partial pressures of carbon dioxide at almost neutral pH. However, addition of fluoride ions to the same solutions results in the formation of apatite. The fluoride increases the crystallinity of the formed apatite as measured by the broadening effects on the x-ray diffraction peaks. Legeros *et al.* also reported that apatites with a high carbonate content had a reduced crystallinity and smaller crystallite size, with increased surface area and solubility. These results are consistent with the caries-inhibiting and caries-potentiating effects of fluoride and carbonate respectively.

Possible Apatite Precursors

Octa-calcium Phosphate. Walter E. Brown strongly advocated a mechanism of apatite formation in which octa-calcium phosphate appears as a precursor stage. Octa-calcium phosphate which is a hydrated calcium phosphate formula may be represented as $Ca_8H_2(PO_4)_6 \cdot 5H_2O$. In Brown's proposed mechanism, three stages occur in the growth of apatite crystals. The first is the formation of an incipient crystallization seed. In the second stage, the seed grows in two dimensions only, length and width, but not in thickness, resulting in a thin blade or ribbon-shaped crystallite. This blade is considered to be a single unit cell thickness of octa-calcium phosphate. The third and final stage resulting in the three-dimensional growth of the crystallite consists of two steps. The first is a precipitation of a single layer of octa-calcium phosphate, one unit cell in thickness, on the crystal followed by a hydrolysis of a unit cell thickness of octa-calcium phosphate to produce a layer of hydroxyapatite two unit cells thick. Fluoride ions would have a profound influence on this system since fluoride converts octa-calcium phosphate to an apatite, as mentioned earlier. Thus, fluoride's effectiveness in reducing dental caries is considered due to its initiation of hydrolysis and the elimination of accidental retention of the more soluble octa-calcium phosphate in the crystal. While octa-calcium phosphate is easily prepared synthetically and has occasionally been reported in studies on the mineralization of bone *in vitro*, no proof has been presented that octa-calcium phosphate is involved in the growth mechanism of enamel crystals or other biological apatitic crystals.

Amorphous Calcium Phosphate. Recent investigations have revealed that an amorphous calcium phosphate phase exists in bone along with the crystalline apatite phase. The presence of this phase and a quantitative evaluation of its percentage of the total bone mineral content have been determined by x-ray diffraction, infrared spectroscopy, and electron spin resonance techniques. In the femur or tibia of several day-old rats, it was discovered that approximately 35% of the bone mineral was in the crystalline apatite form, while approximately 65% was amorphous calcium phosphate. As the animal matured and reached 80 days of age, these percentages were essentially reversed with approximately 65% of bone mineral being crystalline apatite and only 35% being amorphous calcium phosphate. This latter composition was stable and seemed to represent the proportions of apatite and amorphous calcium phosphate in mature bone. Synthetic crystallization studies showed that an amorphous calcium phosphate was formed as a usual initial precipitate. This initial precipitate was metastable and would convert to hydroxyapatite. These two findings led to the conclusion that amorphous calcium phosphate is a predecessor of crystalline hydroxyapatite in bone growth. However, a considerable pool of amorphous calcium phosphate co-exists with the crystalline apatite in the mature bone. Analysis of human enamel indicated that it was 100% crystalline apatite. However, the mineral portion of the dentine was 65 to 70% crystalline, essentially similar in composition to compact bone. Magnesium and carbonate ions stabilize the amorphous calcium phosphate in synthetic preparations and prevent its conversion to the more stable apatite form. In bone and dentine stabilization could possibly be established by binding to an organic component.

Optical Properties

Apatite is optically uniaxial and birefringent, *i.e.*, it has two refractive indices, one for the ordinary ray vibrating perpendicular to the c-axis and another for the extraordinary ray vibrating parallel to c. The extent of birefringence, that is, the difference between these refractive indices, is weak and negative (−0.004). Because of this birefringent property of the enamel, it has been possible to study enamel structure by employing the polarization microscope. Microscopic spaces in the enamel will imbibe aqueous and non-aqueous fluids from solution. These spaces give rise to a positive form birefringence. The increase in submicroscopic spaces during the development of early enamel caries has been investigated by following the increase in form birefringence.

ENAMEL SOLUBILITY

Because the acidogenic theory of enamel caries postulates that the enamel is attacked by organic acids arising from microbial metabolism, there has been considerable interest in the solubility of enamel and hydroxyapatite in acid solutions.

Some investigators have claimed from experimental evidence and theoretical reasoning that hydroxyapatite does not have a thermodynamically predictable solubility product constant based on the mass action law; *i.e.*, it has an anomalous solubility behavior. More recently it has been reported that pure hydroxyapatite, when true equilibrium conditions have been reached, has a true solubility product constant K_{sp} that is consistent with the law of mass action. It can be expressed as:

$$pK_{sp} = 10 \ pCa + 6 \ p(PO_4) + 2 \ p(OH).$$

Values of pK_{sp} in the range of 114.4 to 116 have been determined.

In studies of the dissolution of dental enamel and synthetic hydroxyapatites in acid buffers, it has been observed that a relatively rapid equilibrium is reached where the extent of dissolution is governed by the solubility product for calcium monohydrogen phosphate. This has been interpreted as resulting from a thin layer of monohydrogen calcium phosphate dihydrate which forms on the apatite surface and determines the solubility. The reactions can be shown schematically as:

$$\text{True Hydroxyapatite Equilibrium}$$

$$Ca_{10}(PO_4)_6(OH)_2 \rightleftharpoons 10 \; Ca^{2+} + 6 \; PO_4^{3-} + 2 \; OH^-$$

$$\text{In pH 4 to 6 Buffer solutions}$$

$$Ca_{10}(PO_4)_6(OH)_2 + 8 \; H^+ \rightarrow 10 \; Ca^{2+} + 6 \; HPO_4^{2-} + 2 \; H_2O$$

$$\Updownarrow \; H_2O$$

$$4 \; Ca^{2+} + 6 \; CaHPO_4 \cdot 2 \; H_2O$$

In kinetic studies of acid dissolution of apatite in acetate buffers, equilibrium is not usually reached. The net overall reaction can be expressed as:

$$Ca_{10}(PO_4)_6 \, (OH)_2 + 8 \; H^+ \rightarrow 10 \; Ca^{2+} + 6 \; HPO_4^{2-} + 2 \; H_2O \; (\text{at pH 4 to 6})$$

Several theoretical formulations have been proposed that describe the kinetic rate of this reaction reasonably well.

Variation in Depth of Chemical Components

Since mature enamel is exposed to an environment of saliva supersaturated with calcium and phosphate relative to hydroxyapatite and containing other ions with concentrations different from newly erupted enamel, it is not unusual to find that the composition of the surface enamel differs from that of interior enamel. In a series of papers primarily by Brudevold and co-workers, it has been reported that fluorine, zinc, and lead have a decreasing concentration gradient from the enamel surface toward the enamel junction, while carbonate and magnesium have a gradient in the opposite direction. Further, surface enamel is more mineralized than internal enamel and has a lower water content. The process of mineralization in the enamel involves the displacement of water by minerals. Therefore, the higher mineralization in the surface enamel is expected as a result of exposure to saliva, post-eruptively. Increased mineralization of the surface area results in a reduction of intercrystalline space. This space restriction, together with electrostatic charge repulsion from charges on the surface of crystallites, restricts ion movement as the intercrystalline spaces decrease from mineralization. Certain substituents such as strontium and copper are essentially uniformly distributed throughout enamel. These substances appear to be deposited at the time of enamel formation and are not subject to change subsequently. Substances such as carbonate and magnesium, which are found in an increasing gradient from the outer enamel surface towards the dentino-enamel junction, also appear to be deposited in the enamel at the time of formation. The gradient arises from surface loss of these components during exposure of the enamel to the oral environment.

PRISM STRUCTURE

Prism Dimensions

Anatomically mature enamel consists of a series of prisms or rods approximately 4 to 6 microns in diameter running from the dentino-enamel junction to the outer enamel surface. The prisms are composed of apatite crystallites in a hydrated organic matrix which is principally protein. The crystallites are aligned with their long axes approximately parallel to the long axis of the prism, although in certain regions they diverge quite significantly. During the past several years a new concept of prism architecture has been evolving. It appears to be supplanting the more traditional concept of enamel structure involving prisms, interprismatic substance, and prism sheaths. For the sake of completeness, both concepts of the enamel anatomy will be presented.

Traditional Concept of Enamel Structure

The traditional picture of enamel microanatomy has been derived from optical microscopic studies, including polarization microscopy, supplemented by microradiography. Since enamel is a highly calcified tissue, most of the common histological stains will not stain undecalcified enamel. Decalcification of the enamel leaves only a delicate organic matrix which is difficult to retain. Even in those cases where the organic matrix can be preserved, without association with the corresponding mineral phase, it does not truly represent the enamel structure. Thus, most optical studies have been conducted with ground enamel sections of 30 microns in thickness or greater. This represents a width of at least 5 to 7 prisms and can result in optical artifacts and difficulties of interpretation. Only within the last several years have techniques for the convenient preparation of enamel sections of 4 to 8 microns in thickness been developed.

The typical appearance of enamel as seen in the optical microscope in both transverse and longitudinal sections is shown schematically in Figure 7–5. As mentioned earlier, the primary constituent of the enamel is the enamel prism. These prisms are sometimes roughly hexagonal in transverse section, but are often either round or arcade-shaped, the latter arrangement being similar to a pattern of fish scales. Each prism is surrounded by a prism sheath, a region with a higher concentration of organic material at the perimeter of the prism. The prisms do not lie immediately adjacent to each other, but are separated by the interprismatic substance. In certain regions of the enamel, no interprismatic substance can be demonstrated.

Prisms pursue a spiraling path from the dentino-enamel junction to the outer surface of the enamel. In a transverse section the spiraling course of the prisms results in the appearance of layers of the enamel formed in which all prisms run in the same direction. This gives rise to the appearance of the Hunter-Schreger bands which are found in the inner half of the enamel. In polarized light microscopy, enamel prisms appear to be segmented

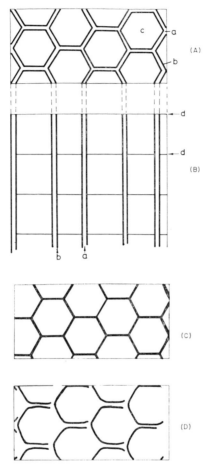

FIG. 7–5. Diagrammatic representation of prisms, prism sheaths and interprismatic substance. (A) Cross-cut prisms: *a*, interprismatic substance; *b*, prism sheaths; and *c*, prism core. (B) Longitudinally cut prisms. Between the cross striations (*d*) are the prism segments. (C) Cross-cut prisms with no interprismatic substance. The prism sheaths are close to each other. (D) Cross-cut prisms with prism sheaths open on one side. Thus the interprismatic substance is in immediate contact with the prism core. The form of the prisms varies according to the relation of the axes of adjacent prisms or groups of prisms. The horseshoe form can therefore vary a great deal in details. (Gustafson, G., and Gustafson, A.-G.: Microanatomy and Histochemistry of Enamel. In *Structure and Chemical Organization of Teeth*, A. E. W. Miles (Ed.), New York, Academic Press, 1967, p. 83.)

(Fig. 7–6). This segmentation has been called cross striation as the prisms appear to be divided by regular transverse lines into segments about 4 to 6 microns in length. Since this is about the same width as the prisms, the segments are practically box-like in appearance. The cross striations appear to be richer in organic material than the prism interior and less radiopaque. In many cases they seem to be mineralized to the same extent as the prism sheath with which they sometimes appear to be continuous. Some investigators believe that the prismatic segments or "boxes" represent periodic accretions from the Tomes' processes during the formation of the enamel matrix from the ameloblast.

Often throughout the enamel one finds a line of prism segments which is less calcified than neighboring prism segments (Fig. 7–7). These lines, often called striae of Retzius or Retzius' lines, represent variations in the degree of mineralization of the prism. Normal or incremental Retzius' lines represent essentially normal periodic variations in calcification. Pathological Retzius' lines, which are broader, result from disturbance in the mineralization. The neonatal line of birth is an example of this type of line. Retzius' lines rarely run transversely to the enamel prisms, but are usually at an oblique orientation. The Retzius' line is formed by a front or stage of ameloblastic activity where calcification was slightly disturbed. As the ameloblasts do not progress in the direction of the prisms, but at an angle to them,

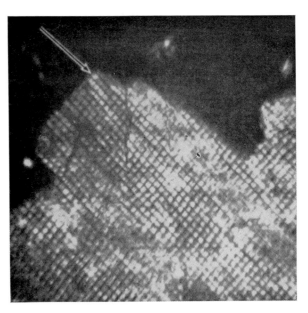

Fig. 7–6. Ground section of human enamel in polarized light (crossed polars). The prisms are divided into negatively birefringent square segments. Arrow indicates the direction of the prisms. × 420. (Gustafson, G., and Gustafson, A.-G.: Microanatomy and Histochemistry of Enamel. In *Structure and Chemical Organization of Teeth*, A. E. W. Miles (Ed.), New York, Academic Press, 1967, pp. 75–134.)

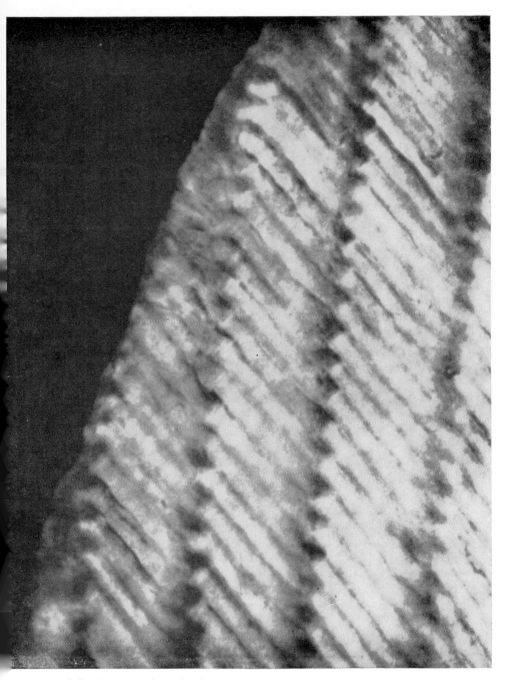

Fig. 7–7. Incremental Retzius' lines ending on the surface of human enamel. The lines show a step-like appearance. The inner (right-hand) side of each line is demarcated sharply by lines transverse to the prism axes but on the other side towards the outer enamel surface the demarcation is much less sharp and less segmented. The lines are first isotropic and then slightly negatively birefringent. × 1100. (Gustafson, G., and Gustafson, A.-G.: Microanatomy and Histochemistry of Enamel. In *Structure and Chemical Organization of Teeth*, A. E. W. Miles (Ed.), New York, Academic Press, 1967, p. 91.)

the Retzius' line represents a plane perpendicular to the direction of amelo-blastic growth.

Retzius' lines are important in determining the progress of the carious lesion in the enamel since Darling has shown that caries tends to spread mainly along the striae of Retzius.

Recent Concept of Enamel Structure

During the past few years, a new formulation of the microanatomy of dental enamel has arisen based largely on electron microscopy. A review of this work can be found in the paper by Nylen.

In the electron microscopic studies it was possible to distinguish enamel crystallites and it was observed that sudden changes in the orientation of the crystallites at the boundaries between prisms served to define the cross-sectional shape of the individual prisms. In cross section, the prisms have an appearance somewhat like keyholes. The prisms are approximately 5 microns in diameter at the round head, and about 9 microns from the top of the head to the extremity of the tail. The prisms are always oriented so that the head of the prism cross section points toward the occlusal surface of the tooth and the tail toward the cervical region of the tooth. Within a single prism, all crystallites are not parallel. In the head region of the prism, the long plate-like crystallites are oriented roughly with their long axes in the direction of the prism axis, but in the tail region the crystallites lie almost perpendicular to the prism long axis (Figs. 7–8 and 7–9).

Meckel, Griebstein, and Neal (Fig. 7–10) have constructed a three-dimensional model of keyhole enamel prisms that shows the varying aspect of prisms for differing angles of the plane section. Essentially all these patterns corresponding to the three-dimensional construction were found in various electron microscopic investigations of actual enamel sections.

In this formulation there is no requirement for an interprismatic substance and no evidence that such a substance exists. The tail extension of one prism between adjacent prisms in the next row would be interpreted as an interprismatic substance in optical microscopy. The prism sheath between the prisms is actually a region of abrupt discontinuity in crystallite orientation. This can be seen clearly in Figure 7–11.

Recent work provides an explanation of the varying crystallite orientation within the prism. Previous workers had generally accepted the concept of a 1-to-1 ratio between the number of prisms and the number of ameloblasts. It had further been accepted that during development one ameloblast formed one prism. New studies reveal that in human enamel each prism is the result of the secretory activity of four ameloblasts. Under this proposal crystallite orientation in enamel is controlled by two major factors: (1) crystallites grow at right angles to the surface of the mineralizing front wherever possible, but (2) where there is a relative movement between the surface of the ameloblast and the surface of the mineralizing front, the

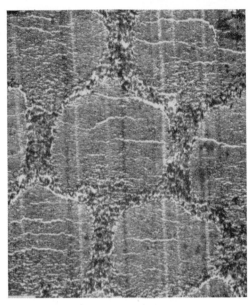

FIG. 7–8. Electron micrograph of a section cut from a human deciduous molar. The plane of sectioning was perpendicular to the long axis of the enamel prisms. × 5000. (Meckel, A. H., Griebstein, W. J., and Neal, R. J.: Structure of Natural Human Dental Enamel as Observed by Electron Microscopy, Arch. Oral. Biol., *10*, 775–783, 1965.)

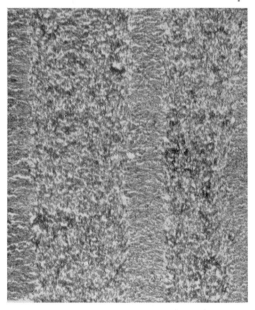

FIG. 7–9. Electron micrograph of a section cut from a human permanent incisor. The plane of sectioning was parallel to the long axis of the enamel prisms and passed across the head and tail regions of adjacent prisms. × 5000. (Meckel, A. H., Griebstein, W. J., and Neal, R. J.: Structure of Natural Human Dental Enamel as Observed by Electron Microscopy. Arch. Oral. Biol., *10*, 775–783, 1965.)

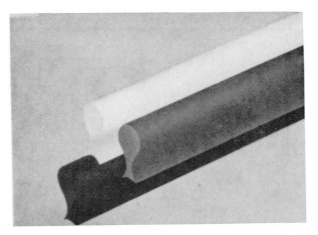

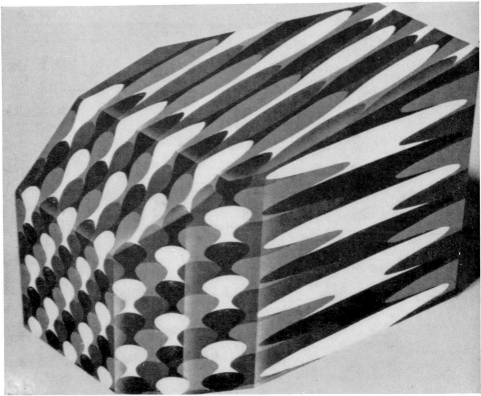

Fig. 7–10. Model of human dental enamel prepared by cementing together individual model prisms as shown above. Note the variety of patterns formed by milling the surfaces of the model at different angles to the prism axes. (Meckel, A. H., Griebstein, W. J., and Neal, R. J.: Structure of Natural Human Dental Enamel as Observed by Electron Microscopy. Arch. Oral. Biol., *10*, 775–783, 1965.)

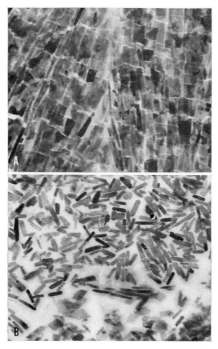

Fig. 7–11A. Electron micrograph of longitudinally sectioned prisms from hypomineralized human enamel depicting the relationship between 2 prisms from adjoining layers. The orientation of the longitudinally cut crystals differs between the 2 prisms so that a more continuous space, identified as the prism sheath, results where the 2 crystal groups abut. × 25,000.

Fig. 7–11B. A portion of a prism sheath separating 2 enamel prisms in a transverse section. The large coherent spaces characteristic of the interface between prisms in this hypomineralized enamel are much more evident in a cross than in a longitudinal section. The hexagonal shape of the crosscut crystals and their relative orientation to each other are also revealed in this type of section. × 50,000. (Nylen, M. V.: Recent electron microscopic and allied investigations into the normal structure of human enamel, Int. Dent. Journal, 17, 719, 1967.)

crystallites tend to be oriented in the direction of this movement. Thus, in the head of the keyhole, the crystallites are oriented in the direction of the prism long axis and perpendicular to the Tomes' process of the ameloblast. On the cervical side of the prism the crystallites are oriented essentially perpendicular to the prism long axis and also perpendicular to the plane of slippage between the Tomes' process surface and the mineralizing front.

DENTINE

Mineral Phase

Dentine is always less mineralized than enamel but has a higher mineral content than either bone or cementum. The mineral fraction of dentine ranges from approximately 68 to 79% by weight as contrasted with approximately 97% by weight in enamel. The crystallites of dentine are considerably smaller than those of enamel. The average thickness is approximately 20 to 35 Å and lengths are usually 200 to 300 Å, although crystallites up to 1000 Å have been measured. The volume of an individual enamel crystallite is approximately 200 times that of a dentine crystallite. Since chemical reactions are confined to the surface of the apatite crystals, the smaller size of the dentinal crystal associated with a correspondingly larger surface area makes dentine less stable than enamel. The Ca/P ratio in dentine usually, but not always, has been found to be lower than that in enamel from the same tooth, and exhibits more variability. As mentioned earlier, amorphous calcium phosphate (ACP) has been reported in dentine. Approximately 35% of the dentinal mineral phase was found to be ACP, about the same fraction as in compact bone.

Dentinal Structure

Dentine, unlike inert enamel, retains a vital cellular component, the odontoblast, as it matures. However, dentine, like other connective tissues, consists primarily of extracellular substance and only a small amount of cellular material. The extracellular component occurs primarily in the form of a densely mineralized collagenous matrix enclosing tubular structures. This mineralized dentinal matrix forms the body of the tooth, protects the dental pulp, and provides attachment and underlying support for the protective enamel covering and the cementum. In mature dentine in the transverse section (Fig. 7–12) it is possible to demonstrate the following structures:

1. Intertubular dentine
2. Outer hypomineralized layer
3. Peritubular dentine
4. Inner hypomineralized layer
5. Dentinal process of the odontoblast.

Not all these structures can be easily demonstrated in a single section. It will be noted that the inner hypomineralized layer cannot be seen in Figure 7–12.

The intertubular dentine consists of a mineralized collagenous framework extending among the dentinal tubules. The collagenous fibers exhibit a typical 640 Å cross banding. The arrangement and distribution of the collagenous fibrils can be seen in a section from the matrix of demineralized dentine (Fig. 7–13). This photograph shows that the collagenous fibrils of the matrix are arranged in a trellis-like framework, while some of the fibers appear to be running tangentially to the dentinal tubules. The presence of oblique longitudinal and cross-sectional views of fibrils indicates that they follow a random course relative to the tubules.

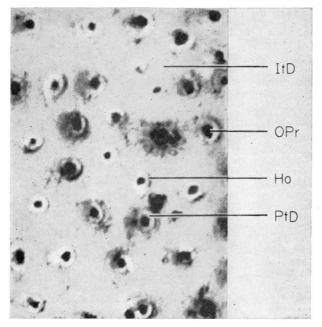

Fig. 7–12. Ground transverse section of human dentine stained with silver nitrate and reduced in sunlight. *OPr*, Odontoblast process; *Ho*, outer hypomineralized layer; *PtD*, peritubular dentine; *ItD*, intertubular dentine. × 1500. (From Bradford, E. W.: Microanatomy and Histochemistry of Dentine. In *Structure and Chemical Organization of Teeth*. A. E. W. Miles (Ed.), New York, Academic Press, 1967, p. 20.)

The tubular portion of mature dentine consists of the inner odontoblastic process, which is separated from the peritubular dentine by an inner hypomineralized layer. The peritubular dentine likewise is separated from the intertubular dentine by the outer hypomineralized layer.

The odontoblastic process is the cytoplasmic extension from the odontoblast through the tubule. Near the vicinity of the predentine-pulp border, the odontoblast process has been clearly shown to be an extension of the odontoblast cytoplasm with continuity of the plasma membrane extending into the dentinal tubule. At this level the odontoblast process still retains some cytoplasmic organelles, including the endoplasmic reticulum and mitochondria. In progressing from the predentine-dentine border into the more mature dentine, the fine structure of the odontoblast process has proven difficult to study because of the high mineral content of mature dentine. In the predentine region, the diameter of the odontoblast process is approximately 5 microns. In the mineralized dentine the odontoblastic process is reduced to about 2 microns and continuity of the cytoplasm cannot always be demonstrated. In studies employing demineralization and fixation of the mature dentine, some dentinal tubules display collagenous fibrils. Others were empty or showed aggregates of granular material in the tubule lumen.

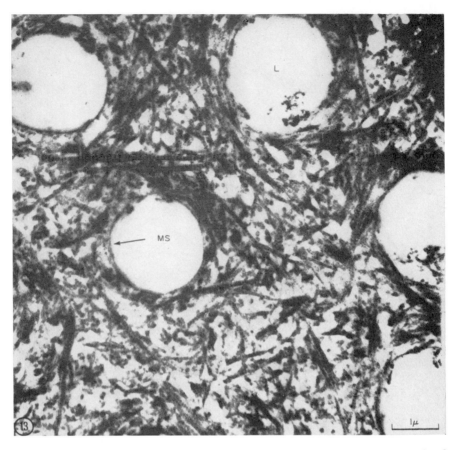

Fig. 7–13. The collagenous fibrils appear in longitudinal, oblique and cross-sectional views in matrix obtained from the vicinity of the predentine-dentine border. A membranous structure (MS) surrounds the lumen (L) of the canal, stained with phosphotungstic acid (approx. × 17,800). (Johansen, E.: Comparison of the Ultrastructure and Chemical Composition of Sound and Carious Enamel from Human Permanent Teeth, in *Tooth Enamel*, M. V. Stack and R. W. Fearnhead (Eds.). Bristol, John Wright & Sons, 1965.)

Peritubular dentine is a hypermineralized material laid down between the intertubular dentine and the odontoblast process. This tissue is presumed to be laid down or secreted by the odontoblast itself. With maturation of the tubule there is a reduction in the diameter of the odontoblast process from 5 microns to approximately 1 to 2 microns at the intermediate dentine level with a corresponding increase in the thickness of peritubular dentine. The peritubular dentine appears to be the most densely mineralized phase of dentine, having a specific gravity of 2.4 as compared with a specific gravity of 2.1 to 2.2 for dentine overall. The collagenous fibrils in the peritubular dentine are narrower than those in the inner tubular dentinal areas. Peritubular fibrils have diameters in the range of 250 to 500 Å, as compared with the 600 to 700 Å fibril width found in intertubular dentine.

Material is continually deposited on the walls of the tubules in the formation of the peritubular dentine until the lumen of the tubule is nearly or completely obliterated. Until complete closure occurs, the highly mineralized peritubular dentine is separated from the remainder of the odontoblast process by the hypomineralized layer. Because the intertubular dentine is formed prior to the peritubular dentine at any given plane, the two tissues are separated by a narrow zone of hypomineralized tissue. This zone is called the outer hypomineralized layer.

SELECTED REFERENCES

Brown, W. E.: Crystal growth of bone mineral, Clin. Orthop., *44*, 205–220, 1966.

Carlstrom, Diego: X-ray crystallographic studies on apatites and calcified structures, Acta Radiol. Supp., *121*, 59, 1955.

Johansen, E.: Comparison of the Ultrastructure and Chemical Composition of Sound and Carious Enamel from Human Permanent Teeth, in *Tooth Enamel*, Bristol, John Wright & Sons, 1965, pp. 177–181.

Legeros, Ragull Z., Trautz, Otto R., Legeros, John P., Klein, Edward and Shura, W. Paul: Apatite crystallites, effect of carbonate on morphology, Science, *155*, 1409–1411, 1967.

Miles, A. E. W.: *Structural and Chemical Organization of Teeth*, Vol. II, New York, Academic Press Inc., 1967.

Nylen, M. V.: Recent electron microscopic and allied investigations into the normal structure of human enamel, Internat. Dent. J., *17*, 719–733, 1967.

Stack, M. V. and Fearnhead, R. W.: *Tooth Enamel*, Bristol, John Wright & Sons, Ltd., 1965.

Trautz, O.: X-ray diffraction of biological and synthetic apatites, Ann. New York Acad. Science, *60*, 696–712, 1955.

Chapter **8**

Bone Apposition and Resorption

DON M. RANLY, D.D.S., Ph.D.

The maxilla and mandible serve as the foundation for the soft tissues of the face and oral cavity. In addition, the roots of the teeth are fixed in the sockets of these bones by periodontal ligaments. Like other bones of the body, the maxilla and mandible are characterized by a growth pattern that attains an ultimate configuration and size in the adult. It should be stressed, however, that at no time in the life of an individual do the shape and architecture of these bones become static. Instead, the addition of new bone matrix (bone apposition) and its removal (bone resorption) are a continuing process. Under physiologic conditions, the resorption and apposition of bone are called remodeling, a vital process during the period of craniofacial growth. Of lesser magnitude but of great importance is the remodeling of bone following the initial and continuing eruption of teeth and drift due to proximal attrition.

In contrast to the orderly remodeling of the normal growth and aging process is the shift toward resorption seen in a number of pathologic conditions. The bone destruction observed in periodontal disease, apical infection, traumatic occlusion, and many other situations constitutes a major reason for the great loss of teeth in the human population.

On the other hand, bone remodeling is used to advantage by the orthodontist. The correction of tooth position with applied forces is made possible by the adaptive potential of bone cells.

Some time in the future patients suffering from bone loss may be treated by some means of bone induction which would entail selective stimulation of bone-forming cells. Unquestionably, a knowledge of bone formation and resorption is essential to an understanding of craniofacial growth and the processes of tooth eruption. Without this background there can be but little appreciation for the processes involved in bone destruction, and little chance for a rational approach to its prevention and treatment.

THE OSTEOBLAST

Morphology and Location

The osteoblast was considered responsible for the manufacture of bone matrix when first described by Gegenbaur in 1864, and during the last three decades solid evidence has emerged supporting this view. As the role of the osteoblast has become known, its morphologic description has become increasingly less precise. This paradox has emerged because the osteoblast is a transitional cell, modulating or differentiating from precursor cells to engage in bone synthesis. The fully developed osteoblast is not capable of mitosis and has a limited life span. Deposition of new bone involves the recruitment of more primitive cells and the modulation of their activity toward synthesis. As a result, the structure of the osteoblast parallels the rise and fall of its functional activity, and any description of the cell must note its location and/or stage of differentiation.

The osteoblast is a surface cell, lining the bone either as the deepest layer of the periosteum, or as a pseudoepithelium around trabeculae or within the canals of the haversian system. Ordinarily the osteoblastic layer is one cell thick, and in the periosteum the cells of the layer next to the osteoblasts are less well-differentiated precursors. Osteoblasts can assume a variety of shapes including ovoid, columnar, and pyriform. When carpeting the surfaces of newly formed trabeculae they tend to be columnar in shape and are oriented perpendicular to the bony surface.

When bone formation is active, most of the osteoblasts are highly polarized in that the nucleus is situated distant from the bone matrix. Inactive osteoblasts, in contrast, are thin and squamous-like, with a flattened nucleus occupying a central position in the cell.

When viewed with the light microscope, an actively synthesizing osteoblast features a large nucleus with one nucleoli and an extensive granular endoplasmic reticulum which gives it an intense cytoplasmic basophilia. When stained with ordinary dyes there is a large, clear area at the center of the cell, near the nucleus, called the juxtanuclear vacuole. This structure is now thought to be associated with the Golgi complex.

With electron microscopy, the organelles of the osteoblast easily distinguish the osteoblast from the other bone cells. The osteoblast is mononucleated, whereas the osteoclast is characterized by multiple nuclei. The osteoblast has an elaborate endoplasmic reticulum and a well-developed Golgi apparatus, whereas neither organelle is prominent in the osteoclast or osteocyte. The osteoblast contains many mitochondria, but the osteoclast has a plethora of these structures (Fig. 8–1).

The impression proffered by ultramicroscopic examination of the osteoblast is one of intense synthetic activity. The endoplasmic reticulum becomes extensive, the granularity increasing with maturity because of the accumulation of free and bound ribosomes. Additional granules are pro-

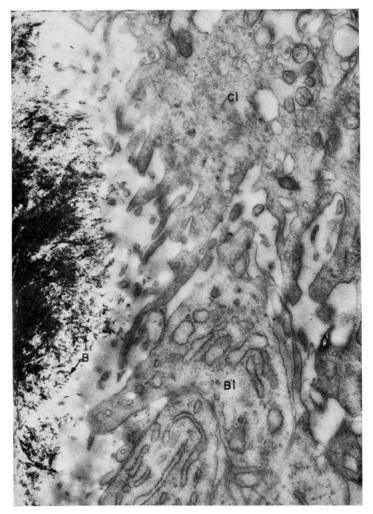

Fig. 8–1.   An osteoclast (Cl) is shown at a site of junction with an osteoblast (Bl). The underlying bone (B) shows a resorption zone.   Note the characteristic cytoplasmic constituents of each cell.   (From Dudley, H. R., and Spiro, D.:   The Fine Structure of Bone Cells.   J. Biophysic Biochem. Cytol., *11*, 647, 1961, with permission.)

vided by the development of protein-containing cisternae or dilatations in the endoplasmic reticulum.

In keeping with this synthetic image the osteoblast features a prominent Golgi apparatus.   This structure is composed of "stacks" of granular membranes arranged in lamellar order.   Single membrane vesicles are scattered throughout the Golgi region.

The osteoblast has intimate contact with its neighbors.   Fine cytoplasmic processes extend out to make contact with such structures from other osteocytes and other osteoblasts. It was debated in the past whether such cell contacts were continuous or contiguous. The electron microscope has revealed no specialization of the membranes such as macula adherens or zonula occludens. Thus each osteoblast is functionally and morphologically a separate entity.

Evidence of Function

Irrespective of biochemical data, the location, morphology, and histo-chemistry of the osteoblast provide overwhelming evidence for its role in bone synthesis. The prominent endoplasmic reticulum, large Golgi apparatus, abundant mitochondria, and conspicuous nucleoli suggest the ultimate in capacity for protein synthesis.

In recent years, sophisticated studies with labeled precursors have provided direct confirmation of heretofore assumed activities. Tritiated amino acids are rapidly incorporated into osteoblasts. Autoradiographs of serially sacrificed animals disclose a movement of the labeled amino acids out of the cells into the newly formed collagen around the cells. The other component of bone matrix, the mucosubstances, is also synthesized by osteoblasts. ^{35}S-labeled sulfate, ^{14}C-glucose, and ^{3}H-glucosamine are taken up by the cell and passed on to the bone matrix. *In vitro* biochemical studies have demonstrated that matrix components are processed intracellularly by the osteoblast before secretion.

Life History

Just as one description cannot encompass the morphologic variations of osteoblasts, a single life history cannot cover the variety of events occurring among an osteoblast population. In the first place, the precursor cells that serve as the origin of the osteoblasts are apparently ubiquitous. Second, the functions of all osteoblasts are not the same. These differences have become obvious as scientific methodology has improved, but there are probably many subtle variations yet to be determined.

The osteoblast, constantly reduced in number by conversion to osteocytes and incapable of reproduction, must arise from precursor cells. These cells are found in the periosteum, the endosteum, and the periosteal bud invading the cartilage shafts of long bones. Osteoblasts can even differentiate from non-skeletal tissue, the result of which is heterotopic bone.

In the periosteum, the source cell has been named the osteoprogenitor or stem cell. It is a nondescript, fusiform cell located near an inactive bone surface or in layers above actively synthesizing osteoblasts.

Thymidine uptake studies have demonstrated that the population of osteoprogenitor cells undergoes active mitosis. Occasionally, mature osteoblasts incorporate ^{3}H-thymidine but they do not go on to divide. Instead, most of the isotopic precursor in the DNA of osteoblasts is originally

Although there are gross indications that electrical impulses are the transducers for stress, the biophysical study of bone is not yet sophisticated enough to provide real insight into the subtle impulses and cellular responses which would operate in such a system.

THE OSTEOCLAST

Location and History

The osteoclast is the most interesting of the bone cells, for sheer size alone if not for its multiple nuclei, brush border, and enigmatic life history. It was named by Kölliker in 1873 after he concluded that it was the cell responsible for bone resorption. With few exceptions most investigators have implicated this cell in bone removal.

The osteoclast varies in size from moderate to very large. In fact, they have measured $85 \times 105 \mu$ with a calculated volume of 200,000 μ^3. With these proportions they are the largest cells in the body.

Another distinguishing feature is their multiple nuclei which are usually close together, oval, and have one or two nucleoli. The giant osteoclasts may contain 100 or more of these organelles, whereas others on the opposite end of the size spectrum may contain only two or three nuclei.

Osteoclasts are found apposed to a flat surface of bone, wrapped around a trabecula, or occupying an erosion pit. These latter areas are called Howship's lacunae, and empty ones may be observed after the osteoclasts have migrated away.

Another characteristic finding of osteoclastic resorption is the junction of certain areas of the cell membrane and bone. Visible with the light microscope are finger-like projections of cytoplasm with vacuoles concentrated at their base between these projections. This specialization of the cell membrane is called the brush or ruffled border and is the site of bone resorption. Some investigators have claimed that exposed collagen fibrils are another visible component of this zone.

Electron microscopy has revealed even more interesting facets about this cell and quashed much of the controversy and confusion over the relationship between structure and function.

The nuclear material in the nuclei is clumped peripherally, and the membrane is interrupted by numerous pores. Associated with each nucleus is a Golgi network which completely surrounds it. The Golgi network is composed of groups of flattened sacs, and the surrounding vesicles appear to have been derived from the sacs closest to the nucleus.

The rough endoplasmic reticulum is not as prominent in the osteoclast as in the osteoblast. The membranes lie close to each other, but the ribosomes are sparse along them. The vesicles, possibly derived from the ER, can be confused with the numerous vacuoles and vesicles arising from the Golgi apparatus and the brush border. There are many free ribosomes in the cytoplasm.

The mitochondria are more concentrated in the osteoclast than in any other bone cell. They are scattered about the cytoplasm except for the brush border zone. If the number of mitochondria can be correlated to actual energy production, then the osteoclast must be a very active cell indeed.

The arrangement of the centrioles is a unique feature of the osteoclast. Since most cells have one pair of centrioles associated with each nucleus, it is not surprising that a multinucleated cell such as the osteoclast has many pairs of centrioles. However, these centrioles are aggregated into one area of the cytoplasm in a structure called the centrosphere. This structure has not been observed in any other type of giant cell.

In some situations the osteoclast and the bone undergoing resorption appear to form a compartment containing the ruffled border. The compartment is sealed off by an annular ring of modified cytoplasm which is transformed from the normal cytoplasm and which progressively converts to the ruffled border.

The brush border is a complex zone of folds and projections in juxtaposition to the matrix. The cytoplasmic extensions are a fraction of a micron wide but may be several microns long. The spaces between these folds are tortuous and often show matrix debris in them. The spaces terminate as vesicles or vacuoles which have been reported to contain apatite crystal and collagen fibers. Other investigators have interpreted this finding as an artifact of the plane of section, and maintain that all tissue breakdown is extracellular. There are few organelles at the base of the brush border, and the cytoplasmic projections contain no microtubules.

Evidence for Role

By the very nature of Howship's lacunae and the brush border visible with the light microscope, the osteoclast has long been implicated in bone resorption. Research has provided confirmatory evidence within the last few years.

Motion pictures of bone tissue culture have embellished the earlier microscopic work. The osteoclasts were seen to be motile and active, and the matrix seemed to "melt" away when confronted by this cell. In several of these microcinematographic studies, the correlation between osteoclast contact and matrix removal was visually strong.

Proof that the "dissolved" matrix was at least partly phagocytosed by the cell was provided by autoradiographic studies with plutonium. This isotope was incorporated into the bone matrix by the osteoblasts. Autoradiographs made after serial sacrifice demonstrated that the isotope was taken up by the osteoclasts sometime after deposition. The radioactivity was found within the cell, confirming that the matrix, at least in part, was absorbed by the cell.

6

Electron microscopy has resolved the complexity of the brush border. Some investigators have demonstrated convincingly that bone debris becomes located within the spaces between the processes and in the vacuoles at their base. Both mineral and collagen fibrils can be observed in various stages of degradation. The matrix at the brush zone becomes frayed and occasionally appears as if demineralized collagen fibrils are exposed to the cytoplasmic projections. Observations on the uptake of thorium dioxide particles by osteoclasts suggest that absorption of exogenous material occurs by "membrane flow" as opposed to "membrane vesiculation" or endocytosis. The former term describes the binding of particles to the surface of the cell followed by the flow of the membrane into the cytoplasm where the material is transferred to the lysosome. The latter term describes the pinching-off of small invaginations of the plasma membrane.

Life History

Theories on the origin and fate of the osteoclast have been controversial since the cell's identification, and, although there are some persuasive arguments supporting one theory, the matter is not entirely settled.

No mitosis has ever been observed in osteoclasts despite the large number of nuclei. It is generally accepted that the osteoclast must arise from smaller cells by fusion. Because osteoclasts are large multinucleated cells, many investigators have attempted to classify them as a kind of foreign body giant cell. Such a cell might arise by the fusion of macrophages or mononuclear leukocytes.

The osteoclast certainly behaves as an amoeboid-type cell in motion picture studies. Unfortunately, the fusion of precursor cells has not been observed in a clear-cut manner. Portions of an osteoclast have been observed to break off and shuttle to another osteoclast. These *in vitro* findings may be an artifact of the tissue culture environment.

When carbon particles were injected intravenously into experimental animals, macrophages were observed to phagocytize the particles. After 15 days carbon particles were found in the osteoclasts. The investigators argued that the macrophages fused to form osteoclasts, assuming that no particles were released by dying macrophages during the period of the study. Unfortunately, carbon particles are likely to be recycled, which raises serious doubts about this interpretation of these results.

When ^{3}H-thymidine uptake is studied by autoradiography, precursor cells are first seen with the isotope. Hours later some of the nuclei of the osteoclast become labeled. The logical assumption is that precursor cells fuse to form osteoclasts. Exception to this theory can be taken because mononuclear leukocytes as well as other cells are known to incorporate this thymidine. In addition, osteoclasts arise from connective tissue around dead bone implants just as osteoblasts do. Such evidence seems to preclude an ancestry for osteoclasts limited solely to bone cells.

Electron microscopic observation of bone cells from animals sacrificed 1 hour after injections of ^{3}H-thymidine revealed that two types of cells were labeled. A type "A" cell resembled the "osteoprogenitor" cell described by other investigators. A type "B" cell, definitely a precursor, was called a pre-osteoclast. Whether this latter cell ever fused to form an osteoclast was not determined. If this study was interpreted correctly, bone may have two lines of cells. One, a pre-osteoblast that upon differentiation becomes an osteoblast and eventually an osteocyte. The other, a pre-osteoclast, could fuse rather than differentiate to form an osteoclast. Other connective tissue, less specialized than bone, might possess the stem cell capable of forming the two lines present in bone. Heterotopic bone induction suggests that it does.

The life span of an osteoclast is brief. *In vitro* studies disclosed a 1-week survival period under optimal conditions. *In vivo* analysis of the turnover of osteoclasts with ^{3}H-thymidine showed that after 3 or 4 days the osteoclast population with labeled nuclei began to decrease. Others remained, however, up to 2 weeks. The fact that portions of one cell may become components of another confuses the issue.

Equally as mysterious as the origin and life span of the osteoclast is its fate. Despite their relatively gigantic size, no one has determined where they go. Presumably the cell dissociates into smaller pieces which either demodulate or die. It is doubtful that osteoclasts undergo degeneration in their largest state, since no one has reported such a cell with all the prerequisite characteristics such as pyknotic nuclei and multiple vacuoles.

Mechanism of Osteoclasis

The resorption of bone by osteoclasts may involve two simultaneous actions, mechanical and enzymatic. The highly motile cytoplasmic projections at the brush border may physically augment the dissolution of matrix by actually twisting and pushing the denuded collagen fibrils. In a mutant strain of rats characterized by a hereditary absence of incisors, bone resorption is markedly reduced. In these animals some mineral is removed, but virtually no matrix. Their osteoclasts reveal an absence of the ruffled borders and no extracellular lysosomal enzyme release. These observations suggest that mineral and matrix removal are separate processes and that the brush border is necessary for matrix dissolution.

How fibrils become demineralized and how they are handled after separation from the bulk matrix are unknown. Studies on osteoclasts have been handicapped by the inability to isolate a population of these cells. Their numbers are never great in bone, and consequently the differentiation between the activity of osteocytes and osteoclasts is difficult. It might be possible in the future to create large numbers of osteoclasts by treating bone cultures with specific agents.

Since electron microscopy shows a strong correlation between the folds of the brush border and the resorption of bone, it is reasonable to assume that the cell possesses the capacity to demineralize and dissolve the matrix by degrading collagen and protein polysaccharides.

The requirements for bone resorption have been outlined: acid production to demineralize, collagenase, proteases and hyaluronidase to remove matrix, and many lysosomal catheptic enzymes to remove the cells.

Several years ago citric acid and then lactic acid were postulated to play a role in mobilizing mineral. Since then, however, most *in vivo* and *in vitro* studies have failed to demonstrate a stoichiometric relationship between acid production and the release of ^{45}Ca from bone explants. The same correlation could not be found for citric acid. It is possible, if lactate is accompanied by equimolar H^+ ions, that aerobic glycolysis is the mechanism for dissolving mineral. Lactate production is stimulated by parathyroid extract, a substance known to mobilize calcium, and suppressed by calcitonin, a hormone that inhibits mobilization.

Collagenase activity was first discovered in 1962 by the technique of placing bone on reconstituted collagen gels and observing the lysis. Since then the development of more sensitive assays has permitted the study of collagenase in normal and disease states. Collagenase has been characterized from human, mouse, and rat bones. Both human and mouse collagenase were obtained by culturing their bone tissue on collagen gels. Collagenase from rat bones was obtained by direct disruption of bone cells. This difference in the techniques required for collection may be species related or may signal the presence of several types of collagenases in bone.

Rodent bone cells are remarkably reactive to PTH. Collagenase levels rise markedly *in vivo* and in culture in the presence of this hormone. In several studies on humans in which bone resorption was pathological, the collagenase levels were higher than those found in a control population.

There is little doubt that collagenase (or collagenases) is produced by bone cells, but identifying the controlling cell or cells must be resolved with techniques for localizing such activities. Recent tissue culture work suggests that heparin may enhance the action of collagenase in collagen degradation. This evidence corresponds with the well-known fact that an increase in bone mast cells and bone resorption develops in animals fed a calcium-deficient diet. Mast cells synthesize heparin for other physiological needs and its relationship to collagenase may be only a curiosity.

Recently, carbonic anhydrase has been postulated to play a role in demineralization by virtue of its control over the local secretion of hydrogen ions. In tissue culture, inhibitors of carbonic anhydrase have suppressed parathyrin (parathyroid hormone)-induced resorption.

Culture work with embryonic calvaria has demonstrated that parathyroid extract-stimulated resorption of bone is paralleled by a rise of lysosomal acid hydrolases released into the medium. Presumably these enzymes (acid protease, acid deoxyribonuclease, β-glucuronidase, N-acetyl-β-glucosaminidase and β-galactosidase) are released in bulk by exocytosis. Another lysosomal enzyme, hyaluronidase, becomes elevated under the same experimental conditions.

The following working hypothesis probably reflects the current thinking about the resorption process. Increased glycolysis and/or carbonic anhydrase-controlled H^+ secretion creates an acidic condition that solubilizes the mineral and prepares the environment for the release of acid hydrolases. These enzymes in conjunction with one or more collagenases resorb the matrix and degrade cellular elements.

It is likely that osteocytes and osteoclasts possess the same cellular machinery to resorb bone, but the emphasis for each may differ. The osteocytes seem to exert more control over demineralization and remineralization as a process in calcium homeostasis, whereas osteoclasts are more concerned with bulk bone removal.

Stimulus

When osteoclastic stimulation is discussed, two related phenomena are usually implied, i.e., the formation of osteoclasts and their activity in resorbing bone. Most histologic studies have used increased numbers as the criterion for increased osteoclastic action. The elevation of serum calcium cannot be ascribed solely to osteoclasts, nor can the release of collagenase and other enzymes. For these reasons, an increase in the number of osteoclasts does not automatically mean increased osteoclasis. Although it is probably reasonable to assume that osteoclast formation and activity are linked, there could conceivably be stimulators for fusion alone.

There are at least two categories of stimuli: chemical agents and mechanical forces. The former has been the object of intense research for many years and substantial progress has been made. The latter stimulus is mostly speculative.

The chemical agent most associated with osteoclast proliferation is parathyrin (parathyroid hormone). After the administration of parathyroid extract, osteoclast numbers are increased, but with a lag of at least 6 hours. Endogenous secretion of parathyrin requires even longer to statistically increase the population. Although there is no question of the correlation between parathyrin and osteoclast formation, no study has yet demonstrated irrefutably that the activity of osteoclasts is increased by this hormone. This fact, coupled with the knowledge that calcium mobilization under parathyrin stimulus is rapid, suggests that transformation of cells into osteoclasts is not really related to calcium homeostasis. In addition, the ability of the bone under parathyrin stimulation to supply calcium cannot be correlated to the number of osteoclasts.

It is now generally conceded that parathyrin has a dual action: one is to stimulate osteolysis to control serum calcium, and the second is to stimulate the new formation of osteoclasts in order that they will be available for remodeling.

A number of other agents are known to stimulate bone resorption, two of which are vitamin D and prostaglandin E_2. Some factors responsible for stimulating osteoclasts in organ culture have been identified as a result of investigations into periodontal disease. Evidence suggests that in chronic inflammation of the gingiva, mononuclear phagocytes, in some unknown manner, promote the elaboration of detectable osteoclast-activating factor by activated lymphocytes. This factor in turn stimulates osteoclastic resorption, resulting in the loss of supporting structures for the teeth. Complete elucidation of this sequence might someday aid the dentist in treating periodontal disease.

Mechanical forces are known to influence the shape of bones by their effect on bone cells. But, just as in the discussion of osteocytes, the mechanism for controlling the osteclasts' formation, location, activity, and disappearance is unknown. Perhaps the formation of osteoclasts is a continual process controlled by parathyrin. Only the activation of these cells may be related to forces.

During cantilever experiments with whole bones, the convex surface became electropositive and the concave surface became electronegative. *In vivo*, theoretically, the logical cellular reaction to such a displacement would be deposition on the concave surface and resorption on the convex side. Such activity physiologically would enable the long bones, for instance, to adapt to increased loads. In this interpretation electronegativity would be associated with osteoblasts and electropositivity with osteoclasts. Implantation of electrodes into bone lends some support to this theory. The cathode is associated with osteogenesis and the anode with osteoclasis.

Interpreting less convexity as an increase in concavity, and less concavity as more convexity, one investigator has analyzed the apposition and resorption patterns in many bones in the body. Unfortunately, the link between the electrical events observed in whole bone experiments and the actual cellular events remains unknown.

TOOTH MOVEMENT—A MODEL FOR STUDYING BONE APPOSITION AND RESORPTION

Nowhere in an *in vivo* situation is it more possible to elicit bone apposition and resorption at will than in the alveolar processes. By the application of mechanical forces to teeth, it is easy to instigate osteoclastic activity on the pressure side of the tooth socket and osteoblastic activity on the tension side. Not only are the resultant histological and biochemical changes somewhat isolated by the anatomy, but the forces responsible for them can be monitored and analyzed. In effect, the bone supporting the tooth becomes a microcosm of all the factors involved in the study of force and bone remodeling.

The tooth is supported in the alveolus by the periodontal ligament. The ligament is composed basically of collagen fibers attached to the cementum of the tooth and the bone tissue of the socket. The collagen fibers are purported to have three distinct structural zones that are important in their adaptive potential to physiological and orthodontic forces. The outer layer, next to the bone, is composed of coarse mature fibers which penetrate the bone (Sharpey's fibers) and anchor the ligament to the alveolus. The intermediate zone is composed principally of precollagenous fibers and constitutes a dynamic, labile area. The third or inner zone consists of mature fibers partially embedded in the cementum of the tooth. The intermediate zone is the link between the outer and inner fibers and is capable of contributing to either by virtue of its capacity for collagen synthesis.

When a tooth drifts the ligament makes adaptive changes in concert with the bone. On the side of the alveolus toward which the tooth is moving, bone is removed uncovering Sharpey's fibers. Numerous Howship's lacunae are present. Some of the exposed fibers are used as transient outer zone fibers which maintain the integrity of the supporting ligament. In addition, temporary deposition anchors new fibers to the bone. The outer zone of the ligament would necessarily become very wide if not constantly reduced by encroachment of the intermediate zone. On the tension side, new bone apposition buries the outer zone fibers. This zone is in turn kept a constant width by the conversion of the delicate fibers of the linkage zone into coarse mature fibers.

Thus, as the root of a tooth moves through bone, the periodontal ligament does not follow intact, but rather progressively transforms itself as fibers are uncovered on one side and enveloped on the other.

The periodontal ligament is surrounded by relatively impermeable tissue, namely, the cementum, bone, and gingiva. Within this space are housed fibers, cells, blood, and interstitial fluid. Blood vessels pass to and from the space by way of openings in the alveolar bone.

When forces of mastication are placed on the teeth, it is likely that the trapped fluid becomes a biological hydraulic mechanism that spares the ligaments the effects of ordinary occlusal forces. Only when a force is sustained enough to squeeze the fluid out do the ligaments come under tension. Ligaments so stressed can provide signals about the direction of force and initiate the appropriate cellular response to normalize the forces.

When sufficient lateral force is applied to the crown of a tooth, the ligament on one side is stretched (the "tension" side) and the other is shortened or compressed (the "pressure" side). Intravenous infusion of carbon particles (a technique that disclosed discontinuity in the vascular channels) following experimental tooth movement revealed an increase in permeability of the vasculature on the tension side. When the forces were strong, frank disruption of the vessels occurred resulting in the extravasation of red blood cells (RBC). No strangulation of vessels has been observed on the tension side.

Apparently because the vessels remain patent on the tension side, only one prominent method of bone apposition occurs. Osteoblasts deposit matrix on the inner surface of the alveolus, incorporating fibers in the process. ^{3}H-Thymidine uptake studies in experimental tooth movements suggest that the osteoblasts arise from as yet unidentified precursor cells of the periodontal space.

The mechanism for translating the tension on the ligament fibers to osteoblastic activity is unknown. The theory that postulates that the alveolus is deformed sufficiently to elicit a piezoelectric response is most attractive. This theory for tooth movement develops from the general relationship claimed for bone that increased concavity is associated with osteoblastic activity. When the tooth is "pulled" by the appliance, the ligaments are stretched and the alveolar walls come under tension. The geometry of the ligaments suggests that the diameter of the alveolus on the tension side might be lessened. In effect, it could become more concave. The electric signals generated would arouse osteoblasts to "correct" the concavity. This phenomenon would continue until the forces were spent.

This theory is not without support because bone bending has been determined to be a feature of orthodontic tooth movement. Strain-gauge probes placed in post-extraction sockets of orthodontic patients were able to detect changes in bone shape when the adjacent teeth were subjected to clinical forces.

On the pressure side the reaction to tooth movement is more complex. The "compressed" ligament undergoes a typical reaction, called ligament hyalinization, the extent of which depends upon the amount of force. Histologically the ligament appears amorphous and acellular. The loss of the fibrous appearance apparently results from the occlusion of the blood vessels, causing asphyxia and death of the cells. In the electron microscope the collagen fibers show few structural changes as judged by their periodicity. However, the fibers are compacted and deprived of cells by pressure. This hyaline zone is a temporary structure which is resolved by the surrounding tissue once the pressure is removed.

The importance of the hyaline zone is its relationship to the kind of bone resorption that occurs and, ultimately, to the rate of tooth movement. If forces are light, the vessels remain intact, and minimal areas of hyalinization occur. The reaction of the osteoclasts under these circumstances is called a "frontal" response. This is described as resorption of the alveolar plate adjacent to the ligament under pressure.

When the vascular supply is occluded by greater forces, hyalinization becomes a prominent feature. Presumably the ligament cells in these zones are incapable of function and therefore cannot differentiate into osteoclasts. Instead, the bone on the pressure side is removed by "rear resorption," which is bone destruction in the marrow spaces opposite the hyalinized ligament. In addition, the wall of the alveolus is resorbed above and below the compacted area.

The patency of the vessels on the pressure side appears strongly correlated to the type of resorption that occurs. If forces are light and the blood supply intact, unimpeded frontal resorption occurs. For this reason it is difficult to ascribe the stimulation of osteoclasts to anoxia. Furthermore, heavy forces that occlude vessels prevent direct resorption and delay tooth movement. However, it has been suggested that, rather than oxygen deprivation, an increase in oxygen tension might result from ligament compression. If vessels become occluded, the stenosis might cause aneurysms, followed by a bubbling-out of oxygen. It has been noted that high oxygen tension does increase osteoclasis in tissue culture. Unfortunately for this theory in rear resorption, the sites of osteoclastic action are removed from the aneurysms and postulated O_2 increase.

Because of these contradictions, the old theory proposing that tooth movement is related to forces exceeding the capillary blood pressure is difficult to support. Instead, the effects of force, blood supply, and bone resorption appear to be related only by the viability of cells.

The stimulation of the cells of the periodontal space is possibly achieved by another mechanism, such as the piezoelectric effect. Osteoclasis might result from a reaction opposite to that which occurred on the tension side. As the tooth is pulled toward the compression side, the ligaments relax and the wall of the alveolus springs out, allowing its shape to become *more* concave. Increased concavity is a signal for osteoclasis. This process would continue until the force, as before, is dissipated. Whether this theory has any validity remains for future research to answer (Fig. 8–5).

Cell response has long been considered the essential activity in tooth movement. To analyze the mobilization of osteoclasts for bone resorption, precursor uptake studies were performed on animals undergoing tooth movement. ^{3}H-Thymidine was incorporated in a portion of the osteoclasts but only after a delay. These findings suggest that preexisting mononucleated stem cells can fuse to form osteoclasts, and only after some time must precursor cells undergo mitosis to replenish them. Therefore, not all osteoclast formation is dependent on cellular proliferation.

Most studies on tooth movement, including those described in this section, are based on histologic interpretation or a variation thereof, such as autoradiography. Recently, other approaches have been used to investigate this subject. In one study, samples of periodontal ligament were taken from rabbits following experimental tooth movement and assayed for collagenolytic activity on reconstituted gel plates. The investigator determined that this tissue developed collagenolytic activity in proportion to the duration of the force applied.

The collagen-destroying potential was attributed to the development of fresh granulation tissue accompanied by vascularity and osteoclasts. Interestingly, the collagenolytic activity peaked with the osteoclast numbers. Unfortunately, this type of experiment is not sufficiently refined to differen-

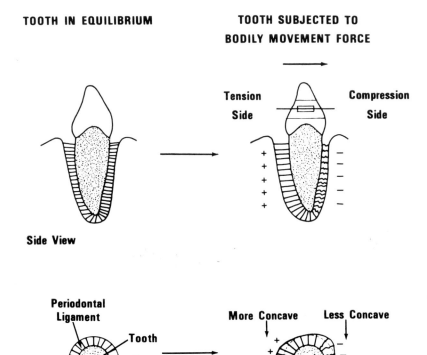

TOOTH IN EQUILIBRIUM

TOOTH SUBJECTED TO BODILY MOVEMENT FORCE

Tension Side

Compression Side

Side View

Periodontal Ligament

Tooth

Bone

More Concave

Less Concave

Top View

FIG. 8–5. Deformation of tooth socket caused by orthodontic force and transferred by the periodontal ligament. The tension side becomes more concave and elicits an osteoblastic response (+). The compression side becomes less concave and responds with osteoclastic activity (−).

tiate between enzymes removing hyalinized ligament or normal ligament collagen and those involved in bone resorption.

Cyclic adenosine-3', 5'-monophosphate (cAMP) has been related to the action of many drugs and hormones. It is thought to mediate the action of parathyrin (parathyroid hormone) on bone cells. To determine if cAMP is a mediator between force and bone resorption, a recent study analyzed the alveolar bone of cats following mechanical tipping of canine teeth. On the compression side the largest increase in cAMP was observed on the seventh day. On the tension side the increase was more moderate, following an initial period of decrease. The implications of this study have yet to be determined, but non-histological studies are beginning to bear fruit.

It would appear from recent research that meaningful data on the relationship between force and bone resorption may soon develop. The tooth and its supporting structures may play a key role in future discoveries.

SELECTED READINGS

BOURNE, G. H. (Ed.): *The Biochemistry and Physiology of Bone, Vol. I: Structure*, New York, Academic Press, 1971.

BOURNE, G. H. (Ed.): *The Biochemistry and Physiology of Bone, Vol. III: Development and Growth*, New York, Academic Press, 1971.

GIANELLY, A. A. and GOLDMAN, H. M.: *Biological Basis of Orthodontics*, Philadelphia, Lea & Febiger, 1971.

FROST, H. M.: *The Laws of Bone Structure*, Springfield, Ill., Charles C Thomas, 1964.

McLEAN, F. C. and URIST, M. R.: *Bone Fundamentals of the Physiology of Skeletal Tissue*, Chicago, University of Chicago Press, 1968.

Chapter 9

Fluoride

EUGENE P. LAZZARI, Ph.D.

In 1901, Dr. J. M. Eager of the U.S. Public Health Service communicated to the Surgeon General a description of the teeth of Italian emigrants embarking at the port of Naples. He noted a high frequency of a dental peculiarity known locally as "denti di Chiaie," which he believed to be due to "volcanic fumes or the emanation of subterranean fires, either fouling the atmosphere or forming a solution in drinking water." Chiaie (key-ĭ-ā) is a quarter of Naples where the natives drink from local wells and "numerous sources of mineral water, sulfurous and ferruginous." Eager also noted that " In Naples it is more often attributed to water than to the air since the Serino water brought in conduits from a distant mountain height has been in use and local wells condemned, the incidence of the disease among infants has greatly diminished."

The year 1901 was also when Dr. Frederick S. McKay arrived in Colorado Springs, Colorado, following his graduation from the University of Pennsylvania Dental School. He immediately noticed that many native patients had permanently brown-stained teeth. Except for inquiries that brought little information from dentists throughout the area, he dropped the matter for the next six years. In 1909, being unable to stimulate much interest by the Colorado Dental profession in the stained teeth, McKay interested Dr. Grune Vardimon Black, Dean of the Northwestern University Dental School, in visiting Colorado. This marked the beginning of serious study to determine the cause of Colorado brown stain, which clinically appears as mottled enamel with brown stain almost always localized in the outer surfaces of the upper incisors and cuspids.

Another dentist in Colorado Springs, Dr. H. A. Fynn, read a paper before the Colorado State Dental Society in 1909 in which he stated: " 87.5 percent of the children born and raised in this city have defects in the enamel." He also concluded that the cause of this defect was probably not the water, since analysis showed the water to be pure, but a lack of calcium in the local food. In their report of 1916, Black and McKay stated that they were convinced "the primary etiological characteristic of mottled enamel was developmental." Furthermore, they believed, as did the populace, the water was in some way responsible either by the presence or by the absence of some waterborne substance. They also stated: "The mottled condition in itself does not seem to increase the susceptibility of the teeth to decay. . . . But when the teeth do decay, the frail condition of the enamel makes it extremely difficult to make good and effective fillings."

In 1925, residents of Oakley, Idaho, and three years later those of Bauxite, Arkansas, changed their public water supply in the belief that mottled enamel was due to an unknown waterborne factor. By 1930, there remained little doubt that an unknown factor in drinking water caused mottled enamel regardless of whether the source was clear mountain streams, springs, artesian wells, blue lakes, deep or shallow wells, or drilled wells. Analyses of the water from areas whose inhabitants had mottled enamel showed nothing particularly unusual for the elements analyzed. These analyses did not include fluoride content.

In 1925, there appeared in the biochemical literature an unheralded and largely unheeded report by McCollum and co-workers on the effect of the addition of sodium fluoride to the incisors of rats. They found that fluoride levels slightly above those occurring in natural foods caused abnormalities in color and position. From 1929 through 1931, further diet studies on dairy cows and albino rats revealed that fluoride had a deleterious effect upon the teeth.

Meanwhile, in July 1930, a study of the mottled enamel problem was begun at the Arizona Agricultural Experiment Station by Dr. Margaret Commack Smith, her husband, Howard V. Smith, and Edith M. Lantz. They performed a survey of the children in St. David and concluded that environmental factors in the area were responsible. Further experiments on white rats supplied with St. David water, both natural and tenfold concentrates, showed gross defects in the incisor enamel including a loss of translucency, a chalky white appearance, and pitting. They regarded these changes as "similar if not identical to the mottling seen in human teeth." A review of the literature made them aware of the work by McCollum and others, which led to their undertaking further sodium fluoride feeding tests in rats. The results were "strikingly similar" to those seen in humans ingesting St. David water. On fluoride analysis, the water was found to contain 3.8 to 7.1 ppm fluoride. This led to the conclusion that mottled enamel was caused by the destructive action of fluoride present in the water supply of communities with afflicted residents.

In 1931, a Dental Hygienic Unit of the National Institutes of Health was formed with the specific mission of resolving the relation of waterborne fluoride to endemic mottled enamel. Standards of classification for the various degrees of severity of mottled enamel were developed, as well as an index of dental fluorosis that would give a numerical weighting to the degree

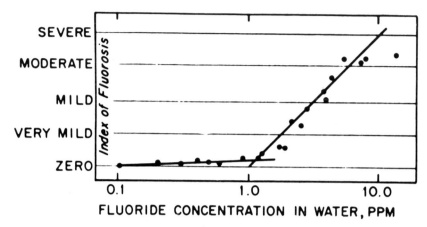

FIG. 9–1. Degree of mottled enamel and fluoride concentration in water. (From McClure, F. J.: Water Fluoridation, The Search and The Victory, Bethesda, Md., National Institutes of Health, U.S. Dept. of HEW, 1970.)

of severity. An analysis of the community fluorosis data obtained is shown in Figure 9–1.

By the middle of the 1930s, the U.S. Public Health Service recognized that information on the epidemiology, developmental and etiological characteristics of dental caries, and dental care requirements of school children was needed. A quantitative evaluation of dental caries was devised to allow comparison among the many groups of children to be examined. A count of the number of decayed, missing, and filled teeth gave the total number of teeth affected by caries, termed the DMF count.

Caries data on 8,257 American Indian children collected from 1928 through 1932 had shown that the severity of caries was greatest in the Northwest and least in the Southwestern States. The Southwest was also known as an area of extensive dental fluorosis. Studies relating fluoride levels in drinking water and the incidence of dental caries were continued throughout the 1930s and early 1940s. Figure 9–2 is a graph of the results of the surveys made in Illinois, Indiana, Ohio, and Colorado. All attempts at correlating the differences in the prevalence of caries with the hardness of the water, the hours of sunshine, or diet failed.

Worldwide studies continuing to the present have shown qualitatively similar results leading to the same conclusion: there is an inverse relationship between dental caries and fluoride content of the drinking water (Fig. 9–3).

In 1945, residents of Grand Rapids, Michigan, began to add fluoride to their drinking water. Many communities today add fluoride to the water to a level of about 1 ppm. In the many studies conducted, no undesirable effects such as fluorosis or other enamel defects have been reported. However, a significant decrease, about 30%, in caries has always been demonstrated. In the period from 1945 through 1971, over 95-million people in the United

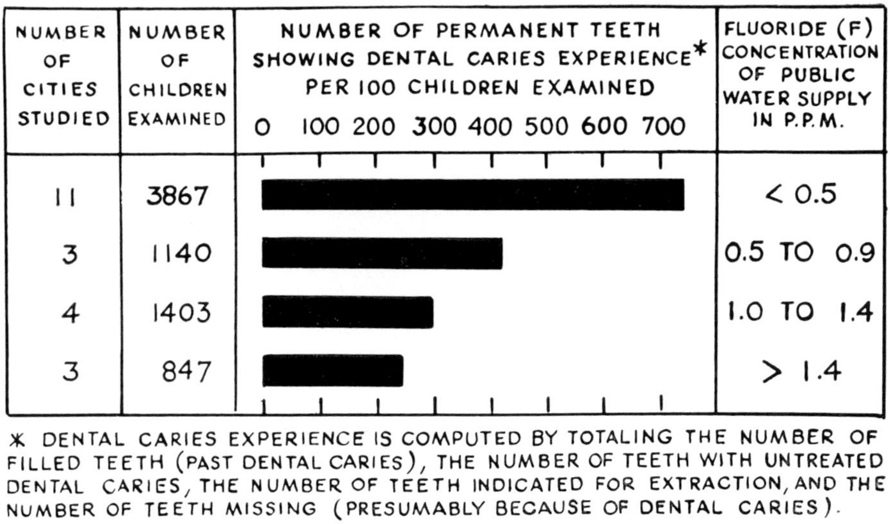

NUMBER OF CITIES STUDIED
NUMBER OF CHILDREN EXAMINED
NUMBER OF PERMANENT TEETH SHOWING DENTAL CARIES EXPERIENCE* PER 100 CHILDREN EXAMINED
0 100 200 300 400 500 600 700
FLUORIDE (F) CONCENTRATION OF PUBLIC WATER SUPPLY IN P.P.M.
11
3867
< 0.5
3
1140
0.5 TO 0.9
4
1403
1.0 TO 1.4
3
847
> 1.4
* DENTAL CARIES EXPERIENCE IS COMPUTED BY TOTALING THE NUMBER OF FILLED TEETH (PAST DENTAL CARIES), THE NUMBER OF TEETH WITH UNTREATED DENTAL CARIES, THE NUMBER OF TEETH INDICATED FOR EXTRACTION, AND THE NUMBER OF TEETH MISSING (PRESUMABLY BECAUSE OF DENTAL CARIES).

FIG. 9–2. Amount of dental caries (permanent teeth) observed in 7,257 selected 12- to 14-year-old white school children of 21 cities in four states, classified according to fluoride concentration of public water supplies. (From McClure, F. J.: Water Fluoridation, The Search and the Victory, Bethesda, Md., National Institutes of Health, U.S. Dept. of HEW, 1970.)

1400
1200
1000
800
600
400
200
DMF TEETH PER 100 CHILDREN
Denmark
Sweden
U.S.A.
1
2
3
4
FLUORIDE CONCENTRATION (PPM)

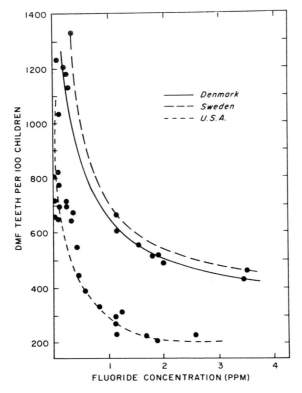

FIG. 9–3. Caries experience of children in Denmark and Sweden, aged 12 and 13, and in the United States, aged 12 to 14, in relation to fluoride content of public water supplies. (From Møller, I. J.: *Dental Fluorose og Caries.* Copenhagen, Rhodos, 1965.)

States, 13-million Soviet citizens, an estimated 6.6-million Canadians, and 4-million Europeans have been receiving fluoridated water. Overall, an estimated 130-million people are drinking artificially fluoridated water.

ENAMEL UPTAKE OF INGESTED FLUORIDE

Much information has been collected about the change in fluoride concentration with enamel depth, largely through the work of Brudevold, Weatherell, their co-workers, and others. Figure 9–4 gives the average fluoride gradient in the enamel of deciduous and permanent teeth from areas with 0.1 and 1 ppm of fluoride in the drinking water. The lower level of fluoride found in the deciduous teeth is due to the shorter period of formation

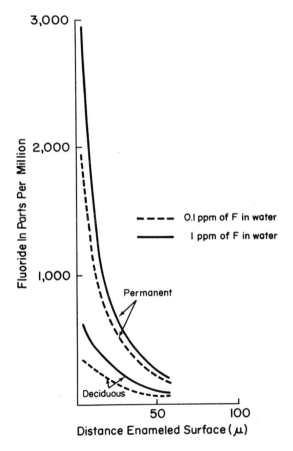

FIG. 9–4. Representative concentration gradients of fluoride from the surface inward in enamel of deciduous and permanent teeth from areas with 0.1 and 1 ppm F in the drinking water. (From Brudevold, F.: Interaction of Fluoride with Human Enamel. In *Symposium, Chemistry and Physiology of Enamel*, Ann Arbor, Mich., University of Michigan Press, 1971, p. 74.)

than is the case for permanent teeth. One study has shown that the teeth of girls have less fluoride in the enamel than those of boys, and this may explain the reports of several investigators that girls are more caries-susceptible than boys. The reasons could be that (1) the teeth of girls erupt earlier by 4 to 5 months, (2) the longer preeruptive time permits greater surface fluoride concentration thus greater caries-resistance, and (3) boys having greater body weight may drink more water than girls.

TOPICAL FLUORIDE

The literature indicates that the saliva fluoride concentration is about 80% that of the ionic fluoride present in the plasma. A subject was found normally to have fluoride levels of 0.014 ppm in the parotid saliva, 0.019 ppm ionic, and 0.091 bound in the plasma. After 3 weeks of a 5-mg daily ingestion of fluoride, the parotid salivary ionic fluoride concentration was 0.11 ppm with a plasma content of 0.112 ppm and 0.073 ppm, free and bound, respectively, 1 hour after the last ingestion. After 3 hours, the salivary level fell to 0.045 ppm, the plasma free ion decreased to 0.055 ppm, but the bound fluoride remained at 0.075 ppm and is seemingly not affected by the amount ingested and is unrelated to the saliva level. These amounts of salivary fluoride appear too low to inhibit caries at the salivary pH, although concentrations of 0.1 ppm fluoride in acid medium will reduce the enamel solubility in *in vitro* experiments.

Nonapatitic systems do not incorporate fluoride into their structure, so it appears that, whenever phosphate is not associated with calcium, fluoride is also missing. This unique property does not include the other halides nor do the other halides clear the kidney as rapidly as does fluoride. About 95% of the total body fluoride is present in the bones and teeth. Even in areas of low fluoride concentration in the drinking water, the bones of adults contain about 500 ppm, with variation depending on the *area*, *type*, and *source* of bone. Some fluoride is also found in human cartilage.

Average values, with much variation, of 100 to 200 ppm of fluoride are found in the enamel of teeth from persons drinking low fluoride-containing water. Dentin from a similar source would contain 200 to 300 ppm. Cementum contains a greater amount of fluoride than any other calcified tissue, as much as 4500 ppm. Pulp contains 100 to 650 ppm and plaque levels are as low as about 100 ppm. The plaque fluoride is bound to a large extent and only 2 to 3% exists in a free ionic form. Urinary calculi have high concentrations of fluoride (2500 ppm), biliary tract calculi are low (20 ppm), and most soft tissues except the aorta (50 ppm) are even lower (1 to 3 ppm).

The deposition of fluoride, regardless of the amount ingested, appears to reach a plateau at about 55 years of age for bone and dentin and at about 35 years for enamel.

Shark enamel is the only biologically calcified tissue that approaches pure fluorapatite and the theoretical fluoride content of 3.8%. The outer surface

Table 9–1.   Ways of Increasing the Fixation of F Applied Topically

---

1. Increase concentration of solution F.

2. Lower pH.

3. Increase exposure time   a. repeated applications

                             b. cover F-exposed enamel with sealer

4. Pretreatment with   a. 0.5% phosphoric acid

                             b. Al^{3+} or other F complexers

5. Use NH_4F rather than NaF at low pH.

From Brudevold, F.: Interaction of Fluoride with Human Enamel. In *Symposium, Chemistry and Physiology of Enamel*, Ann Arbor, Mich., University of Michigan Press, 1971, p. 83.

of human enamel contains 0.2 to 0.3% at the highest level and the only evidence for pure fluorapatite as a constituent is largely circumstantial.

Topical solutions have been found to be most effective when applied according to the approaches outlined in Table 9–1. Of the first three approaches cited, the reasons for increased fluoride concentration and exposure time are obvious. The only factors to be considered are assurance that a maximum fluoride uptake results within a time period that will cause no damage to the surrounding tissue and make the most efficient use of the practitioner. The higher concentration permits the rapid diffusion of fluoride ions into intercrystalline spaces and through the organic film surrounding the enamel apatite crystallites. A study of a 3-minute topical treatment *in vivo* with acidulated phosphate fluoride (1.2% F, 0.1 M H_3PO_4) indicated that the penetration of fluoride does not exceed 50 μ and is nearly depleted after 24 hours. Naturally, repeated application counters this effect and the use of sealers such as cements or adhesive resins prevents the surface ions from interacting with the oral environment.

The use of a solution of low pH aids in the rate of dissolution of apatite crystals and the formation of calcium fluoride. The principal products formed with acidulated phosphate fluoride (APF) solutions on hydroxyapatite are most probably small amounts of fluorapatite (FA) (eq. 1), large amounts of calcium fluoride (eq. 2), and possibly a small quantity of dicalcium phosphate dihydrate (DCPD) (eq. 3). Calcium fluoride and dicalcium phosphate ultimately dissolve in saliva, and the released ions can react further to cause more fluorapatite formation (eq. 4 and 5). The solution rate of dicalcium phosphate is known to be more rapid than that of calcium fluoride, so it may also be more important as a fluoride source.

$$\text{Ca}_{10}(\text{PO}_4)_6(\text{OH})_2 + \begin{bmatrix} \text{H}^+ \\ \text{H}_2\text{PO}_4^- \\ \text{F}^- \end{bmatrix}$$

Hydroxyapatite   APF

$$\longrightarrow \text{Ca}_{10}(\text{PO}_4)_6\text{F}_2 + 2\text{OH}^- \quad \text{(Eq. 1)}$$

$$\longrightarrow 10\text{CaF}_2 + 6\text{PO}_4{}^{3-} + 2\text{OH}^- \quad \text{(Eq. 2)}$$

$$\longrightarrow 6\text{CaHPO}_4 \cdot 2\text{H}_2\text{O} + 4\text{Ca}^{2+} \quad \text{(Eq. 3)}$$

$$10\,\text{Ca}^{2+} + 2\text{F}^- + 6\text{PO}_4{}^{3-} \longrightarrow \text{Ca}_{10}(\text{PO}_4)_6\text{F}_2 \qquad \text{(Eq. 4)}$$

$$10\,\text{Ca}^{2+} + 6\text{HPO}_4{}^{2-} + 2\text{F}^- \longrightarrow \text{Ca}_{10}(\text{PO}_4)_6\text{F}_2 + 6\text{H}^+ \qquad \text{(Eq. 5)}$$

(From Brudevold, F.: Interaction of Fluoride with Human Enamel. In *Symposium, Chemistry and Physiology of Enamel*. Ann Arbor, Mich., University of Michigan Press, 1971.)

Equation 1 is predominant when fluoride concentrations are low.

REACTIONS OF FLUORIDE WITH HYDROXYAPATITE

Incorporation of minor ionic components into the teeth depends upon ion availability, crystallite accessibility, and the metabolic activity of the calcifying tissue. This may involve the following processes:

Accretion

The transport of ions is easily accomplished in the comparatively large volume of water found in the forming tissue cells. During crystallite growth, ions are incorporated by accretion.

Adsorption

Adsorption is a nonspecific uptake on the apatite crystallite surface involving the weak electrostatic force between the ions. It is a rapid, easily reversible process which predominates during the early 1 or 2 hours of fluoride exposure. It appears that the adsorbed fluoride is eventually incorporated into the crystals to a large extent.

Exchange

Replacement of an identical ionic species, such as calcium ion for calcium ion, without altering the crystallite lattice is an example of isoionic exchange. However, a strontium ion in place of a calcium ion or the diffusion of fluoride ions into the crystallite lattice effecting an exchange with the hydroxyl (OH^-) groups (eq. 1) would cause a change in the composition and properties of the crystallites, and is considered an heteroionic exchange.

Recrystallization

A dissolution of the enamel apatite crystallite surface can occur followed by reprecipitation of FA when it is in the presence of fluoride (eq. 4 and 5). Recrystallization is a slow process but is probably responsible for the preponderant amount of fluoride incorporated at the lower pH of 5.5 when compared with neutral conditions. This fact may explain the greater fluoride retention in the enamel when applied as an acidic solution.

Precipitation

The formation of FA may occur spontaneously by precipitation of the calcium, phosphate, and fluoride ions present in the immediate milieu regardless of source. Precipitation leads to crystal growth, and is equally as important as recrystallization in the formation of FA at the acid pH (eq. 4 and 5). For example, studies have shown that 90% of the fluoride ion in calcium fluoride formed in treated human enamel is easily leached out during washing.

Preconditioning the enamel in an attempt to increase the reactivity of the enamel to fluoride is the subject of number 4 of Table 9–1. It is well known that hypomineralized areas have greater amounts of fluoride present than normal enamel. A weak acid etching increases fluoride uptake in slightly demineralized enamel. Pretreatment of human enamel *in vivo* for 1 minute with 0.05 M phosphoric acid greatly increases fluoride uptake. This treatment is believed to form FA by recrystallization and by the dissolution and recrystallization of dicalcium phosphate and the large amounts of calcium fluoride formed. The combined acid–APF-treated enamel has a normal microscopic appearance with less enamel lost than by a pumice prophylaxis. A clinical test using 0.05 M H_3PO_4-APF treatment showed a significant decrease in caries compared to APF alone. Analyses 1 year post treatment revealed that much of the fluoride remained in the outermost enamel, probably as FA, indicating an effectiveness nearly equal to a lifelong ingestion of fluoridated water.

Analysis revealed a direct correlation of fluoride and aluminum concentration in the enamel, which prompted an *in vivo* experiment with a topical pretreatment of 0.01 M and 0.05 aluminum nitrate followed by APF. This resulted in a sixfold fluoride increase bound to the enamel, probably as a phosphate-aluminum-fluoride complex rather than as FA. A 1-year clinical trial with 0.05 M $Al(NO_3)_3$ and APF proved ineffective in reducing caries. Although cations found in the enamel, for example, aluminum, iron, tin, and titanium, are known to complex with fluoride, it is unknown whether they form complexes in enamel.

A 3-minute treatment with 0.62 M NH_4F at pH 4.4 to children's enamel pretreated with 0.05 M H_3PO_4 resulted in a fluoride retention unexceeded by any other fluoride reagent. The effect is pH-dependent, being less detectable at the higher values. The role of the ammonium ion is unknown but probably involves a catalytic effect on the formation of heavy spherical deposits of CaF_2 on the enamel surface.

Accumulation of a majority of the foreign ions in the outer surface area of mature enamel is due to adsorption and heteroionic exchange. The inner enamel gains extraneous ions by both accretion and heteroionic exchange during crystallite formation and prism growth. It is difficult to distinguish which process, accretion or exchange, is responsible for the acquisition of certain ions in the teeth. During tooth formation when the enamel is still hypomineralized, both processes are possible. Fluoride is found in high concentrations in the surface enamel of unerupted teeth and, in general, reflects the level of the ion in the blood, which in turn directly depends upon the amount available from the water and food ingested.

Some ions such as carbonate may have a metabolic source, and the carbonate concentration in the tooth could be due to the change in ameloblastic activity with age. Size of the crystallite may also influence the ability of ions to either penetrate its lattice structure or permit only interaction with the surface. The large citrate ion may fall in this category. As the surface-

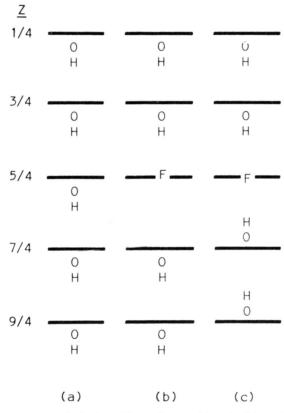

Fig. 9–5. Arrangements in hydroxyl ion column with and without fluorine present. Heavy lateral bars represent positions of calcium triangles viewed edge on. (a), Ordering in uninterrupted OH column; (b), OH-F configuration corresponding to doublet portion of NMR signal. F-H distance is 2.12 A; F is moved off plane of calcium triangle toward neighboring H. (c), OH . . . F . . . HO configuration corresponding to triplet portion of NMR signal. F-H distance is 2.22 A, F remains in plane of calcium triangle, column reversal takes place. (From Young, R. A.: Implication of Atomic Substitutions and other Structural Details in Apatites, J. Dent. Res. Suppl. 53 (2), 198, 1974.)

to-mass ratio of the crystallites decreases, the processes of accretion and ion exchange also diminish.

According to Young, fluoride ions substituting for OH ions tend to locate at the sites they occupy in FA. This location permits hydrogen bonding with the adjacent unsubstituted OH ions, allowing two possible configurations. The OH ions can be aligned with OH pointing in opposite directions (Fig. 9–5b), or in the same direction (Fig. 9–5c). The latter alignment results in a reversal of the normal order of the OH column and leads to a hexagonal instead of a monoclinic structure. The presence of fluoride ions in the structure would probably result in greater bonding energy due to its greater electronegative nature. Substitution of about 8% of the OH ions in HAP by fluoride ions revealed complete dispersal along the column without regions of FA formation. This dispersed arrangement and hydrogen bonding can result in a little fluoride having a large effect especially upon inhibiting OH diffusion. Studies on the diffusion of OH ions along the crystal column showed no observable exchange in structural OH for OD in human tooth enamel at $37°$ C for 813 hours.

Diffusion of hydroxyl ions into the apatite structure is probably an important factor in the rate of dissolution; small amounts of fluoride would block OH passage and should reduce the penetration rate.

MECHANISM OF CARIES INHIBITION

The mechanism by which fluoride reduces dental caries is not entirely understood. Several theories have been advanced to explain this phenomenon.

Solubility

In vitro measurements show that the solubility of enamel by acid dissolution is reduced in enamel previously exposed to fluoride. Many studies have been conducted on the solubilities of hydroxyapatite and fluorapatite as model compounds in order to prove whether solubility alone is responsible for the cariostatic efficiency of fluoride.

The principles of solubility that apply to other substances are also applicable to the equilibrium between the fluids interacting with the enamel surface, either fluorapatite or hydroxyapatite, and the aqueous oral environment. Dreissens has recently discussed the theory, experimental evidence, and consequences of the complicated equilibria involved in the reaction of fluoride ion with hydroxyapatite.

The equilibrium between solid hydroxyapatite crystals (S) and its liquid solution (L) can be represented as:

$$Ca_2[CA_3](PO_4)_3 \, OH(S) \rightleftarrows 5Ca^{2+} (L) + 3PO_4^{3-} (L) + OH^- (L). \qquad (1)$$

If a sublattice is defined as a set of equivalent sites in the crystal, then the formula on the left indicates that all OH^- ions occur in one sublattice, all PO_4^{3-} ions in a second sublattice, 60% of the Ca^{2+} ions in a third, and 40% of the Ca^{2+} in a fourth sublattice.

The solubility product expression for pure hydroxyapatite is:

$$K_{HA} = [Ca]^5 \ [PO_4]^3 \ [OH], \qquad (2)$$

which can be expressed as the negative logarithm in the form:

$$-LogK_{HA} = 5pCa + 3pPO_4 + pOH. \qquad (3)$$

The expressions for other pure ternary compounds, such as fluorapatite, are stated similarly. It must also be noted that:

1. The rates of dissolution and precipitation are relatively fast, and equal.
2. The reactions occur at the crystal surface.
3. Solid state diffusion through the crystal is unnecessary.

The occurrence of secondary reactions results in the formation of many complexes, the most important of which are HPO_4^{2-}, $H_2PO_4^-$, $CaHPO_4$, $CaH_2PO_4^+$, $CaOH^+$, CaF^+, HF, and HF_2^-. This largely explains the pH dependency of HA solubility and to a lesser extent the effect of ionic strength.

The bioapatites are not pure ternary apatites for they contain varying amounts of Na^+, Cl^-, F^-, Mg^{2+}, Zn^{2+}, Pb^{2+}, CO_3^{2-}, and so forth, which complicate the thermodynamic aspects of the process. In a consideration of the incorporation of F^- ions by HA crystals from an aqueous solution, a very slow process, the obvious equilibrium reaction, assuming equal ratios of ions in both phases, would be:

$$[Ca^{2+}]_2 \, [Ca^{2+}]_3 \, (PO_4^{3-})_3 \, OH_X \, F_{1-X} \, (S) \rightleftarrows 5Ca^{2+} \, (L) + 3PO_4^{3-} \, (L)$$
$$+ \, xOH^- \, (L) + 1{-}x \, F^- \, (L).$$

It appears that there are two "apparent solubility products" connected by the equilibrium for ionic exchange,

$$OH^- \, (S) + F^- \, (L) \rightleftarrows OH^- \, (L) + F^- \, (S),$$

and results in the relation for the overall equilibrium constant of

$$\log K_{exch} = \log K_{FA} - \log K_{HA}.$$

The degree of F^- ion uptake by HA after equilibration depends upon the pOH, and the pF, and the relative solubility products of pure FA and HA.

Dreissens further concludes that F^- ions stabilize the enamel crystals by the apparent diminutions of Na^+ and CO_3^{-2} incorporation and conversion of the enamel carbonatoapatite into hydroxyapatite. A combination of these factors is estimated to lower the solubility product of enamel apatite, K_{HA}, by 5 to 10 orders of magnitude.

Brudevold, McConn, and Grøn have reported results of the solubility of fluorapatite, dicalcium phosphate dihydrate, and hydroxyapatite in centrifuged whole saliva over the pH range of 3.1 to 7.4. An average value for fluorapatite was a K_{sp} of 1×10^{-7} or pK_{sp} of 7.0 down to pH 4.4. The same results were obtained for dicalcium phosphate, synthetic hydroxyapatite, and the same hydroxyapatite containing 0.12% fluoride obtained by soaking in an aqueous KF solution for a month. At the lower pH levels of 3.11 to 3.5, a value of 8.0×10^{-11} was obtained, which compares favorably with the K_{sp} of 7.8×10^{-11} given for calcium difluoride in the literature. Therefore they conclude the "activity product," $A_{CA}^{2+} \cdot A_{HPO4}^{2-}$, would be the controlling factor at the lower pH. The assumption that a solubility difference exists is not a valid one and does not explain the mechanism of fluoride protection according to these investigators.

Other investigators, using aqueous buffer systems on pooled powdered enamel, have reported a solubility product constant, K, of $(Ca^{2+})^{10} (OH^-)^2 (PO_4^3)^6 = 5.5 \times 10^{-55}$, whereas fluorapatite was given as $(Ca^{2+})^{10} (F^-)^2 (PO_4^{3-})^6 = 2.63 \times 10^{-60}$, indicating it to be a less soluble substance. The literature values for log K_{HA} scatter over the range -49 to -58 and those of log K_{FA} over -58 to -61. These observations, though valid, may not apply in the case of surface enamel, which in comparison contains only one-tenth of the fluoride present in FA and which may also have little or no FA structure present.

Poole and associates observed that, when enamel prisms cut perpendicularly are acid etched, the centers are hollowed out, producing a honeycomb pattern as seen by scanning electron microscopy. A possible explanation is that the crystallites vary in orientation; one area of the prism might dissolve more rapidly than another. Measurements of fluorapatite dissolution show a small difference in the chemical solubility with respect to the prism plane, however a five times greater velocity of penetration into etch pits occurs in the c-axis than perpendicular to it. Crystals of hydroxyapatite have been studied similarly. The dissolution of hydroxyapatite crystals is highly anisotropic in 5 M citric acid at $37°$ C. The acid penetrates into the crystals parallel to the c-axis with a velocity of about 60/nM/sec, whereas perpendicular to the c-axis dissolution is negligible. Another factor could be that the differing orientation of the crystallites in enamel may present different surface areas which vary in their solubility rates.

Remineralization

In 1912 Head reported that enamel artificially softened by acid is partially rehardened by immersion in saliva. More recent studies have confirmed this observation, especially when solutions of calcium and phosphate ions are used, resulting in 90% of the hardness being recovered. In early enamel caries, the visible stages are known as the translucent zone, the dark zone, and the body of the lesion. Arrested caries has a broad dark zone believed to be due to a remineralization in the lesion. This mineralized enamel is less porous and contains dense collections of foreign crystals which are larger and more plate-like than the HA crystallites of enamel. The presence of sodium and chloride ions increases the range of pH over which solutions of HA are able to reharden buffer-softened enamel, whereas other ions, such as $P_2O_7^{4-}$, HCO_3^-, SO_4^{2-}, CrO_4^{2-}, Mg^{2+}, and Zn^{2+}, appear to have an inhibiting effect. Figure 9–6 is a graph of the effects of fluoride in studies of this type, which shows fluoride having a fourfold increase in the rate of rehardening and a nearly complete return of hardness.

In supersaturated solutions of calcium and phosphate, octacalcium phosphate formation is kinetically favored but, in the presence of greater than 0.01 mM of fluoride, hydroxyapatite is predominantly formed. Fluoride ion at 0.4% has the ability to prevent HA from converting to dicalcium phosphate even at a pH as low as 2.0.

Human saliva, both resting and stimulated, is always saturated with calcium (Ca = 5.8 mg%, 2.2 to 11.3) and phosphate (P = 16.8 mg%, 6.1 to 71) with respect to HA. Resting saliva is undersaturated, whereas stimulated saliva is saturated with respect to brushite, dicalcium phosphate dihydrate, and octacalcium phosphate. Calculus may therefore include a number of different calcified minerals, including hydroxyapatite, octacalcium phosphate, whitlockite, and brushite. The crystal structure of

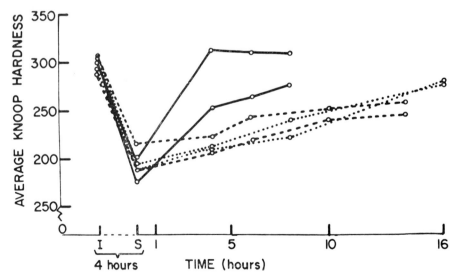

Fig. 9–6. Effect of fluoride on rehardening rates. Softening solution: acetic acid (1.0 mM, pH 5.5); rehardening solutions at 37° C: (————) Ca:P 1.67; [Ca] 1.5: [F] 0.05; I_{pH} 7.3, (- - - -) Ca:P 1.67; [Ca] 1.5; I_{pH} 7.3, (. . . .) Ca:P 1.00; [Ca] 1.5; I_{pH} 7.25. (From Koulourides, T.: Effect of Fluoride on Rehardening Rates. In *Art and Science of Dental Caries Research*. R. S. Harris (Ed.). New York, Academic Press, 1968, p. 368.)

remineralized enamel is little understood although it is now known from electron probe analysis that the Ca:P ratio is about 2.1, the same as normal enamel. Recent measurements of a model remineralization system show that fluoride increases the rate of deposition and is incorporated probably as fluorapatite or fluorohydroxyapatite.

If remineralization does exist, how is caries possible? Saliva and its components are not available to all areas of the oral cavity, especially those deeply grooved and fissured tooth surfaces or those covered with dense masses of microorganisms and their products. There is an irreversible limit in enamel demineralization after which remineralization is not possible even with prolonged exposure to remineralizing solution.

Diffusion Inhibition

An essential feature of the apatite structure is the c-axis-oriented column of OH^- ions with an associated triangle of calcium ions. The OH^- ions are about 3.44 Å apart, whereas the intercolumn distance is about 9.43 Å. This structure should permit easy movement of OH^- along the column and less motion between adjacent columns. Experimental evidence points to a mechanism in which there is an interchange of ions with vacancies in the crystals of both FA and HA. It has been suggested that fluoride ions in the HA of enamel block the OH^- diffusion within the columns and decrease the rate of dissolution. Tse and co-workers raise two problems associated with the incorporation of fluoride ions into HA. Fluoride ions have a one-dimensional diffusion path into the crystal and a vacancy mechanism that permits movement back and forth along the path but no change in relative position, therefore a random mixing is impossible. This would require a net flux of vacancies to the crystal surface. The second problem is that in the event fluoride ions can diffuse into the crystal, the ions could leave by the same mechanism at essentially the same rate. Their theoretical calculations show that the OH^- migration energy in pure HA along the c-axis column is 2.1 ev and that of an OH^- ion adjacent to an F is 2.2 ev, essentially equal. There is no blocking effect by the fluoride ions in HA to the movement of OH^- ions according to their model system.

Enzyme Inhibitors

Jenkins raised the possibility that fluoride ions arising from the dissolution of the fluoride-containing enamel surface act as an enzyme poison, thus reducing the amount of acid released by the bacteria in the plaque. This could play a role in the overall mechanism, but is unlikely to be predominant considering the many *in vitro* experiments that have shown a decrease in enamel solubility in the presence of fluoride and in the absence of microorganisms.

SELECTED REFERENCES

BRUDEVOLD, F.: Interaction of Fluoride with Human Enamel. In *Symposium, Chemistry and Physiology of Enamel*, Ann Arbor, Mich., University of Michigan Press, 1971.

DREISSENS, F. C. M.: Fluoride incorporation and apatite solubility, Caries Res., 7, 297, 1973.

JENKINS, G. N.: Art and Science of Dental Caries Research, Robert S. Harris (Ed.). New York, Academic Press, 1968, pp. 331–354.

JONGEBLOED, W. L., BENG, P. J. VAN DEN, and ARENDS, J.: The dissolution of single crystals of hydroxyapatite in citric and lactic acids. Calcif. Tissue Res., 15 (1), 1–9, 1974.

McCLURE, F. J.: Water Fluoridation, The Search and the Victory. Bethesda, Md., U.S. Department of HEW, National Institutes of Health, 1970.

MORENO, E. C., and ZAHRADNIK, R. T.: Chemistry of enamel subsurface demineralization in vitro, J. Dent. Res., 53, 226, 1974.

POOLE, D. F. G., and SILVERSTONE, L. M.: Remineralization of Enamel. In Hard Tissue Growth, Repair and Remineralization, New York, Elsevier, 1973, pp. 35–52.

TSE, C., WELCH, D. O., and ROYCE, B. S. H.: The migration of F^-, OH^- and O^{2-} ions in apatites. Calcif. Tissue Res., 13, 47–52, 1973.

WEATHERELL, J. A., and ROBINSON, C.: The Inorganic Composition of Teeth. In *Biological Mineralization*. I. Zipkin (Ed.). New York, John Wiley & Sons, 1973.

YOUNG, R. A.: Implication of atomic substitutions and other structural details in apatites. J. Dent. Res. Suppl., 53 (2), 193, 1974.

ZIPKIN, I.: Fluoride. In *Calcified Structures in Biological Mineralization*. I. Zipkin (Ed.). New York, John Wiley & Sons, 1973, p. 487.

Chapter 10

Biochemistry of the Dental Pulp

ERNEST BEERSTECHER, JR., Ph.D.

The first chemical studies of pulp by Wurtz in 1856 were unknown to the dental world until emphasized by Magitot in 1878. The first entire work on the chemistry of pulp by Whitslar in 1889 had only this single study on which to depend. Commendably, it pointed out the need for study of living rather than dead and decomposing material and the problems that the pulp's small size and inaccessibility presented to the chemist. Hodge's study in 1936 of pulpal lipids was perhaps the first dependable work on pulp chemistry. Hertz as early as 1866 had proposed that the intertubular substance of dentine was the chemically changed and calcified intercellular substance of the pulp cells, but this received little experimental verification before the histochemical studies on alkaline phosphatase in odontogenesis by Engel and Furuta (1942), Bevelander and Johnson (1945), and Greep, Fischer and Morse (1948). This, then, was the background to Bruckner's work on alkaline phosphatase in pulp (1949) and Pincus' study on pulp respiration (1950), which introduced the extensive literature which developed over the past 25 years.

HISTOLOGY AND FUNCTION

The dental pulp, although anatomically removed from the other soft tissues of the oral cavity, is inextricably related to them by considerations of structure, function, composition, pathology, and therapeutics, and its biochemical nature must therefore be considered in the light of this relationship. Histologically, the pulp is remarkably similar to the connective tissue of the gingiva, and this similarity is supported by all except a few biochemical considerations. Both tissues are concerned with the support of odontoblastic activity and the nutrition of adjacent mineralized connective tissue. The nutrition and innervation of the pulp are via channels that traverse the periodontium, which provide an inevitable common source of pathogenesis. The permeability of the dentine provides for appreciable nutritional interchange between these tissues and thus a certain degree of symbiosis and mutual responsiveness. Indeed, the aim of root canal therapy must, ideally, be directed toward stimulation of periodontal (cemental) closure of the apical foramina of the pulp chamber.

While the study of pulp chemistry evolved as an approach to odonto-genesis, there can be little doubt that present emphasis is directed toward achieving more effective pulp therapy. The pulp is remarkably sensitive to its environment, and although it it seemingly well insulated, it is normally influenced and injured by a constant succession of both physical and chemical factors. Extremes of heat and pressure are easily transmitted to it and may bring about not only traumatic damage, but also chemical injury through ionic changes and changes in the molecular configuration of its macromolecules. Direct chemical injury may occur from filling materials acting either as enzyme poisons after diffusion to the pulp or electrochemically to modify its ionic balance. Other drugs used in cavity preparation and pulp therapy [*e.g.*, $AgNO_3$, NaF, ZnO-Eugenol, $Ca(OH)_2$] may act similarly or as outright protein precipitants. In addition, microorganisms may attack the pulp on all perimeters, creating biochemical damage in much the same manner as they do in other connective tissues (*i.e.*, by toxin production; by hydrolysis of macromolecules of cells, fibers and ground substance; by modification of low molecular weight organic substances to form noxious substances such as amines; and by changes in pH). The study of the biochemistry of the pulp is thus a prerequisite to the establishment of any system of dentistry or pulp therapy based upon "sound biological principles."

Histologically, the pulp has been described as "primitive connective tissue." Most of the chemical details of its structure may be deduced from a consideration of the biochemistry of the closely related gingival connective tissue so they will not be repeated in this chapter. The pulp is a loose or fluid tissue in a highly dynamic state. It contains relatively few cells: fibroblasts concerned with fiber production and odontogenesis, mesenchymal cells possibly concerned with mucopolysaccharide production, and histiocytes concerned with defense mechanisms. Dispersed among these are a few vascular elements, nerves, and lymphatic channels. Among the cells is a network of fibers, largely collagenous. All these formed elements are suspended in the ground substance composed of pulp fluid of vascular origin to which indigenous mucopolysaccharides have been added.

It is most remarkable that so simple a tissue serves so well the several functions for which it is responsible. These may conveniently be listed as:

1. Architectural—the elaboration of collagenous fibers and of dentine.
2. Nutritive—nourishes the nerve fibers and dentine (and in a more restricted sense, perhaps, even the enamel and periodontium).
3. Sensory—a source of pain receptors.
4. Protective—through inflammation and by secondary dentine formation.

In order to achieve this efficiency, each structural unit must serve at least one or more vital functions and these must be highly integrated. It is proposed, therefore, that the often-cited defenselessness of the pulp rests in the fact that a disturbance in any one function is rapidly reflected in the whole organ, there being a conspicuous lack of relief mechanisms compared with other tissues.

These various considerations bring about a critical point with regard to the biochemistry of the dental pulp. The architectural, sensory, and protective functions of the pulp are performed by the cells, which are sparse in proportion to the great mass of ground substance. They contribute negligibly to the chemical composition, but virtually all to the pulp metabolism. The nutritive function of the pulp and the preponderance of its mass lie in its extensive extracellular material, which accounts for its chemical composition, but not for its metabolism. This is more true of pulp than almost any other tissue and bespeaks a significant need to cite quantitative metabolic data on the basis of some function of the total cellular mass. This varies greatly throughout the various histologically distinguishable zones of the pulp organ. It is for this reason that the discussion which follows concerns itself respectively with the pulp cells, the fibers, and the ground substance with its integrative functions.

BIOCHEMISTRY OF THE ODONTOBLASTS

The biochemistry of the fibroblast and its modifications have been so extensively investigated that it is essential in this chapter to limit the discussion to those facets pertaining specifically to the pulp. These are primarily concerned with its respiration and its odontoblastic activity.

Ribonucleic Acid (RNA)

One of the major functions of the odontoblast is the synthesis of collagen fibers. Whenever cells synthesize any protein, the pattern for that particular protein is transmitted from the chromosomal DNA in the nucleus to *ribosomes* in the endothelial reticulum of the cytoplasm in the form of templates consisting of ribonucleic acid (RNA). This material, which characterizes actively synthesizing cells, is believed to give such cells their characteristic basophilia, and active odontoblasts tend to be more basophilic than inactive ones for this reason. The RNA is at a maximum when collagen is being synthesized and declines when the cells become quiescent, as after secondary dentine formation. RNA increases as odontoblasts differentiate from fibroblasts and is absent when collagen synthesis is impaired, as in ascorbic acid deficiency (scurvy).

Alkaline Phosphatase

Alkaline phosphatase is involved in the cleavage of phosphate ion from organic ester linkage in the calcification process. Large amounts are found

Table 10–1. The Cholesterol Content of Dental Pulp*

Tissue sample		Mean % cholesterol
BOVINE:	Embryonic pulp	0.067
	Young pulp	0.069
	Mature pulp	0.078
	Gingiva	0.112
HUMAN*:	Young and mature	0.163
	Most mature	0.218
	Mature	0.245
	Gingiva†	0.200

* Modified from Fisher and Stickley. Human samples pooled.
† Hodge (1933)

in pulpal odontoblasts, particularly when active in calcification, but also when the pulp is in the inflammatory state, presumably as a reflection of secondary dentine depositing activities. Some acid phosphatase* also occurs in the ground substance of the pulp localized along the collagen fibers.

Lipids

The peculiar carbohydrate metabolism of pulp cells is one that favors fatty acid synthesis, and immense fat globules are seen in some more or less isolated fibrocytes (e.g., chondrocytes). The material may function either as a storage form of energy or in the synthesis of neural material. Hodge found human pulp to contain (on a moist weight basis) 0.91% lipids, 0.70% phospholipids and 0.11% cholesterol. By comparison, he found human *gingiva* to contain 0.20% cholesterol. In searching for some pulp constituent that might show progressive changes during tooth maturation, Fisher and Stickley studied the cholesterol content of both human and bovine pulp (Table 10–1). They found increases with age in both cases, with human somewhat higher than bovine material. It is of some interest that in comparing other human and bovine tissues, only liver and adrenal gland have higher cholesterol values. These tissues, like the pulp, are noted for their phosphogluconate metabolism and for their steroid synthesis and secretory activity. The increased sterol content with age, as in plasma and other tissues, is of unknown significance.

Proteases and Peptidases

Pulp has been demonstrated to contain a variety of enzymes capable of hydrolyzing to utilizable fragments (amino acids) the ever accumulating

* Acid phosphatase also liberates phosphate ion from phosphate esters, but functions better at a pH of about 6 than at the higher pH levels (9) at which the more common alkaline phosphatase functions best. Both function at normal tissue pH levels, but are distinguished clinically by the pH levels at which they are measured in the laboratory.

debris of degenerate collagen fibers and other cell wastes, and of activating certain special cellular processes. The presence of such proteases has been demonstrated in the pulp by histochemical techniques. Preparations from pulp odontoblasts have been found to contain a variety of proteases and dipeptidases capable of digesting hemoglobin and reducing collagen to its free amino acids. Kroeger *et al.* found mouse, rat and dog pulp to contain a polypeptidase which hydrolyzes and inactivates the smooth muscle-stimulating substance obtained from the pulp of stimulated teeth.

Glycogen

Glycogen is generally found in high concentrations in those areas where calcification mechanisms exist, presumably serving as a source of glycolytic alcohols which may form phosphate esters and thus maintain high phosphate concentrations in solution. Glycogen granules have been demonstrated in pulp odontoblasts. They disappear during active calcification and appear again in the quiescent state as might be expected from their function.

Carbohydrate Metabolism of the Pulp

Carbohydrate metabolism in the dental pulp must serve a number of special purposes other than that of the energy-producing function common to all cells. Prominent among these is (1) the provision of materials for synthesis of the mucopolysaccharides which constitute the major portion of this organ, (2) the synthesis of carbon skeleton for the large amounts of glycine, proline, and hydroxyproline necessary for collagen synthesis, and (3) the provision of organic alcohols for the phosphate ester formation in the calcification process. While the synthesis of these carbohydrate derivatives has not been demonstrated to occur exclusively within the pulp (some may be supplied by the blood), it is most probable that a major fraction is endogenous in nature. In addition to the above considerations, the rapid production of collagen places a high demand upon the pulp for pentose used in RNA synthesis.

Studies on the respiration of the pulp contribute materially to the explanation of how these manifold demands are met. These may be summarized as follows:

1. The sparse cellular population of the pulp accounts for the respiration of its entire mass so that, on a weight basis, its oxygen consumption at rest is low by comparison with other tissues.
2. Its respiratory quotient (RQ) (CO_2/O_2) is about 0.90 in most species studied.
3. The oxygen consumption is highest during dentinogenesis ($Q_{O_2} = 2.04$), falling to lower values (0.47) in the later quiescent state.
4. The oxygen consumption is higher in bovine pulp than in human pulp, perhaps because of continuing odontogenesis.

Table 10–2. Effect of Some Common Dental Material
on the Oxygen Consumption of Pulp*

Material	Q_{O_2}
Normal pulp	0.55
ZnO-Eugenol	0.42
Calcium hydroxide	0.42
Eugenol	0.31
Amalgam	0.33
Zn phosphate cement	0.32
Adrenalin	0.34
Procaine	0.16

* Bovine dental pulp. Concentrations varied so as to simulate reasonable clinical exposure. Adapted from Fisher *et al.*, 1957.

Certain observations suggest that the carbohydrate metabolism in pulp differs from that in most other tissues. In *in vitro* studies, despite the fact that carbohydrate reserves may be limited and rapidly depleted within the pulp, the tissue continues to respire for 8 to 12 hours without requiring added glucose or using cellular lipid or protein reserves (but possibly using reserves from the matrix). It has been demonstrated that some form of anaerobic glycolysis is more important in pulp than in most other tissues. Further, pulp produces a great deal of acid under aerobic conditions which may act as a controlling factor in its metabolism. These various data indicate the existence in pulp of a vigorous phosphogluconate (pentose phosphate) shunt type of carbohydrate metabolism in addition to the usual glycolytic pathway and citric acid cycle. This shunt system provides for relative anaerobic function, supplies large amounts of ribose, leads to fat accumulation, and has been shown to parallel collagen synthesis in pulp.

Because of the manifold functions that pulp serves, inhibition of its respiratory system might well be expected to have dramatic results. Fisher *et al.* have shown that a great many materials frequently employed in clinical dental procedures do have the property of depressing the oxygen uptake of the pulp. Some of their results are summarized in Table 10–2. The results reflect to some extent the water solubility of the various agents and the proximity to the pulp that they might achieve. A variety of similar observations suggest that data of this nature may be valuable criteria in the experimental evaluation of various new clinical therapeutic agents.

BIOCHEMISTRY OF THE PULP FIBERS

Most of the known facts regarding the fibrous network of the dental pulp indicate that it is similar to that of gingival connective tissue. Therefore only a few salient points will require special attention. The fibers are synthe-

7

sized by the odontoblasts and are of two main types. Collagen predominates in the matrix, and elastin is found predominantly in the walls of the larger afferent vascular channels. The two proteins are the only known source of hydroxyproline in living material and are further characterized by high concentration of proline and glycine. In the relative amounts of these three amino acids and of others, they differ greatly.

The collagenous fibers account for an integral portion of the nitrogen content of the pulp. The nitrogen content does not vary among different species, but it may increase slightly with age. In general, collagen synthesis (and therefore the fibrous content) does not appear to increase appreciably with age, but only as a response to irritation. Studies of collagen fiber synthesis by fibroblasts measured by ^{15}N-labeled amino acid uptake show that both synthesis and breakdown proceed at a rate similar to that of liver and less than that of gingival mucosa.

BIOCHEMISTRY OF PULP GROUND SUBSTANCE

The ground substance of pulp resembles in general that of gingival connective tissue. It is composed of dental pulp fluid (exudate) derived from the blood plasma and containing added colloidal mucopolysaccharides originating in the cellular elements of the pulp. A fluid portion of the ground substance also leaves the pulp by its lymphatic system and in lesser amounts via the dentine, cementum, and enamel. The ground substance has a higher calcium and phosphate content than plasma exudate due to the binding of these substances by the mucopolysaccharides. The calcium and fluoride content tends to increase with age, and the fluoride content is higher in geographical areas where the fluoride content of drinking water is high. Parathormone administration tends to increase the citrate content of the pulp, which may account for some of the decalcification that occurs. It also increases the number of phagocytes present in the pulp, however, which may effect the same result.

In general, pulp contains the same amounts of glucose and other low molecular weight metabolites as does blood plasma. It contains only about one-fifth the protein content, however, as is characteristic of other filtrates. The protein is composed largely of albumin and α_1, α_2, β and γ globulins in proportions similar to those in blood plasma. Pulp fluid differs from dentinal and enamel fluid in having a much higher protein content than the latter two which are ultrafiltrates.

The colloidal mucopolysaccharides of the ground substance increase its viscosity while permitting it to remain readily diffusible to nutrients. They consist of two high molecular weight linear polymers.

1. Hyaluronic acid, composed of alternating units of glucuronic acid and N-acetylglucosamine.
2. Chondroitin sulfate B, composed of alternating units of iduronic acid and N-acetylgalactosamine sulfate. No other chondroitin derivative

is known with certainty to be present in the pulp, although a sialic acid derivative may be present.

These glycosaminoglycans (GAGs), common to all ground substance, occur in human pulp in concentrations of about 0.55 mg/gm wet tissue weight.

The precise functions of the mucopolysaccharides of the pulp are not all known with certainty but several are assured. It seems established that they stabilize collagen fibrils into fibers by chemically cross-linking the collagen molecules. In lathyrism, caused by consuming excessive amounts of certain peas or artificially by the administration of amino-acetonitrile, mucopolysaccharide synthesis is depressed, and collagen is not converted into insoluble collagen fibers. Mucopolysaccharides are also involved in calcium binding in mineralizable areas and in this manner participate in the calcification mechanism. Finally, being hydrophilic colloids, they are involved in water binding and retention permitting sol-gel interconversions. This fact is believed to be associated with the observed effects of certain endocrine substances on connective tissue.

The dental pulp is a unique tissue from a biochemical standpoint in view of its remarkable adaptation of a few cell types to perform a variety of functions. In addition to a conventional glycolytic system, it contains a pentose phosphate shunt respiratory system permitting it to function under varying degrees of ischemia, to synthesize carbon skeletons for mucopolysaccharides and collagen synthesis, and to contribute large amounts of ribose directly to RNA synthesis. The pulp has a highly organized structure but retains a permeable and fluid nature. Its respiratory enzymes and state of mucopolysaccharide aggregation are exceedingly sensitive to environmental influences.

SELECTED REFERENCES

FISHER, A. K., SCHUMACHER, E. R., ROBINSON, N. P., and SHARBONDY, G. P.: Effects of dental drugs and materials on the rate of oxygen consumption in bovine dental pulp, J. Dental Res., *36*, 447–450, 1957.

FISHER, A. K. and SCHWABE, C.: Effects of procaine concentration and duration of contact on oxygen consumption in bovine dental pulp, J. Dental Res., *41*, 484–490, 1962.

————: The endogenous respiratory quotient of bovine dental pulp, J. Dental Res., *40*, 346–351, 1961.

FISHER, A. K. and STICKLEY, J. J.: The cholesterol content of some bovine and human oral tissues, J. Dent. Res., *39*, 1037–1040, 1960.

HALDI, J. and JOHN, K.: Sulfanilamide and penicillin in the pulp fluid of the dog, J. Dent. Res., *44*, 1386–1388, 1965.

HALDI, J., LAW, M. L., and JOHN, K.: Comparative concentration of various constituents of blood plasma and dental pulp fluid, J. Dent. Res., *44*, 427–430, 1965.

LEBLOND, C. P.: Elaboration of dental collagen in odontoblasts as shown by radio-autography after injection of labelled glycine and proline, Ann. Histochem., *8*, 43–50, 1963.

ROTBLAT, N. D. and YAEGER, J. A.: Dental pulp citrate during the development of abnormally mineralized dentine, Arch. Oral Biol., *10*, 617–623, 1965.

SHAZER, D. O. DE: Glucose-6-phosphate and 6-phosphogluconic dehydrogenase in bovine dental pulp, J. Dental Res., *41*, 986–996, 1962.

STARK, M. M., MYERS, H. M., MORRIS, M., and GARDNER, R.: The localization of radioactive calcium$_{45}$ hydroxide over exposed pulps in rhesus monkey teeth, J. Oral Therap. & Pharmacol., *1*, 290–297, 1964.

TEN CATE, A. R.: Alkaline phosphatase activity and formation of human dentine, Arch. Oral Biol., *11*, 267–268, 1966.

WHITSLAR, W. H.: A study of the chemical composition of the dental pulp, Dent. Regist., *43*, 581–586, 1889.

Chapter 11

The Periodontium

PAUL B. ROBERTSON, D.D.S., M.S.

The periodontium consists of a group of interrelated structures designed to support and protect the teeth. This system has both epithelial and connective tissue components, detailed in Figure 11–1. The connective tissues include alveolar bone (a), cementum (c), periodontal ligament (p), and the gingival lamina propria (l). These structures are covered by stratified squamous gingival epithelium (e).

The surface anatomy of the gingiva in health is thoroughly considered in a number of other texts. Briefly, the gingiva may be divided into two parts: the *free gingiva* (fg) and the *attached gingiva* (ag). The transition from one to the other is occasionally demarcated by a narrow depression, the *free gingival groove* (fgg), which corresponds roughly to the bottom of the *gingival sulcus* (s). The color of normal free and attached gingiva is usually described as a pale

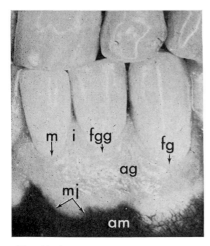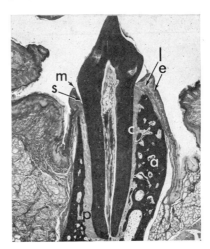

Fig. 11–1. The normal periodontium. See text for explanation. (Courtesy of Dr. B. M. Levy.)

pink, but in fact, may present a broad range of hue depending on the extent of pigmentation, degree of keratinization and vascularity, and overall thickness of the epithelium. The *interdental papillae* (i) fit tightly into the interproximal spaces and attach firmly to the teeth and alveolar bone. The gingiva slopes coronally to end in a thin edge at the *gingival margin* (m) and then plunges apically for a short distance (1 to 3 mm) to form the *gingival sulcus* (s). The attached gingiva is clinically delineated from *alveolar mucosa* (am) by the *mucogingival line* or *junction* (mj).

GINGIVAL EPITHELIUM

The gingival epithelium varies considerably in thickness with an average depth of 12 to 14 cells. This stratified squamous epithelium presents a basal layer of cells (*stratum germinativum*) which rests on the basement membrane. Progressively superficial to the basal cells are the *stratum spinosum*, characterized by intercellular bridges or "prickles," the *stratum granulosum*, distinguished by deeply staining basophilic keratohyalin granules, and the *stratum corneum*, or keratinized layer consisting of acidophilic cells in which nuclei are not discernible (orthokeratinization) or are pyknotic (parakeratinization), or a mixture of both. In man, the sulcular epithelium is not keratinized.

Ultrastructurally, the epithelial cells of gingiva present morphological features similar to those of cells of other tissues (Fig. 11–2). The double membrane-enclosed *nucleus* (N) contains deoxyribonucleic acid (DNA) and is responsible for control of cellular activity and cell division. The denser appearing bodies in the nucleus, the *nucleoli* (n), contain ribonucleic acid (RNA). *Ribosomes* (r) are cytoplasmic sites of protein synthesis. *Mitochondria* (M), found adjacent to the nucleus, are involved principally in production of aerobic energy. The *Golgi complex* (Go) appears as layers of membranes that collect products of cell metabolism for eventual secretion outside the cell or for storage within the cell. The Golgi complex appears to have a role in the production of hydrolytic enzyme-containing *lysosomes*. *Melanin granules* and *keratohyalin granules* (k) are observed in the basal and prickle cell layers of gingival epithelium. Epithelial cells appear to be held together by variations of complex structures termed *desmosomes* (d), which consist of a collection of dense fibrillar material (attachment plaque) associated with the plasma membranes of adjacent cells plus structures that lie between each attachment plaque. An analogous structure, the *hemidesmosome* and its *internal basement lamina*, is responsible for the attachment of gingival epithelium to the tooth surface. The internal basement lamina appears to be a product of epithelial cells, and present evidence suggests that this structure is biochemically similar to certain glycosaminoglycan complexes found in intercellular spaces. Filamentous bundles of *tonofilaments* (t) course throughout the cytoplasm, and in some areas short tufts of tonofilaments appear to insert into desmosomes of the basal cells.

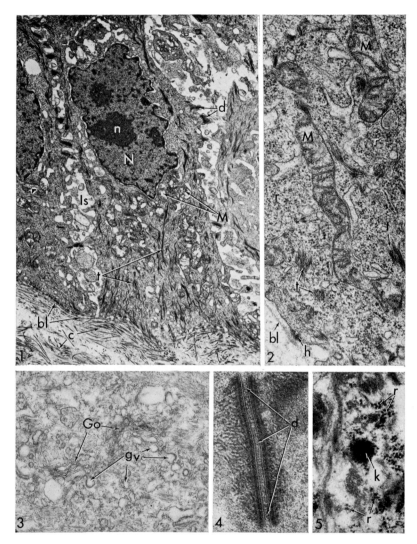

Fig. 11–2.   Electron micrographs of human gingival epithelium.   1, Basal cell showing attachment to underlying connective tissue. Nucleus (N); nucleolus (n); desmosome (d); mitochondria (M); tonofibrils (t); collagen fibrils (c); basal lamina (bl); intercellular space (Is).   ×7425.   2, Portion of basal cell showing elongated mitochondria (M), ribosomes (r), tonofibrils (t), basal lamina (bl), and hemidesmosome (h).   ×36,000. 3, Golgi complex (Go) in perinuclear region showing Golgi sacs and vesicles (gv). ×36,000. 4, High-power view through desmosome (d) between cells in spinous layer.   ×110,000. 5, Keratohyalin granule (k) typically surrounded by ribosomes (r).   ×68,000. (Courtesy of Dr. George Rose.)

Stratified squamous epithelium has access to blood supply only in the area of the basement membrane. Cells in the more superficial layers must depend on the passage of nutrients through or between deeper cell layers. It is therefore assumed that energy production in gingival epithelium is mediated primarily through anaerobic glycolysis. This theory is consistent with the decreasing concentration of mitochondria from the basal to the surface cell layers. One measure of aerobic metabolism is the volume of oxygen consumed per unit time, or Q_{O_2}. Average values of oxygen consumption, expressed as milliliters per gram dry weight per hour for oral epithelium (Q_{O_2} = 1 to 3), are considerably lower than those observed in liver (Q_{O_2} = 12 to 14), cardiac muscle (Q_{O_2} = 18), and kidney (Q_{O_2} = 20 to 25). Another measure of metabolism is the use of tissue lactate dehydrogenase and malate dehydrogenase activity ratios. Lactate dehydrogenase activity (pyruvate–lactate) reflects anaerobic glycolysis, whereas malate dehydrogenase (malate–oxaloacetate) is an indicator of Krebs cycle activity. The ratio of lactate to malate dehydrogenase activity in oral epithelium is twice that in surrounding muscle tissue, lending further support to the concept of anaerobic glycolysis as the predominant mode of energy conversion in gingival epithelium.

About two-thirds of the stratum corneum is composed of insoluble proteins collectively termed *keratins*. The marked resistance of keratins to a wide variety of biochemical agents is related in great measure to their sulfur content, most of which is a function of covalent disulfide bonds characteristic of cystine (Fig. 11–3). In addition, salt linkages and hydrogen bonding further contribute to the stability of the structure. The process of keratinization appears to depend on both tonofilaments and keratohyalin granules. Although the exact contribution of each is not known, it is generally agreed that keratohyalin acts as an embedding matrix for tonofilaments, which are the precursors of the insoluble keratin protein in the stratum corneum. The formation of keratin was once thought to be a function of nutritional deprivation and subsequent cell degeneration. Present evidence, however, suggests that the process is actually a form of cytodifferentiation, involving organization of tonafilaments into definite bundle systems, progressive increases of

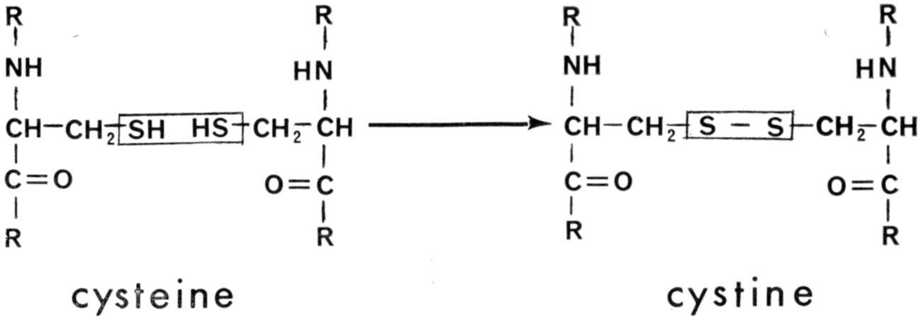

Fig. 11–3. Oxidation of two cysteine polypeptide residues to yield one cystine residue.

disulfide linkages, concentration of keratin precursors in upper cell layers, and tissue dehydration as the keratin layer is formed.

CONNECTIVE TISSUE

The connective tissues of the periodontium can be roughly divided into *mineralized* and *unmineralized*. The unmineralized connective tissues are comprised of the lamina propria of the gingiva and the periodontal ligament. The two major chemical components of these tissues are *collagen* and *glycosaminoglycans*, the structure and metabolism of which are discussed in detail in Chapters 2 and 3.

Fullmer has described formic acid-soluble resistant fibers, termed oxytalin fibers, which are relatively abundant in the human periodontal ligament. Histochemically, the material is stained by resorcin-fuchsin and orcein after oxidation by peracetic or performic acid. Oxytalin fibers are digested by elastase, but only after oxidation. The difficulty in obtaining uncontaminated (collagen-free) material has impeded chemical characterization of oxytalin, and several investigators have suggested that oxytalin fibers are either immature elastin fibers or collagen fibers in early stages of degradation.

The mineralized connective tissues of the periodontium consist of cementum and alveolar bone.

Cementum has many of the properties of bone and serves to anchor fibers of the periodontal ligament to the tooth. Deposition of cementum is continuous throughout life. The cementum has an average thickness of 16 to 60 μ at the coronal portion and 150 to 200 μ at the apical portion of the root. Owing to the difficulty in obtaining sufficient quantities of cementum for chemical analysis, little information is available on its exact composition. The data that have been reported suggest a close similarity to bone, and amino acid analysis of cemental collagen appears consistent with that of collagen from other tissues. Cementum does not appear to have an internal blood supply, but probably receives nourishment by diffusion from the adjacent periodontal ligament.

The composition and metabolism of bone are discussed in Chapter 8.

PERIODONTAL DISEASE

The majority of tooth mortality results from the loss of the integrity of the periodontium and, in particular, the degradation of periodontal connective tissue associated with inflammatory periodontal disease.

It is accepted that the initiating agents in inflammatory periodontal disease are products of microorganisms which live on and about the teeth. These microorganisms and their immediate environment form a tenacious gelatin-like substance termed *plaque*. A variety of systemic conditions, including metabolic and hormonal disturbances, malnutrition, and stress, may modify the clinical manifestations or progression of plaque-induced periodontal pathology, but experimental simulations of such conditions do not initiate the characteristic lesion. Mechanisms by which microorganisms induce destruction of the periodontium are not fully delineated, nor have specific organisms been shown to cause human periodontal disease. Nevertheless, the literature strongly supports the view that inflammatory periodontal diseases are of microbial origin and will not occur in the absence of microorganisms.

It may be convenient, though oversimplified, to visualize inflammatory periodontal disease along a continuum, with initial inflammatory changes localized to the gingiva (gingivitis) at one end and apical migration of epithelium, loss of alveolar bone and periodontal ligament, and resulting tooth mobility (periodontitis) at the other. The initial subclinical lesion is characterized by changes in the microcirculation, including vasodilation and

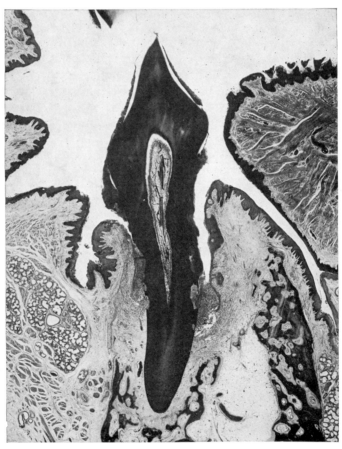

FIG. 11–4. Periodontitis. The gingival epithelium has migrated down the root surface forming a "pocket." The tooth surface is covered with calcified and uncalcified microbial plaque. A dense inflammatory infiltrate is observed in the lamina propria. Extensive loss of alveolar bone is apparent. (Courtesy of Dr. B. M. Levy.)

increased vascular permeability. Emigration of polymorphonuclear leuko-cytes quickly follows and clinical changes in the color, contour, and consistency of the gingiva become apparent. As the inflammatory lesion progresses, destruction of collagen fibers within the gingiva can be demonstrated. As one moves down the continuum, lymphocytes and plasma cells dominate the inflammatory infiltrate, and the process involves the deeper supporting structures with proliferation of gingival epithelium along the root of the tooth, forming an epithelium-lined "pocket." The lesion advances along vascular pathways at the expense of alveolar bone and periodontal ligament, eventuating in tooth mobility and impending tooth loss (Fig. 11-4).

It has been estimated that over 90% of the world's population manifests some degree of inflammatory periodontal disease, and therein lies the difficulty in describing the normal or baseline biochemistry of the periodontium. Much of the tissue for biochemical studies has been obtained at time of operation from human patients under treatment for periodontal disease or from animals exhibiting various forms of periodontal pathological change. The problem is further compounded by the difficulty in obtaining sufficient material for analysis necessitating, in many investigations, the use of pooled tissue extracts or homogenates. The net result is that the literature reflects, in great measure, the biochemistry of periodontal disease rather than the biochemistry of the normal periodontium. The following discussion is concerned with some of the biochemical phenomena encountered along the continuum of periodontal disease. A discussion of gingival fluid, collagen metabolism, the chemical mediators and modifiers of inflammation, and the immune response, as they pertain to the pathologic alteration of the periodontium, is included.

GINGIVAL FLUID

Histologically healthy human gingiva exhibits essentially no fluid emanating from the gingival sulcus. Inflamed gingiva, however, consistently demonstrates the presence of fluid, the quantity of which is proportional to the severity of the inflammation. Filter paper strips placed at the entrance of the gingival sulcus show the presence of fluid before clinical signs of inflammation are present. Accordingly, fluid height on paper strips is used as a sensitive method for the assessment of gingival health.

It appears likely that crevicular fluid originates from the gingival microcirculation and is modified by cells in the area of the sulcus. A number of investigations, therefore, have been directed at the composition of gingival fluid as a reflection of cellular and chemical changes in gingival tissue with varying stages of disease. The cellular elements of gingival fluid consist principally of desquamated epithelial cells, a variety of microorganisms, and leukocytes. The latter cells, composed of approximately 96% neutrophils, 2% lymphocytes, and 2% monocytes, have been shown to increase in direct proportion to the degree of gingival inflammation. As might be expected, the numbers and types of cells in gingival fluid have a profound influence on its chemical composition.

Enzyme studies have received particular attention because of their potential role in tissue degradation. A number of hydrolytic enzymes have been demonstrated in gingival fluid. Of these, acid phosphatase, alkaline phosphatase, β-glucuronidase, lysozyme, and cathepsin D have generated the most interest. Acid phosphatase, the classic lysosomal marker, is found at substantially higher concentrations in gingival fluid than in serum. Cimasoni suggests that about half of the acid phosphatase activity in whole gingival fluid may be a product of bacteria. Alkaline phosphatase, β-glucuronidase, lysozyme, and cathepsin D consistently demonstrate greater enzyme activity in gingival fluid than in serum and have been positively correlated with inflammatory periodontal disease.

Several studies on the concentration of electrolytes have been reported. The results vary in a fairly wide range from laboratory to laboratory, probably in part because of differences in fluid collection methods, differences in degree of gingival health at time of collection, and circadian periodicity. Average reported concentrations of potassium, for example, vary from 69 mEq/L to 9.5 mEq/L. In general, however, it would appear that gingival fluid contains significantly higher amounts of sodium and potassium than serum, and both tend to increase with gingival inflammation. More conclusive are results on sodium : potassium ratios in gingival fluid. If the fluid passes from the microvasculature to the sulcus through tissue that is physiologically intact, one would expect essentially the same quantities of sodium and potassium as those found in serum. As the number of damaged cells encountered by the fluid increased, a corresponding decrease in the sodium : potassium ratio should result owing to the accumulation of intracellular potassium. This appears to be the case, as a number of studies have shown that potassium concentrations in gingival fluid are two to 10 times as great as that recovered in serum. The Na : K ratios in extracellular fluids average approximately 28.1, whereas Na : K ratios reported for gingival fluid range from 2.1 to 17.1. Several investigations have shown that the Na : K ratio is negatively correlated with the severity of periodontal disease.

Cimasoni presents data from several investigations suggesting that the protein content of gingival fluid is qualitatively similar to that of serum. Immunoglobulins A, M, and G have been identified in gingival fluid, and Montgomery has demonstrated components of the kallikrein–kinin system after topical application of endotoxin or bacterial plaque. In addition, gingival fluid has been shown to contain appreciable amounts of fibrinogen, a protein rarely found in vascular fluids except in cases of inflammation.

COLLAGEN METABOLISM

In the healthy periodontium, well-organized groups of collagen fibers originate in the cementum and pass into the lamina propria (gingival fibers) or into alveolar bone (periodontal ligament fibers), giving tone to the gingiva and supporting the teeth in their bony sockets. One of the primary consequences of inflammatory periodontal disease is the overall loss of these collagen systems. A number of investigations have demonstrated a significant reduction of total collagen content, ranging from 50% to 70%, in tissues manifesting chronic periodontal disease. Such substantial losses of collagen may be a function of increased collagen degradation, decreased collagen production, or a combination of both.

Extracellular and intracellular mechanisms proposed for collagen degradation generally involve increased levels of hydrolytic enzymes that are active against collagen. Since native collagen in an undenatured state is markedly resistant to nonspecific proteases, a concerted effort has been directed toward the investigation of specific collagenases. Collagenases fall into two broad groups. One group is elaborated by microorganisms that do not contain collagen. The second group, the tissue collagenases, are produced in higher organisms with collagen as a major component of their tissues. Seifter and Harper have defined a collagenase as an enzyme capable of causing hydrolytic scission of peptide bonds in the characteristic helical regions of undenatured collagen. This definition includes enzymes making only one cleavage per collagen molecule, as in the case of most tissue collagenases, and those making multiple scissions, typical of bacterial collagenases.

A number of microorganisms found in dental plaque have been shown to elaborate collagenase. These include *Clostridium histolyticum*, *Mycobacterium tuberculosis*, *Pseudomonas aeruginosa*, and *Bacteroides melaninogenicus*. Bacterial collagenases may promote up to 200 cleavages per collagen alpha chain, appear to require calcium, and have an optimal pH ranging from 6.8 to 8.0.

Tissue collagenase from a vertebrate source was first described by Gross and Lapiere in studies of tadpole metamorphosis. Tadpole tissues were incubated in a salt solution on a surface of collagen gel and collagenolytic activity was demonstrated by an expanding area of lysis. The enzyme thus derived is active from pH 7.0 to 9.0, requires calcium, and is inhibited by EDTA, cysteine, and heating to 60° C. The tissue collagenases cleave the collagen molecule only once, three quarters of the distance from the amino terminal of the molecule. The helical structure appears to persist for both pieces, but their denaturation temperature is significantly lower than that for native collagen, rendering the pieces more susceptible to spontaneous denaturation and/or nonspecific protease activity at physiological temperature. Fullmer has demonstrated a collagenase with characteristics similar to those found in the tadpole enzyme in culture fluids of human gingiva and alveolar bone. The gingival collagenase has a broad range of activity from pH 7.0 to 9.5, has a molecular weight of approximately 40,000, and is inhibited by serum. An analogous enzyme can be extracted from culture media of isolated cells including fibroblasts, macrophages, and platelets. A collagenase has been extracted directly from the lysosomal fraction of polymorphonuclear (PMN) leukocytes.

Several investigations have demonstrated higher levels of collagenase in culture media of inflamed gingival tissue than in media of normal tissue. In addition, dental plaque, sterilized by irradiation or membrane filtration, appears to stimulate macrophages, resulting in an increase in cell size, substantial increase in numbers of lysosomal granules, and release of acid hydrolases and collagenase into extracellular fluids.

A number of sources of collagenase appear to be available in the periodontium and the increased activity of this enzyme in periodontal disease is certainly plausible. The overall loss of collagen may also be related to a decrease in collagen production. Page and co-workers have followed the course of incorporation of ^{14}C-proline into hydroxyproline and its eventual loss from collagen in a variety of tissues. The specific activity of hydroxyproline in collagen was significantly greater in gingiva than in any of the other tissues analyzed. These observations are consistent with the hypothesis that collagen in periodontal connective tissue is metabolized at an extremely high rate and, assuming constant degradation, minor alterations in production may yield a net loss of collagen.

HORMONES

Three hormones, estrogen, progesterone, and prostaglandins, have received particular attention in regard to their role in periodontal pathologic alterations. A clinical relationship between estrogen–progesterone levels and gingival inflammation was observed well before the physiological activity of these hormones was established. Clinical terms such as "pregnancy gingivitis," and "pubertal gingivitis" are scattered throughout the dental literature. Significant increases in the severity of gingivitis during puberty, pregnancy, and administration of oral contraceptive agents have been described. Formicola has demonstrated localization of ^{3}H-estradiol in mucosa and gingiva of ovariectomized rats in significantly higher concentrations than in the submaxillary gland, uterus, liver, kidney, and skin, 1 hour after injection. In addition, the estradiol remained in the tissue for at least 4 hours without significant decrease. Histological studies of gingival tissues from pregnant females have demonstrated a reduction in keratinization, increased epithelial glycogen, and decreased connective tissue glycoprotein.

Although alterations in hormone levels may be associated with variations in gingival tissue, present evidence suggests that estrogen–progesterone changes will not initiate inflammatory periodontal disease. Rather, they appear to modify or exaggerate tissue responses to bacterial plaque.

The prostaglandins are a group of unsaturated cyclic fatty acids that exhibit diverse biological activities including vascular dilatation, increased capillary permeability, and stimulation of osseous resorption. The prostaglandins have been divided into five broad subgroups on the basis of structure and function: prostaglandins (PG) A, B, E, F, and 19-hydroxy. Elevations of prostaglandin E levels have been observed in both experimentally

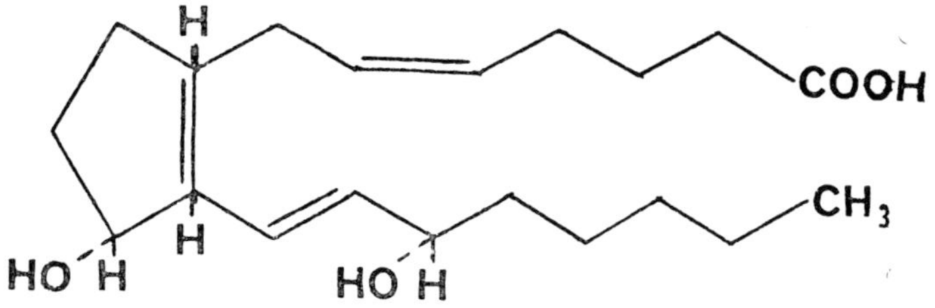

FIG. 11–5.   Prostaglandin E$_2$.

induced and naturally occurring inflammation.   Goodson and co-workers have shown that levels of prostaglandin E$_2$ (PGE$_2$) are elevated in gingival tissues from patients with advanced periodontal disease, and furthermore, that concentrations of PGE$_2$ measured in purulent exudates are sufficient to stimulate bone resorption (Fig. 11-5).

THE IMMUNE RESPONSE

In recent years, a great deal of attention has been directed toward the immunological response (Chapter 16) as one mechanism by which plaque products may cause the tissue destruction associated with periodontal disease. This concept is based on the premise that plaque antigens are capable of inducing B-cell production of antibodies or T-cell and B-cell production of pharmacologically active lymphokines.   Plaque antigen–antibody complexes, once formed, may initiate a chain of biochemical reactions collectively termed *complement*, resulting in a wide range of biological effects which include mass cell degranulation and histamine release, chemotaxis, phagocytosis and lysis of cell membranes, as well as the production of mediators by activation of lymphocytes. Lymphokines that may have particular relevance to periodontal disease include macrophage-migration inhibitory factor (MIF), lymphotoxin (LT), osteoclast-activating factor (OAF), and chemotactic factor (CTX).   Macrophage-migration inhibitory factor appears to facilitate the accumulation of macrophages in the periodontal tissues where they may function in processing additional antigen for presentation to lymphocytes as well as in releasing a variety of tissue destructive lysosomal hydrolases. Lymphotoxin is cytotoxic for cultured human fibroblasts and therefore may contribute to a decrease in collagen production. Osteoclast-activating factor has been shown to induce osteoclastic resorption of bone in organ cultures and may be important in the loss of alveolar bone characteristic of advanced periodontal disease.

Although immunological mechanisms have not been clearly defined, a number of observations lend support to the participation of the immune response in periodontal disease.   The presence of lymphocytes and plasma cells in inflamed periodontal tissues is consistent with the concept of a localized immune response. IgG-, IgA-, IgM-, and IgE-containing plasma cells have been identified in gingiva. IgG-containing cells appear to be most numerous. Moreover, several studies have demonstrated an increase in IgG-, IgA-, and IgM-staining cells in inflamed as compared to healthy periodontal tissues. Dental plaque and specific microbial antigens appear to stimulate peripheral blood lymphocytes from patients with inflammatory periodontal disease to undergo blastogenesis. Lymphocytes from clinically normal individuals are unresponsive to these antigens. The degree of lymphocyte stimulation seems to be correlated with the extent of periodontal destruction. Endotoxins are important constituents of microbial plaque. These lipopolysaccharides stimulate lymphocytes, and appear to elicit a greater response in cells from patients with periodontal disease than in those from disease-free controls.

Macrophages and polymorphonuclear leukocytes may be localized to the periodontium by several immune mediators. Among other functions, these cells are repositories for lysosomal enzymes capable of effecting much of the tissue degradation in periodontal disease. Lysosomal enzymes are synthesized in ribosomes, packaged in the Golgi complex, and collectively appear in the cytoplasm enclosed by a lipoprotein membrane. This membrane-bound assortment of enzymes has been defined as a *primary lysosome*, which may secrete its contents outside the cell or may store enzymes for use in extracellular digestion of material engulfed by the cell. The stability of the lysosomal lipoprotein membrane is apparently affected by a number of chemical agents. The inclination of this membrane to release its enclosed enzymes is inhibited by such "stabilizing agents" as cortisone, prednisone, and salicylates. Release of enzymes, on the other hand, appears to be facilitated by such "labilizing agents" as vitamin A, endotoxin, progesterone, and antigen–antibody complexes.

Granules isolated from polymorphonuclear leukocytes and macrophages have been found to possess many of the properties of lysosomes. It is generally agreed that phagocyte granules are responsible for intracellular digestion of material engulfed by these cells, and in the event that phagocyte granules become discharged in the extracellular spaces, digestion of tissue components could occur there as well.

Individual lysosomes may vary in size, enzyme content, density, and sedimentation coefficient. A number of investigations have made use of these differences to separate lysosomes into definitive types. Fractionation of rabbit polymorphonuclear leukocytes into at least two granule types (A and B), for example, can be accomplished by centrifugation of the granules through increasingly higher concentrations of sucrose. The A and B granules not only show differences in their location in the sucrose gradient, but also differ with respect to the enzymes they contain.

Over 35 enzymes have been identified in the lysosomal fraction of a number of cell types. The positive correlation of several of these hydrolases to gingival inflammation has led to the speculation that much of the glycosaminoglycans and collagen degradation observed in periodontal disease might be mediated by lysosomal enzymes.

This discussion has moved rather generally along a continuum from periodontal health to advanced periodontal disease, pausing occasionally to briefly view a few of the biochemical phenomena along the way. Some attempt has been made to relate several areas of biochemistry to an almost universal human affliction, periodontal disease, and several conclusions pertaining to the biochemistry of the periodontium can be drawn. First, the chemical nature of periodontal glycosaminoglycans or collagen or bone does not appear to differ appreciably from that of other tissues; there are no major differences in the chemical nature of pharmacologically active mediators of periodontal inflammation. The differences are concerned with the unique tooth–soft tissue interface, the close juxtaposition of various connective tissues to the oral cavity and the environment in which the system resides. Such an environment gives comfort to a variety of microorganisms that constantly subject the tissues of the periodontium to metabolic by-products. Periodontal disease results from the ensuing war between microbial products and host defenses fought within the close confines of the periodontium. It should be clear that a knowledge of the biochemistry of structures common to the periodontium is critical to solve the problems involved in the pathogenesis of periodontal disease and in many areas this knowledge does not, in fact, exist.

Second, the concept that inflammatory periodontal disease is simply the result of "irritation" by bacterial products acting directly against the structures of the periodontium is no longer tenable. Certainly the loss of sulcular epithelial integrity may, in part, be due to the activity of bacterial products such as hyaluronidase, chondroitinase, various proteases, and hydrogen sulfide, but the majority of periodontal destruction, particularly loss of connective tissue, appears to be mediated by host mechanisms in response to bacterial products. A case in point is the resorption of alveolar bone. It has been demonstrated that soluble extracts of human bacterial plaque stimulate resorption of bone in tissue culture. If the bones are devitalized by heating prior to culture, thereby eliminating the possibility of osteoclastic activity, no resorption is stimulated by plaque extracts. Thus, the plaque extracts do not act directly against bone, but rather set in motion a series of host events that stimulate osteoclasts to resorb bone.

Finally, it would appear that the host effector mechanisms participating in periodontal destruction are multifactorial, rather than the independent activity of a single pathological pathway or hormone or enzyme. The previous discussion dealt with a number of chemical mediators of periodontal disease. Bacterial enzymes may damage the integrity of sulcular epithelium facilitating the ingress of bacterial products. Early inflammatory changes including increased vascular permeability and emigration of leukocytes may be mediated by a number of chemical effectors. Continued challenge by plaque toxins sets in motion a variety of host systems that mediate overall loss of collagen and resorption of alveolar bone. In response, the sulcular epithelium migrates along the root of the tooth forming a pocket in which the microflora continues to thrive. The contribution of each system may vary with the stage of disease, the nature of the microbial flora, and the status of the host. Once established, the severity, extent, and direction of the inflammatory lesion may be modified by a number of factors including hormone levels, host nutritional factors, establishment of particular types of microorganisms, and perhaps excessive forces generated by occlusion. The exact interrelationships remain cloudy. Nevertheless, it is clear that degradation of the biochemical components of the periodontium is initiated by bacterial plaque, and at present the prevention of such degradation must be based on the prevention of plaque.

SELECTED REFERENCES

CIMASONI, G.: The Crevicular Fluid. In *Monographs in Oral Science*, Volume 3. H. M. Myers (Ed.). Basel, S. Karger, 1974.

FORMICOLA, A. J., WEATHERFORD, T., and GRUPE, H.: The uptake of ^{3}H estradiol by the oral tissues of rats. J. Periodont. Res., *5*, 269–275, 1970.

FULLMER, H. M.: Metabolic Hydrolysis of Collagen. In *Metabolic Conjugation and Metabolic Hydrolysis*, Volume 2. W. Fishman (Ed.). New York, Academic Press, 1970, pp. 301–343.

GOODSON, J. M., DEWHURST, F. E., and BRUNETTI, A.: Prostaglandin E_2 levels and human periodontal disease. Prostaglandins, *6*, 81–85, 1974.

GOLDMAN, H. M., and COHEN, D. W.: *Periodontal Therapy*, 5th ed. St. Louis, C. V. Mosby Co., 1973.

GRANT, D. A., STERN, I. B., and EVERETT, F. G.: *Orban's Periodontics*, 4th ed. St. Louis, C. V. Mosby Co., 1972.

MELCHER, A. H., and BOWEN, W. H.: *Biology of the Periodontium*. New York, Academic Press, 1969.

PAGE, R. C., and SCHROEDER, H. E.: Biochemical aspects of the connective tissue alterations in inflammatory gingival and periodontal disease. Int. Dent. J., *23*, 455–469, 1973.

RANNEY, R. R., and MONTGOMERY, E. H.: Vascular leakage resulting from the topical application of endotoxin to the gingiva of the beagle dog. Arch. Oral Biol., *18*, 963–970, 1973.

SEIFTER, S., and HARPER, E.: The Collagenases. In *The Enzymes*, Volume III. P. D. Boyer (Ed.). New York, Academic Press, 1971, pp. 649–697.

Chapter **12**

Saliva

IRA L. SHANNON, D.D.S., M.S.
RICHARD P. SUDDICK, D.D.S., Ph.D.

MECHANISM OF SECRETION

The physiological mechanisms underlying the secretion of saliva may be broadly divided into two categories: the secretion of organic nonelectrolytes (proteins and the like), and the secretion of fluid and electrolytes. The biochemist, physiologist, and morphologist are concerned with an understanding of how function is related to structure in all organs, cells, and organelles. It may be helpful to consider the secretion of saliva in relation to Figure 12–1, a schematic version of the secretory parenchyma of salivary glands. It must be emphasized, however, that there are variations in these structures from gland to gland and from species to species.

There are three basic structures to consider when discussing secretion. The first of these is the acinus, a ball of cells, which when cut in section shows the large pyramidal cells arranged in a circle around a minute lumen (Fig. 12–1). The narrow portion of the cell that faces the lumen is known as the apex, and that membrane bordering the lumen is the apical membrane. The opposite pole of the cell faces the interstitial fluid; it is known as the basal portion and the membrane, as the basal membrane. The lateral membranes of adjacent cells lie extremely close to each other and adjacent to the lumen and are tightly joined by structures known as tight junctions. The junctional structures are sometimes called terminal bars or desmosomes. During certain stages of activity, the lateral membranes of these cells become less closely apposed to each other giving the appearance of channels or canaliculi which appear to course between the cells, but only as far as the tight junction. Thus, it appears that the only way substances may enter the lumen of the gland is by coursing through the acinar cells or perhaps by moving through the lateral channels and then through the minute gap of the tight junction or perhaps in some way through the matrix of the tight junction structure.

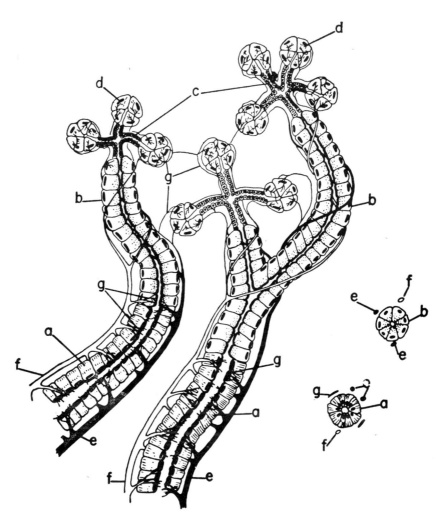

Fig. 12–1. Schematic drawing of the relationships of the vasculature to the secretory tubules and acini in the rat submaxillary gland as described by Suddick and Dowd (1969). Each tubule is supplied by one parallel artery (f). In the striated duct region (a) numerous capillaries cross the tubule transversely (g). Such capillaries become fewer as more distal tubular regions are reached. The intercalated ducts (c) connect the granular tubules (b) with the acini (d) and all seem to be served by a common capillary bed. This bed consists of long terminal capillary loops which vary in their proximity to the different structures. Blood returns from the common acinar-tubular areas and separate striated duct capillary beds by way of two veins (e) (observed in cross-sections of the tubules). Points of inception of these veins and their confluence with the larger veins which accompany the central collecting (or intraglandular excretory) ducts could not be ascertained from this study.

The acinar units are connected to a short duct structure known as the intercalated duct. These ducts are composed of small cuboidal cells with no remarkable or highly characteristic cytological features. The intercalated ducts are connected to the secretory tubules which in turn join the intralobular collecting ducts. The latter collect fluid from other secretory tubules within the lobule before joining a centrally located excretory duct which carries the secretions from the gland to the oral cavity. The major salivary glands develop as invaginations of the oral epithelium beginning about the sixth week *in utero*. The simple epithelial infolding gradually deepens and branches. In some species in which the glands of a newborn animal (*e.g.*, a rat) have been examined, the glands lack acini. The acinar elements develop during the first few weeks after birth. The acini develop like buds from the terminal end of the intercalated ducts during the development of the gland. Thus, the intercalated ducts from several acini join at one secretory tubule.

The secretory tubules are composed of tall columnar epithelial cells with distinctive cytological features. Several different types of cells occur in the secretory tubules, and these tubules have been subcategorized according to the appearance of the two main types of cells. One of these cells has a characteristic striated appearance in the basal portion, probably due to a heavy concentration of mitochondria when viewed with the light microscope. The other is known as the granular duct cell because of the appearance of numerous granules in the cell, predominantly in the apical half of the cell. The secretory ducts of the parotid glands of man and many other species appear to be composed entirely of striated ducts, whereas the secretory ducts of the submandibular gland in most mammals contain both granular and striated cells, both arranged as distinctive segments. The granular duct segment in these circumstances appears closest to the acini.

To gain another perspective on the processes of secretion associated with the structures, it should be mentioned that the entire acinar–tubular structure is composed of a sheet of epithelial cells tightly bound to each other, and that this sheet of cells is rolled into a blind-ended tube. Thus, the contents of this tube in any part of the gland are always separated from the interstitial fluid and plasma within the gland by this continuous layer of cells. The processes of secretion then involve two principal activities. One is the biosynthesis of materials within the cells of the gland and the export of these products into the lumen. The other process involves the transfer of water and electrolytes across this continuous sheet of cells into the lumen. These are two completely distinctive biological processes and an understanding of secretion in exocrine glands requires information on both these processes.

Protein Secretion

More than 20 different proteins, identifiable by electrophoresis, have been found in human parotid saliva. The most well-known protein in saliva, of course, is the enzyme amylase. Amylase initiates the breakdown of starch molecules into the alpha-limit dextrins and amylose. Several of the proteins isolated from saliva have been characterized as proteases. It is not clear whether any of these digestive enzymes perform a significant and important digestive role in animals.

The experimental results on rats which have had their salivary glands removed suggest that the major function of the salivary glands, as far as the intake and assimilation of food, is to provide a lubricant and a medium in which the food can be mixed and partially dissolved so that it can be swallowed. Perhaps the major function of the proteins and glycoproteins in saliva relates to the protection of the mucous surfaces of the mouth and pharynx against drying, infection, and damage during the mastication of hard foods. These aspects of salivary function will be discussed later.

There is abundant evidence to associate the secretion of proteins with the acinar cells and, specifically, with certain intracellular organelles and inclusions in these cells. The acinar cells of the pancreas are analogous in this respect. In fact, much of the basic research on the process of protein secretion has been done on pancreatic tissue, and many of our ideas about protein secretion from salivary glands are only inferential from experiments performed on the pancreas. In fact, when we speak of protein synthesis and secretion we cannot really be sure that each of the individual proteins found in the secretions has been synthesized and secreted by the process described here. This process begins with the uptake of amino acids through the basal membrane of the acinar cell. About 60% of the volume of these cells is occupied by elements of the rough-surfaced endoplasmic reticulum (RER). The RER is characteristically arranged in a series of more or less parallel interconnected, flattened saccules or cisternae located primarily in the basal half of the cell (Fig. 12–2). In cross section each cisterna is seen to be bound by a unit membrane, about 70 Å in width, which separates the cisternal cavity from the surrounding cytoplasmic matrix or cell sap. The outer or cytoplasmic surface of the RER membrane typically is studded with ribosomes known as the attached polysomes. Numerous free polysomes also reside in the cytoplasmic matrix between segments of the RER.

In the typical resting acinar cell, the apical cytoplasm is populated with numerous spherical mature storage granules, each bounded by a smooth-surfaced unit membrane approximately 80 to 100 Å in thickness. These storage granules contain material of high electron opacity and are believed to be identical with the zymogen granules observed with the light microscope. Between these two poles of the cell in the supranuclear region are the elements of the Golgi complex. These consist of stacks of laterally placed, flattened saccules bounded by a smooth-surfaced unit membrane about 80 Å wide. Peripheral to these stacks are small smooth-surfaced vesicles about 45 to 60 nm in diameter. Centrally located in the complex are a number of immature zymogen granules or condensing vacuoles. The unit membrane of these vacuoles possesses an irregular scalloped profile. The vacuoles contain

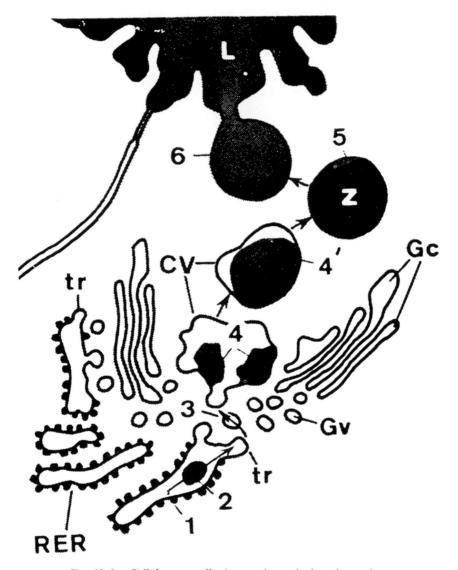

Fig. 12–2.   Cellular organelles in protein synthesis and secretion.
(See text for details.)

material of variable electron density.   The acinar cell thus contains a number of discrete membrane-bound sections which comprise the synthetic machinery and storage compartments for the secretory products.   In addition, the cell is highly polarized, with the synthesizing machinery located basally and the storage elements apically.   The Golgi complex lies in an intermediate position and is believed to perform the function of processing the protein products of the RER into the storage granules.

The sequence of protein synthesis and secretion may be outlined in the following steps (Fig. 12–2):

1. After the uptake of amino acids across the basal membrane of the acinar cells, synthesis of exportable proteins occurs in association with polysomes attached to the outer surface of the cisternae of the RER. Actually, only the synthesis of a few proteins has been clearly established to occur in this manner, and work on salivary gland proteins has been limited to amylase. It can be reasonably predicted, however, that the synthesis of all exportable proteins of salivary gland origin occurs in the same manner.

2. There is a transfer (tr) of the secretory proteins into the cisternae of the RER, and a movement of these proteins through the cisternal space. The transfer of the proteins from the outer polysomal surface into the cisternal space probably occurs during the course of the growth of the proteins, and thus segregation of the proteins within the space occurs upon completion of the synthesis of a particular polypeptide chain. At least in the pancreatic cell, the processes of elongation of the chain and discharge into the space are not dependent on energy other than that involved in peptide bond formation and discharge of amino acids from transfer RNA. Instead, these processes of cisternal transfer seem to be governed by the structural relationships between the ribosome and the cisternal membrane.

3–4. The secretory proteins apparently move through the cisternal space to the transitional elements of the RER. These elements are part rough-surfaced, part smooth-surfaced portions of the cisternae of the RER that abut on and feed into the Golgi peripheral region. These transitional elements bud off the cisternae by membrane fusion to become free vesicles in the cytoplasm and are indistinguishable from the population of vesicles comprising the Golgi peripheral region. It is believed that these Golgi vesicles (Gv) move across this region and fuse with preexisting empty condensing vacuoles or with each other. This, then, represents the initiation of the storage process of the secretory proteins.

5. The condensing vacuoles (Cv) become transformed into zymogen granules (Z) by the filling and concentration of their secretory protein content. Radioautographic observations of pancreatic cells demonstrate that the condensing vacuoles begin to accumulate large amounts of label about 20 minutes after a pulse dose of radioactively labeled amino acids. Thereafter they become progressively more electron-opaque and more heavily labeled as secretory proteins accumulate within the granules. The typical mature zymogen granule is highly electron-dense and has a smooth circular profile. In addition to segregation and concentration of secretory proteins, the Golgi complex (Gc) may mediate the addition of sugar residues to the polypeptide backbone of some of these products. Many of the salivary proteins or glycoproteins in the Golgi complex and other cell types seem to be responsible for the synthesis of polysaccharide moieties.

6. The last step in protein secretion consists of discharge of the content of

the zymogen granule into the acinar lumen (L). This involves movement of the granule to the cell apex where its limiting membrane fuses with the apical membrane of the acinar cell resulting in release of the granule content into the duct lumen. This process is sometimes called exocytosis.

It is now pertinent to examine the means by which reflex stimulation of the gland cells results in secretion of proteins, and thus with the steps for protein synthesis which have been outlined above. It seems certain that nerve processes make connections with or are in close proximity to the basal membrane of the acinar cells. It is not certain whether such nerve processes are sympathetic or parasympathetic. However, the preponderance of evidence suggests that the cells are innervated by both divisions. Whatever the effects of nerve stimulation on synthesis and secretion of exportable proteins are, they seem to be on the expulsion of the zymogen granule content into the gland lumen and not directly on the previous steps in the synthesis and transport in the cisternae of the RER and Golgi complex. Thus, effects of nerve stimulation probably permit the increased activity in the first phases of amino acid uptake, protein synthesis, protein movement through the RER, packaging in the Golgi complex, and renewed zymogen granule generation, by means of removal of the end product of the entire process through this primary initiation of zymogen granule expulsion. None of these steps appears to require energy derived from glycolysis, but the initial steps at least are highly sensitive to any inhibitor that interferes with mitochondrial energy production. The latter is a finding derived specifically from studies on the pancreas and whether it is entirely applicable to salivary acinar cells is not yet known.

Equally interesting are the energy requirements for movement of the zymogen granules toward the apical membrane and for the fusion of the granules with the expulsion of their contents into the glandular lumen. It is not necessary to postulate a translational structure for granule expulsion. The laws of diffusion indicate, for example, that in an aqueous medium a particle 2000 Å in diameter separated from the cell membrane by 100 Å will reach the membrane in 0.13 msec, and a particle of the same size will traverse a distance of 5 μ in 33 sec. Calculated times for zymogen granules 1 μ in diameter traversing the same distances are 0.65 msec and around 50 sec. The latter corresponds to the distance from the center of the Golgi region to the apical membrane of the cell. These calculations are based on an assumed intracellular viscosity of 0.06 poise and simply describe the possible course but give no indication of the probability of such events. During secretion, significant amounts of water move through the cells from the basal membrane toward the apical membrane and into the lumen. Thus, diffusional forces alone would not be required to cause net movement of the large zymogen granules toward the apical membrane.

From electron microscopic studies, a number of investigators have reported on the fusion of the zymogen granule membrane with the cell membrane so that a direct opening into the lumen is formed. Whether or not this is always true before release of the zymogen granule content, the granule membrane or the fused membranes must be modified in order to release the zymogen content. As a result of nerve stimulation, a factor in the fusion process itself probably modifies the apical cell membrane resulting in the dissolution or rupture of the membranes.

The other major process concerned with secretion of saliva is the way the large volumes of water and electrolytes are moved from the interstitial side of the epithelial sheet to the lumen of the gland. There are reasons to consider that these processes are governed by quite separate mechanisms from those governing protein secretion. The only factor both probably have in common is the required mediation by the autonomic nervous system for their effects to be realized. Since there is some controversy concerning the basic energy that drives fluid secretion, it is well to begin by considering this question in its historical perspective.

In his famous experiment on dog submaxillary secretion carried out nearly 125 years ago, Ludwig found that the intraductal pressure of the submaxillary gland will rise near or above the femoral artery pressure when the duct is occluded. From this, he concluded that secretion is an active process within the gland and is not the result of glomerular-like ultrafiltration of fluid driven by the hydrostatic pressure differential between the intraglandular capillaries and the ductal lumina. In 1961 Langley and Brown repeated this basic experiment on dog parotid gland. They found similar results and agreed with Ludwig's interpretation. Since then it has been the underlying assumption of virtually all studies conducted on the mechanisms of secretion of electrolytes and fluid in the salivary glands that the driving energy for the movement of water across the cells is due to the movement of one or more of the osmolytes found in the secretory fluid. Since the osmotic pressure of saliva secreted from virtually any gland at virtually any rate of flow can be accounted for on the basis of the sum of the concentrations of sodium, potassium, chloride, and bicarbonate, it has also been widely assumed that the active transport or selective transfer of one or more of these ions is responsible for the osmotic gradient that pulls water across the secretory cells.

Most investigators seem to assume that the acini are the sites where most or all of the fluid of secretion is transferred. Although the evidence to support the fact that these cells are primarily responsible for protein secretion is irrefutable, there is no direct evidence to support the assumption that they are responsible for most of the fluid secretion. This assumption probably arose simply because the acinus is the anatomical end point of the branching tubular secretory structure. In order to obtain direct evidence that most fluid is transferred in the acinar units, one would have to be able to demonstrate quantitatively the amount of fluid transferred in a single acinus per unit time, and to multiply this by the number of active acinar units in a gland. This value would have to equal approximately the amount of fluid secreted. The only types of experiments in which techniques that permit sampling of fluid within the glandular tubular structures are employed are the micropuncture experiments. In these experiments, extremely minute glass micropipettes (diameter of the tip is 6 to 12 μ) are inserted into the tubular structure, usually at the junction of two or more intercalated ducts as they drain toward a striated duct. Fluid samples sufficient for analyses (about 0.1 nl) can be obtained in this manner without applying negative pressure. Analyses of sodium, potassium, and chloride can be performed with such small volumes. It is not possible to determine how much fluid is transferred in the acinus or in the clumps of acini draining toward the pipettes. Thus, it is simply not possible to state with certainty that most of the fluid of secretion enters the tubular structure in the acini of the gland.

Good evidence indicates other elements of the tubular structure of the gland are capable of elaborating significant amounts of fluid and electrolytes. It is suggested that the secretory tubular structures or perhaps even more distal ductal elements are able to elaborate the fluid and electrolytes of secretion. Related to the question of location of fluid transfer is the matter of the cytological appearance of the cells in the different elements of the gland.

In contrast to acinar cells, which appear to be specialized for protein secretion, there are other cells in the body that appear to be specialized for transfer of fluids. Again, these are epithelial sheets of cells which line organs such as the stomach, small intestine, large intestine, gallbladder, and choroid plexus. Perhaps the most appropriate organ to compare to the salivary glands, as far as the cytological features of the component cells, is the kidney. Cells of other organs such as the gallbladder, which are similarly responsible for such luminal to interstitial fluid transfer, also appear similar to these types of cells. As a generalization, organ epithelial cells that appear to be involved in water and electrolyte transfer functions seem to present a characteristic appearance involving many if not all of the features cited.

Saliva: A Hypotonic Fluid

Part of the great interest in saliva as a physiological fluid arises from the fact that it is hypotonic with respect to the other fluids in the body, *i.e.*, plasma, interstitial fluid, lymph, aqueous humor, cerebrospinal fluid, and the cytoplasmic fluid in cells in general. It has been of considerable interest to investigators to try to unravel the mechanisms by which the parotid gland is able to elaborate a fluid that is hypo-osmotic to other body fluids. In human parotid saliva, for example, osmolarity rarely exceeds 120 mOsm per kilogram during the highest levels of physiological secretion, and levels much lower than this predominate at lower levels of secretion, reaching values as low as 60 mOsm per kilogram. In comparison, the osmolarity of blood plasma is approximately 290 mOsm per kilogram. The major question is how these glands are able to elaborate a fluid across the tubular epithelial sheet and maintain it against this osmotic gradient.

A Hypothesis for Secretion of a Hypotonic Fluid. The most broadly promulgated theory to explain this phenomenon has come from the interpretations of investigators using the various micropuncture experiments. Most of these experiments have produced similar results and have been performed by similar techniques. Authors have usually stated that the micropuncture samples have been withdrawn from the "acinar-intercalated duct region," or from the intercalated ducts. In the various studies, samples also were withdrawn from other sites, including the main excretory duct into which microcannulas were inserted deep to the gland, so that the fluid collected had passed through the secretory tubular region and perhaps through other collecting duct structures as well.

The interpretation of the results of micropuncture experiments is that the acinus elaborates a primary secretory fluid that is isosmotic to plasma and isotonic in its major electrolyte content. The secretory fluid collected at the orifice of most mammalian parotid and submandibular glands is markedly hypo-osmotic, and its electrolyte profile is much different from that collected by the micropuncture techniques at the intercalated ducts. Since the fluid collected from the latter sites is isosmotic to plasma, the main point of interpretation of these experiments is that the glands elaborate a primary isosmotic fluid in the acinus, and that this is modified by subsequent resorptive processes as this fluid passes out through the tubular structures. It is further assumed that the tubular structures are relatively impermeable to water and that the resorptive processes are capable of extracting ions in excess of water molecules, thus rendering the fluid hypotonic. The ions that appear to be resorbed and cause the saliva to become hypotonic are sodium and chloride. In certain glands this type of evidence suggests that potassium is secreted by the tubules in at least a partial exchange for the resorption of sodium so that the potassium concentration, which is essentially plasma-like at the acinus (around 4 to 5 mEq/L), becomes more concentrated in the tubular structures, perhaps reaching values of 10 to 20 mEq/L. If all of the prior assumptions upon which these interpretations are based are accepted, then, these ideas on secretion of fluid and electrolytes are perfectly reasonable. However, without any direct evidence it seems unwise to accept the major primary assumption that the acinus is the primary site for secretion of essentially all the fluid entering the parenchymal tubules of the salivary glands.

An Alternate Hypothesis for Secretion of a Hypotonic Fluid. Experiments have proved that the blood flow to the submaxillary gland of the rat is essential for the secretion of fluid. The results suggest that a hydrostatic pressure differential across the secretory epithelial cells generated by the intravascular hydrostatic pressure is required for normal secretion, and/or that an immediate dynamic relationship is necessary between the various fluid compartments in the fluid supply required for secretion, *i.e.*,

vascular fluid → interstitial fluid → cellular fluid → secretory fluid.

Although hydrostatic pressure and fluid supply could be involved, the precisely parallel decline of venous outflow, which reflects the decline of intraglandular vascular pressure, together with the decline in fluid secretion, provides strong circumstantial evidence that the intraglandular vascular pressure is the crucial element. If this is true, then fluid secretion should be regarded as being dependent upon vascular pressure, and vascular pressure may be the primary energy source for fluid secretion. It could represent a type of water filtration process through cellular structures that heretofore has not been defined.

When the submaxillary ducts and the venous outflow from the submaxillary gland are isolated and cannulated in rats, the secretory pressures produced during active secretion, as well as the venous pressures produced, can be measured and manipulated during active secretion or during quiescence. When the pressures are increased, a stepwise and directly proportionate decrease in both venous outflow and secretory flow rate occurs. In addition, the actual secretion of fluid always ceases just below or near the same pressure at which venous outflow ceases. This is true under a wide variety of conditions of the experimental animal. From this type of data the actual work, kinetic or potential, of secretion can be calculated in ergs. It should be evident that the work output of glandular blood flow and secretory fluid production are directly proportional under widely different conditions and at widely different hydrostatic back pressures. These experiments, considered with those described previously, provide convincing evidence that a hydrostatic pressure differential across the secretory epithelial tubes from the direction of the interstitial fluid to the lumen is an essential component of the physiological process of fluid and electrolyte secretions in rat submaxillary glands.

Whether or not this concept can be extrapolated to other salivary glands is uncertain. However, it appears to be an attractive concept to explain the entire process of secretion of the hypotonic fluid common in the major salivary glands of mammals. It is believed that the secretion of hypotonic fluid takes place in the striated duct region of salivary glands and that the vascular hydrostatic pressure provides the energy for fluid secretion.

FACTORS IN SALIVA FLOW RATE

Although it is the mixed whole saliva that constantly bathes the teeth and oral soft tissues, the heterogeneity of this fluid makes it most difficult to study biochemically. In addition to the fluid contributions of all the oral glands, mixed saliva contains exfoliated mucosal cells, blood cells, bacteria, food debris, and countless other contaminants. Therefore, the study of whole saliva is of virtually no value in clarifying the confusion related to salivary gland secretory processes. For these reasons, as well as others, much research on human saliva has been conducted on secretions of the individual salivary glands. Accumulated secretion presents the problem of emanating from all the glands and being derived from both serous- and mucous-type cells. Consequently, the easily collected fluid from the serous parotid gland has been studied extensively. The bulk of this chapter will be devoted to a discussion of this specific fluid.

Methods of Collection

In 1832, Misterlich studied parotid secretion in a patient with a parotid fistula. Direct cannulation of Stensen's duct was first performed by Ordenstein in 1860. He pointed out, however, that fluid tended to leak around the cannula and that the cannula frequently slipped from the expanding duct. In 1910, Carlson and Crittenden listed several undesirable factors associated with collecting parotid saliva by cannulation. They introduced a significant innovation by employing a collection device based upon the principle of surrounding "the opening of Stensen's duct with a metal cup which communicates with the exterior by means of a metal tube; surrounding this inner cup and fixed to it is an outer larger one communicating with the exterior by means of another metal tube." Vacuum produced in the outer cup held the device in place and parotid fluid was free to flow through the outlet tube under virtually physiological conditions.

Present devices continue to be based on the original Carlson and Crittenden concept of stabilizing the device by negative pressure and placing no direct vacuum on the duct orifice.

The two most important problems associated with collecting parotid fluid from human beings are cap dislodgment and the extravasation of tissue fluid and/or blood into the collection device and, ultimately, into the sample being collected.

In certain experimental situations, it is highly desirable for the subject to have the ability to collect his own saliva. Such is the case when the subject is to undergo prolonged periods of complete isolation or when multiple samples are to be collected in a pattern, such as hourly throughout the night. A device developed to meet this specific requirement has been employed by pilots of jet aircraft and by subjects during exposure to physical stresses, vibration, acceleration, deceleration, and centrifugal forces. It is of interest that both the American and Russian astronauts have been fitted with these devices, and that the devices were employed for saliva sampling during the Apollo-Soyuz program.

In automating saliva collection, an automatic sample receptacle that can divide the collection interval into precise time increments is used. In the hospital, an automatic collector has been found invaluable in taking samples during the night. Another use is in sampling patients undergoing hemodialysis on the artificial kidney. A series of 12 test tubes rotate to position under the collection tube so that sampling intervals can be timed exactly; the duration of each sample collection is controlled by a variable timer.

Sources of Whole Saliva

Saliva originates primarily from the three pairs of major salivary glands: the parotid, submandibular, and sublingual glands. Histologically these glands are usually described as purely serous, mixed serous and mucous, and purely mucous, respectively. The exact details of functional innervation are not completely clear. It is well established that parasympathetic stimulation elicits a relatively profuse flow from all three glands, but the results of sympathetic stimulation are not nearly so well delineated. This point will receive additional attention later.

Additional fluid flow is produced by oral minor mucous glands that occur in many areas of the mouth and have been classified as minor sublingual, lingual, labial, buccal, palatine, and glossopalatine glands. These minor mucous glands contribute 7 to 8% of the total volume of saliva under resting and stimulated conditions.

Another possible source of oral fluid, first suggested in 1817 by Serres, is the flow of fluid from the gingival crevice into the mouth. Formerly, crevicular fluid was thought to originate from glands encircling the roots of the teeth. It now appears clear that crevicular fluid flow is nonexistent when there is no gingival inflammation and that it can be disregarded as a fluid source under physiological conditions.

A small body of literature has accumulated on the contributions of the major salivary glands to the volume of whole saliva. The consensus is that parotid glands contribute a larger percentage as stimulation is increased and a higher volume of whole saliva is produced. Paraffin stimulation increases parotid flow sixfold, whereas the extra-parotid (all other than parotid) saliva increases to less than double the resting rate.

Schneyer and Levin studied whole saliva flow in 23 subjects under reduced exogenous stimulation and found that the parotid glands contributed approximately 26% of the total flow. Stimulation by acid on the tongue increased the parotid contribution to 34%. Calculations based upon this study suggested the surprising conclusion that 45% of the whole saliva might have been derived from the small mucosal glands.

Studies on two subjects revealed that parotid flow accounted for 18.4% and 30.8% of unstimulated flow. In a single subject, the contribution of the parotid glands increased markedly in reflexly stimulated saliva.

Enfors found an unstimulated flow mean of 0.031 ml/min from a single parotid gland in 71 subjects, and the mean flow for a single submandibular gland in 54 subjects was 0.101 ml/min. Under citric acid stimulation he found that, in most cases, the greater response was elicited from the parotid glands. With 6% acid the parotid glands produced approximately two-thirds of the whole saliva.

Resting submandibular flow is about three times that of the parotid glands. As stimulation increased, the prominence of parotid flow became evident. At half-maximal flow the rates from the two glands were approximately equal, but with maximal flow the parotid glands contributed about two-thirds of the total saliva.

Other research into the source of whole saliva has involved comparisons of parotid and extra-parotid contributions. Collectors were placed over the orifices of both parotid glands and the combined flow was directed into a single graduated tube. The remaining saliva, the extra-parotid, was expectorated into a second graduated tube. All subjects were healthy young adult men, and collections were initiated at about 7:00 A.M. with the subjects in the fasting state.

An initial experiment involved 11 subjects employing one, three, and five pure gum (size 32) rubber bands as successive stimulants. Flow rate from both pairs of gland increased significantly as the number of bands increased, and the percentile contribution of the parotid glands to whole saliva volume increased from 42.5% to 47.0% and to 51.3%. In a second portion of the study, six pairs of samples were collected from each of 10 participants under the stimulation of 16 mg of pilocarpine HCl administered orally. Collection of parotid and extra-parotid samples began 10 min after parotid secretions were flowing freely, and six consecutive 10-min pairs of samples were taken

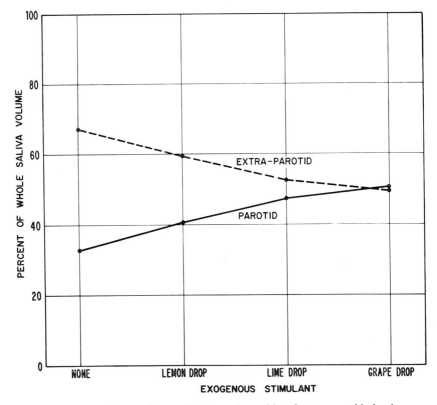

FIG. 12–3. Percentile contributions of parotid and extra-parotid glands to whole saliva volume (63 subjects).

from each subject. Parotid flow increased by 148.0% and extra-parotid flow increased by 84.2%. As flow rate increased, the percentile contribution of the parotid glands increased from 40.7% to 48.1%.

Another experiment involved the collection of both parotid and extra-parotid flow. During the first 90-min period the oral fluids were collected without exogenous stimulation. Each subject then provided a series of three 10-min stimulated sample pairs, parotid and extra-parotid, elicited with peppermint, cherry, and grape sour candy drops, in that order. Figure 12-3 outlines the contributions of parotid and extra-parotid glands to whole saliva volume on a percentage basis. As rate of flow increased, the extra-parotid percentage dropped from 67.1% to 59.3%, to 52.8%, and to 49.6% of total flow. The parotid contribution thus increased from 32.9% to 40.7%, to 47.2%, and to 50.4% in the sample pairs.

Thus we may conclude that in the resting state the greater portion of the whole saliva originates from extra-parotid sources. As increasing intensities of exogenous stimulation are applied, the parotid glands respond more strongly than the other glandular sources and, at a moderate rate of flow, they produce the major portion of the whole saliva. Experiments at high rates of flow have induced a parotid output in man that accounted for approximately two-thirds of the total saliva volume. This represents essentially a complete reversal of the situation found when measurements were made at the resting level of gland function.

Right Versus Left Gland Flow

The controversy concerning whether or not there is a true right or left salivary gland dominance in man can best be exemplified in findings of Korchin and Winsor and of Lashley. Korchin and Winsor collected unstimulated parotid saliva and found a significant left gland dominance in males and right gland dominance in females. They also studied subjects with exogenous stimulants and found that the same pattern of glandular dominance persisted. Dominance of hands, feet, eyes, and ears was not correlated in any way with gland dominance. On the other hand, Lashley collected unstimulated parotid saliva samples and found that the quantity of secretion from the two glands was almost exactly the same. Stimulation on one side induced a more copious flow from the gland on that side but bilateral stimulation affected both glands equally.

In 1928, Winsor found that when stimulation was applied evenly there was an agreement he termed "phenomenal" in the rate of functioning of the two sides. More recent studies, including ours, have shown no significant differences in the flow rate of the right and left glands with or without exogenous stimulation.

Systemic State of Hydration

There is considerable evidence to suggest that dehydration decreases the rate of human salivary flow. One study reported that 70 hours of water deprivation decreased parotid flow to one-sixth of its normal level. The ingestion of 1 L of water reinstituted normal flow patterns. The hydration, seasonal changes, and environmental temperatures of the body have been found to affect parotid flow. There was a decrease in rate of flow when male subjects moved to a hotter climate and, as the men became acclimatized, parotid flow increased somewhat, but in no case did it return to the original rate of flow. Other experiments indicated that parotid secretion was halted when water consumption was cut in half, permitting the conclusion that salivary flow is restricted under any condition that stimulates the body to conserve water.

Dehydration is an important etiological factor in acute suppurative parotitis, because it decreases flow rate to the point at which retrograde invasion of the parotid gland by oral bacteria is possible. Dehydration decreases the stimulated rate of gland function, but overloading the tissues with water by forced ingestion has no effect on salivary flow.

A compilation of flow rate data for different months, along with a statement of mean temperature over 2 years, is presented in Table 12–1. Flow rate was high in January, dropped to a low plateau in May, June, July, and August, and increased progressively to the high level by December. Differences among the months were highly significant.

A reciprocal relationship was noted between seasonal temperature and seasonal flow rate. The results of this study support an interrelationship between heat, dehydration, and depression of salivary flow rate. These observations become even more significant when it is realized that this was not a single group of subjects sampled repeatedly over a long period. Rather,

Table 12–1.   Parotid Fluid Flow Rate Responses and Mean Temperatures during Different Months (3868 Subjects)

Month	Number of Subjects	Mean Temperature	Parotid Flow Rate (ml/min) Mean	S.D.
Jan.	137	48.6	0.046	0.045
Feb.	432	51.2	0.040	0.036
Mar.	495	63.6	0.044	0.037
Apr.	365	72.6	0.039	0.031
May	225	77.6	0.031	0.027
June	304	82.9	0.030	0.030
July	438	85.8	0.033	0.029
Aug.	387	86.0	0.031	0.026
Sept.	298	80.6	0.035	0.026
Oct.	485	70.2	0.038	0.030
Nov.	189	62.5	0.044	0.032
Dec.	113	49.0	0.046	0.039

these differences are clearly evident even though different subjects are studied in each day of the 2-year experiment. The obvious conclusion is that the summer heat in San Antonio, Texas, where the exposure to cold is mild, led to a relative dehydration and that this systemic change produced, in turn, the lowered rate of parotid gland function.

It is thus evident that dehydration produces a significant decrease in salivary flow rate, but little work has been done to investigate the effect of hyperhydration on the rate of gland function. When 125 subjects were made to ingest either 0, 500, 1000, 1500, or 2000 ml of water in a 10-min period, the 4-hr urine excretion rates were 64 ml (S.D. = 22), 195 ml (S.D. = 114), 442 ml (S.D. = 197), 1026 ml (S.D. = 22), and 1072 ml (S.D. = 193), respectively. Figure 12–4 presents salivary flow rates before and at 1 and 2 hours after water ingestion, with salivary flow elicited by sucking on a grape sour candy drop. Under these conditions there was no significant effect of forced ingestion of fluid at any level.

Highly significant effects were noted, however, when the saliva samples were collected without exogenous stimulation (Fig. 12–5). For the groups receiving 0 to 500 ml of water, rate of flow during collection of the second sample was not significantly increased from the control value. For subjects ingesting 1000 ml or more, increases in the second sample were highly significant. These results clearly indicate that overloading the tissues with water exerts a significant effect on unstimulated salivary flow rate but not

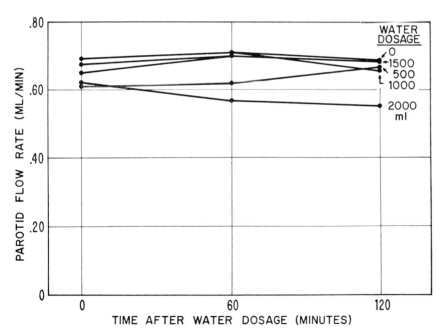

Fig. 12–4.   Effect of water ingestion on stimulated parotid flow rate (65 subjects).

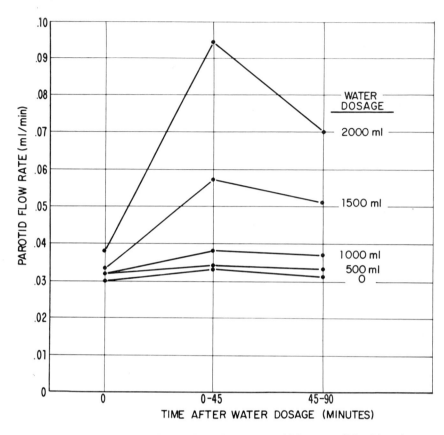

FIG. 12–5. Effect of water ingestion on parotid flow rate (25 subjects.)

on stimulated rate of flow. This result with stimulated flow is in accord with the consistent observation that the parotid gland may be stimulated at a high level for prolonged periods (certainly as long as 3 hours) with no decrease in rate of flow. Thus, normally there is a sufficient interstitial source of fluid to support long-term near-maximal flow, and evidently increasing the water load in the tissues does not elevate the level of output. It is reasonable to speculate that there is a theoretical point of interstitial tissue hyperhydration that, if exceeded, would increase salivary gland flow, but it was not reached even by the 2000-ml doses employed in this study.

Mental Exercise

There is no agreement as to the role of mental effort in the control of salivary gland function. Several investigators have placed subjects under conditions of strenuous mental exertion and attempted to correlate salivary flow rate patterns with the mental exercise. Some have found that such mental exertion increases the output of saliva. Others conclude that such periods of concentration either bring about decreases in flow, exert no significant effect at all, or increases or decreases in flow may result, depending upon the normal flow rate pattern of the individual subject.

In 1872, it was reported that mental stimulation did not alter the flow pattern appreciably in a woman patient with a parotid fistula. Research early in this century indicated that the quantity of saliva was smaller during mental activity than during repose, and that this could be interpreted as evidence that mental exercise was directly inhibitory in this regard.

Later experiments showed an unmistakable increase in parotid flow rate during a 20-min period while subjects were squaring three-place numbers as compared to a control period. Erotic emotion was found to decrease the rate of flow. Winsor noted that multiplying three-place numbers without visual aid brought about a definite decrease in parotid flow rate. In a later study he measured parotid flow rate while subjects underwent differing forms of mental exercise: solving mechanical puzzles, mirror drawing, threading needles, adding columns of figures, multiplying two-place numbers, crossing out vowels in printed material, and taking mental and achievement tests. There was a definite reduction in flow rate during any period of more or less intense attention. The extent of this inhibition was attributed to the type, duration, and intensity of the mental activity, and the inhibition was explained in terms of the restraining influence of the cerebral cortex.

Korchin found that the tasks assigned to elicit mental activity could, at times, bring about an inhibition in flow rate and, at other times, either increase parotid flow or not affect it at all. He believed that a crucial factor was the variation in the direction of the tension gradient between the control period and that during the mental activity.

Winsor and Korchin measured parotid flow rate while subjects were reading or working mathematical problems, and noted that mental activity may be accompanied by either an enhanced or an inhibited secretion rate, depending in part upon whether the problem allowed for greater or lesser release from the tension or mental activity involved in the control period. In general, subjects with a low normal rate of secretion exhibited a marked increase in flow rate while reading or engaged in arithmetical tasks, whereas subjects with high normal rates showed a partially inhibited flow while performing the same tasks.

More recent experimenters have concluded that about 10 times as much saliva was secreted during silent reading as during the periods of concentrated mental exercise, that mental excitation produced an increased salivary flow, and that parotid flow decreased in some instances when subjects were made to think of food with the suggestion that this inhibition might be due to the mental concentration involved.

From three experiments in 1969, I found no indication that mental exertion was in any way related to the rate of parotid gland function in healthy young adult men in the fasting state. The same type of mental exercise was employed in all three experiments. Subjects were instructed to add columns of whole numbers, four digits wide and four digits long, to complete as many problems as possible within the allotted time, but not to sacrifice accuracy for the sake of speed.

The first experiment involved the collection of two samples of unstimulated parotid saliva from each subject. Flow rate responses for the resting collections are outlined in Figure 12–6. In the control group (no mathematical problems), the flow rate means were 0.048 ml/min (S.D. = 0.038) and 0.047 ml/min (S.D. = 0.035). In the group working mathematical problems during the second collection interval, the means were 0.046 ml/min (S.D. = 0.026) and 0.047 ml/min (S.D. = 0.032). When the problems were solved during the first collection interval, the means were 0.046 ml/min (S.D. = 0.033) and 0.046 ml/min (S.D. = 0.028). Analyses of variance were performed on these data and no significant differences of any type were identified.

Subjects were then studied in an experiment with paraffin ($\frac{1}{4}'' \times \frac{1}{4}'' \times \frac{1}{2}''$ block) as an exogenous stimulant. The control group flow rate means were 0.224 ml/min (S.D. = 0.157) and 0.213 ml/min (S.D. = 0.125). When problems were solved during the second collection, the means were 0.236 ml/min (S.D. = 0.122) and 0.186 ml/min (S.D. = 0.105). Mental exercise did not exert a significant effect on parotid flow rate elicited by paraffin stimulation.

The third experiment was identical to the paraffin phase except that the eliciting agent was a 3-gm stick of sugared chewing gum. The gum bolus was renewed at 5-min intervals. Chewing gum provided flow rate means for the control group of 0.511 ml/min (S.D. = 0.252) and 0.501 ml/min (S.D. = 0.236). For those solving problems during the second sampling,

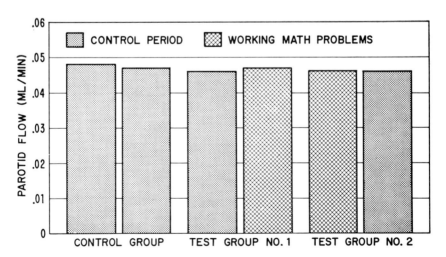

Fig. 12–6. Effect of mental exercise on parotid flow rate (no exogenous stimulation).

the means were 0.603 ml/min (S.D. = 0.230) and 0.602 ml/min (S.D. = 0.235). With the problems presented during the first collection period, the means were 0.521 ml/min (S.D. = 0.327) and 0.493 ml/min (S.D. = 0.275). Again, there was no significant effect of mental exertion on the rate of parotid gland function.

Although these results are not offered as positively ruling out cerebral factors as mediators of parotid gland function, it seems fair to interpret the results as conclusive for the experimental conditions imposed.

Suggestion, Sight, Sound, and Olfaction

Whether or not verbal suggestion exerts an influence on salivary gland function is controversial. It has been suggested that giving a stimulating solution a false identity significantly alters the rate of salivary flow. Other investigators have found that suggestions, either verbal or visual, exert no influence upon salivary gland function, or only vaguely discernible influence. A single example will suffice to demonstrate the several experiments that we have conducted in this area. In one of my experiments, 50 subjects participated in two sampling sessions, each subject providing four parotid fluid test samples at each session. The same gustatory stimuli, distilled water and 1.0% citric acid, were utilized at each session, but the suggestion varied for each sample.

The flow rate results are presented in Figure 12–7. The null hypothesis that suggestion does not influence parotid flow rate was tested with an analysis of variance approach. One factor was subjects and the other was

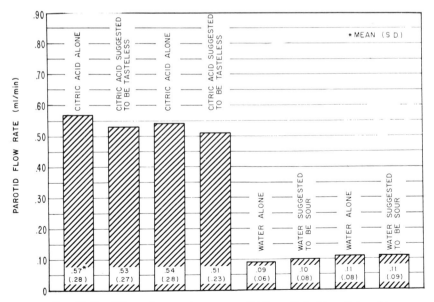

FIG. 12–7. Effect of suggestion on parotid flow elicited by citric acid and by water (N = 50).

treatments (introductory, stimulus suggested correctly, stimulus suggested incorrectly). Neither the suggestion that citric acid was tasteless nor that water was sour exerted a significant influence on the rate of the parotid salivary flow when compared to results for stimulation without suggestion.

Some investigators have found that suggestion may significantly affect rate of parotid secretion. One set of experiments measured parotid secretion rate in a group of 12 subjects selected as being relatively nonamenable to suggestion. The parotid secretion rate was greater when subjects received citric acid without suggestion than when citric acid was suggested to be sweet. The latter, in turn, was greater than the rate obtained when citric acid was suggested to be tasteless. The flow rate obtained when sucrose was suggested to be sour was greater than that for sucrose without suggestion, whereas sucrose suggested to be tasteless evoked the lowest secretory rate in this triad.

Other researchers presented water and citric acid sequentially to 16 subjects with and without direct verbal suggestions that water was sour and citric acid was tasteless. Half of the subjects had been rated as "highly suggestible" and half as relatively "nonsuggestible." Direct verbal suggestion significantly altered parotid gland secretion rates in both groups of subjects.

One group of experimenters summarized three experiments measuring the effect of verbal or symbolic stimulation on parotid flow rate and concluded that the parotid gland response to gustatory stimuli can be influenced by verbal suggestion but that the mechanisms involved remain obscure.

The results of these studies do not support the conclusion that suggestion influences rate of flow from the stimulated parotid gland. No direct comparisons with all studies can be made since experimental designs differ so distinctly.

Table 12–2. Parotid Flow under Varying Experimental Conditions

| | *Parotid Flow (ml/min)* | | | | | |
| | *Control Sample* | | *Test Sample* | | *Control Sample* | |
Experimental Conditions	*Mean*	*S.D.*	*Mean*	*S.D.*	*Mean*	*S.D.*
Watching lemon cut and squeezed	0.065	0.044	0.063	0.038	0.074	0.041
Cutting and squeezing lemon (nose clamp and gloves)	0.071	0.048	0.074	0.048	0.081	0.038
Cutting and squeezing lemon (nose clamp)	0.066	0.023	0.075	0.037	0.074	0.031
Sniffing cut lemon	0.066	0.037	0.114	0.062	0.060	0.039

There is also controversy as to whether or not speaking of food, as well as seeing or handling food, will significantly affect the rate of salivary flow. There is evidence in the literature that verbal reference to food and/or the sight of food increases secretion but others have found no increases under these conditions.

Although there is general agreement that olfactory stimulation increases the rate of salivary flow, agreement is by no means universal on whether this is a conditioned response or a true reflex mechanism.

Some experiments in these areas have been primarily involved with either watching lemons being cut, cutting lemons, or smelling freshly cut lemons.

Table 12–2 presents results from one experiment. The flow rate mean for the test sample did not differ significantly from its controls except when olfactory stimulation was a factor. Sniffing freshly cut lemon at 15-sec intervals elicited a significant (P = 0.01) increase in secretion rate.

General Body Factors

There is considerable evidence in the literature indicating that general body factors such as age, weight, height, blood pressure, and pulse rate do not affect the rate of salivary secretion.

In one body weight experiment, a series of three stimulated saliva samples were collected from each of 261 healthy young adult men. Exogenous stim-

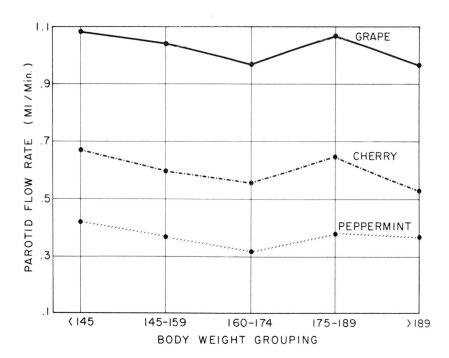

FIG. 12–8. Parotid flow rate for body weight groups (261 subjects).

ulants were, in order, peppermint, cherry, and grape candy drops. Figure 12–8 plots the results for flow rate in this experiment. Although some of the mean flow rates for the weight groups differed statistically, the differences in no way suggested a weight-related pattern.

In another study, a total of 1145 parotid saliva samples from 403 system-ically healthy young adult men were taken to ascertain the correlation be-tween body weight and parotid flow rate. Collections were made in the resting state and under varying degrees of gustatory stimulation. The rate of parotid gland function has been consistently independent of body weight, regardless of the elicitation procedure employed.

In an effort to ascertain the correlation between blood pressure and parotid flow rate, a total of 212 parotid fluid samples were collected from 104 healthy young adults. The rate of parotid gland function was invariably independent of blood pressure, regardless of the elicitation procedure employed.

Figure 12–9 presents the results when both flow rate and blood pressure were studied in 23 subjects. All mean differences, for both flow rate and blood pressure, between standing and sitting, sitting and lying, and standing and lying, were significant except for the sitting and lying diastolic blood pressures.

These studies demonstrate that posture exerts a significant effect upon the rate of parotid gland function and that a change in blood pressure, due to a change in body position, was associated with a change in the unstimulated rate of parotid flow. This study demonstrates that a change in blood pressure

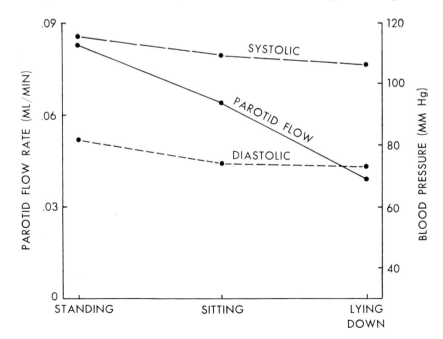

FIG. 12–9. Effect of body position on blood pressure and parotid flow rate.

can occur concomitantly with a change in the secretion of saliva. Blood pressure changes from different postural positions and from sleep vary in the same stepwise direction as the rate of function of the unstimulated human parotid gland. As was pointed out in the first study, however, differences in blood pressure among normal individuals are not related to significant differences in rate of salivary gland function.

As cited previously, it was found that sleep reduced the resting parotid flow rate mean to only 0.003 ml/min, and that in about 40% of the subjects there was no measurable flow at all. This low rate of function supports past results suggesting that the human parotid gland does not secrete spontaneously during sleep.

Light and Darkness

With others we have recently observed that the smoking of cigarettes exerts a significant stimulating effect on the resting salivary flow rate. Figure 12–10 demonstrates this effect on 50 subjects tested in the morning and in the afternoon. In the paper by Barylko-Pikielna and associates reporting the results, they pointed out that wearing of goggles that completely eliminated vision while smoking produced consistent and significant decreases in parotid secretion compared to smoking without visual obstruction. They also observed that resting parotid flow was significantly reduced in all subjects during blockage of vision. Although they admit that it is unclear as to why both resting levels and smoking in the absence of visual stimulation resulted

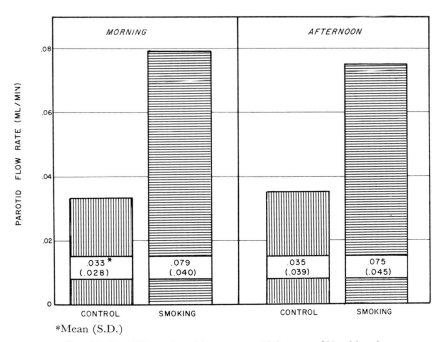

*Mean (S.D.)

FIG. 12–10. Effect of smoking on parotid flow rate (50 subjects).

in lowered secretion rates, they suggest that this inhibition of salivary secretion might occur in the process of interference with mental concentration or
attention that might be operative in blocking of the eyes of a vision-oriented
animal such as man. At present, there is no actual hypothesis developed to
explain the depressant effect of light deprivation on salivary gland function.

Experiments were undertaken to gain an understanding of the nature of
this light deprivation-induced salivary gland depression. In the first experiment, the subjects were five male dental students who had been providing
salivary samples, beginning at 6:30 A.M., 5 days per week for more than
2 years. This information on the subjects is cited to assure that factors such
as emotional stress are not involved in the effects that are to be shown.
Collections were made from the right parotid gland. All subjects were in the
fasting state. During the first 5 days of testing, a 20-min sample was collected from each subject without the blindfold in position. This was followed
immediately by a second 20-min sample during which the subjects were blindfolded. Precautions were taken to assure that light deprivation was complete. During the second 5-day collection period the procedure was reversed, with the subjects blindfolded during the first sampling interval. Thus,
there were 10 pairs of unstimulated flow rate (ml/min) data for each subject.
The overall mean flow rate without the blindfold (N = 100) was 0.057
ml/min (S.D. = 0.027), and 0.014 ml/min (S.D. = 0.014) with the blindfold
in place. The order of wearing the blindfold did not exert a significant

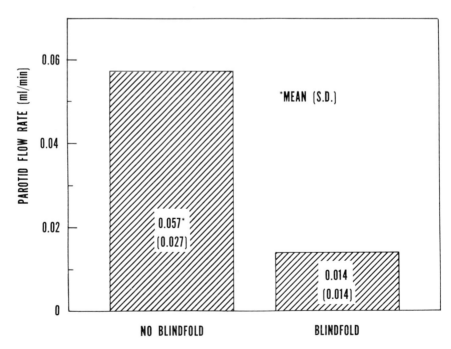

FIG. 12–11.   Light deprivation and unstimulated parotid flow.

effect. Means for unstimulated parotid flow for all collections with and without a blindfold are presented in Figure 12–11. This illustrates the 75% decrease in the rate of parotid gland function associated with light deprivation by blindfolding.

Once more the effect of visual deprivation on salivary gland function in smoking subjects was tested. The experimental conditions were identical to those outlined in the previous unstimulated flow rate light deprivation study, except that the subjects smoked continuously during the collection, both with and without a blindfold in position. When an unstimulated collection was made from these 20 subjects under routine laboratory conditions, except that they were smoking, the flow rate mean was 0.070 ml/min (S.D. = 0.037). When the conditions were identical except that a light-tight blindfold was in position, the flow rate mean fell significantly to 0.051 ml/min (S.D. = 0.038).

Since the possibility was present that the physical use of the blindfold might exert some effect other than light deprivation, supportive experiments were designed to test the light-darkness concept. The mean unstimulated parotid flow rate for five subjects over the full 10 days in routine laboratory light was 0.056 ml/min (S.D. = 0.028). Under identical conditions except with the room darkened, the flow rate decreased significantly (P = .01) to 0.028 ml/min (S.D. = 0.016). There was no significant difference between the two orders of sampling, differences between collection days were not significant, and there was no significant interaction between light, order, and days. Significant differences were found in the flow rate means for each subject for all 10 days in light and in darkness.

The next experiment in this series involved the collection of parotid saliva samples under the stimulus of chewing a 3-gm bolus of sugarless chewing gum. The deprivation of light by blindfolding caused a significant (P = .01) decrease in the rate of stimulated parotid function. Although this depression was significant, it was proportionately much less than that observed with unstimulated parotid fluid. This was suggestive that light deprivation was an active factor in the unstimulated flow but that it did not interfere with the parasympathetically mediated reflex flow. The significance of this observation will become clear later in this discussion.

In the third portion of this experiment, the experimenters were able to depress parotid gland function and derive meaningful inferences as to glandular management of biochemical constituents. The data for this experiment will be presented in the section on Biochemical Constituents of Saliva; however, a comment on what may be the mechanism underlying the effect of light deprivation on salivary gland function is offered now.

Feller and I have completed two additional studies on light and salivary flow. In the first, resting parotid flow rate was monitored under various lighting conditions. Cool-white fluorescent lighting (standard office and laboratory lighting), four narrow-spectrum (UV, blue, green, and red) source lighting, and absolute darkness were imposed on human subjects.

No mean resting flow rate change was observed under any lighting condition other than darkness. With darkness, the rate of flow decreased significantly ($P = .01$). Thus, the entire action spectrum of light is not necessary to induce the normal level of resting parotid secretion.

In the second study, light deprivation was found to decrease human submaxillary flow rate from 0.146 ml/min to 0.045 ml/min, a fall of 69%. It was also found that the parotid flow rate pattern remained constant over a relatively long period of imposed darkness. This suggested no accommodation by the gland. It was also noted that a light intensity as low as 0.1 footcandle was sufficient to maintain the usual level of resting parotid flow. Increasing intensity to 150 footcandles did not significantly increase this rate of flow.

For years there has been an awareness of the importance of the parasympathetic nervous system in the control of parotid gland function. It is known, at the same time, that the parotid gland does receive sympathetic innervation originating at about the T1-T2 level and following the sympathetic chain to the superior cervical ganglion and, from this point, along the blood vessels to the parotid gland. Definite statements can be made concerning parasympathetic stimulation and its effect on both experimental animals and man. Such parasympathetic stimulation invariably brings about both vasodilatation and saliva flow from the parotid gland in all species studied. Such definite statements cannot be safely made concerning the effects of sympathetic stimulation. There is no clear-cut evidence of stimulatory effects on secretion by sympathetic stimulation in the human being. The picture in experimental animals is even more confusing and it might be well to cite an example or two in this regard. Sympathetic stimulation produces flow from the cat submaxillary gland but not from the parotid gland. Conversely, sympathetic stimulation causes flow from the rabbit parotid gland but not from the submaxillary gland. Thus, the function of the sympathetic nervous system varies from species to species and its place in parotid function in man is not completely understood.

All of our flow rate results with light deprivation demonstrate a significant decrease in parotid function. We suggest photic stimulation of retinal receptors is responsible for a component of sympathetic neuronal activity that plays a part in control of human parotid secretion and that, indeed, may play a dominant role in maintaining the resting secretion of the gland. There are two principal reasons for this suggestion. First, specific sympathetic pathways are known to exist from the retina to the parotid gland by way of the superior cervical ganglion. Second, there are several striking similarities in the innervation and light-induced cyclic changes between the parotid gland and the pineal gland. The pineal gland is a neuroendocrine organ controlled by light through nerve fibers that leave the main visual pathway at the optic chiasma and reach the superior cervical ganglion. Both the pineal and the parotid glands are supplied by sympathetic fibers passing directly from this superior cervical ganglion.

There are chemical and electrophysiological similarities that are beyond the limits of this discussion, and recent electron microscopic observations have demonstrated that the adrenergic transmitter norepinephrine reaches all acinar cells as well as myoepithelial cells in the human parotid gland. There is, therefore, reason to believe that the sympathetic nervous system could contribute functional control to secretory potential in the human parotid gland. It was concluded that this suppression of parotid secretion produced by light deprivation is mediated via the sympathetic innervation of the glands and that the pathways and mechanisms involved may well be similar to those established for the pineal gland.

BIOCHEMICAL CONSTITUENTS OF SALIVA

Although it is not possible to deal at length with each of the biochemical constituents of saliva, some of the more general types of measurements made with this fluid can be discussed. Figure 12–12 demonstrates the highly significant positive correlation between the rate of gland function and the specific gravity of parotid saliva. My laboratory routinely employs peppermint, cherry, and grape candy drops, in that order, to provide the ascending order of gland function shown by the solid line on the graph. If specific gravity of these samples of parotid fluid is measured, a highly significant positive correlation exists between these two variables. That is, as the rate of stimulated gland function increases, the actual weight of dissolved substances per unit volume of saliva also increases in a stepwise fashion. This applies only to stimulated collections. The lowest stimulated flow rate mean shown in this figure, that for the peppermint-elicited collections, is less than 0.40 ml/min. The normal rate of unstimulated flow for a large group of subjects falls at approximately one-tenth of this level, approximately 0.04 ml/min. This information is included to demonstrate that, even at the low stimulated rate of flow shown in the peppermint samples, the gland is working at a tremendously increased level of function.

In another specific gravity experiment, peppermint-, cherry-, and grape-stimulated collections were made exactly as in the previous experiment. The only difference was that the stimulated collections were preceded by the collection of a 45-min nonstimulated sample from all participants. It was immediately evident that the positive correlation between flow and specific gravity noted in stimulated collections is completely reversed when the gland is allowed to flow at its resting level. In other words, as the unstimulated rate of gland function is increased significantly by the use of peppermint stimulus, there is an inverse change in specific gravity that constitutes a highly significant negative correlation between these two variables at these two flow rates. Again, this is exactly the opposite of the relation noted in stimulated parotid saliva.

To emphasize this relationship, Figure 12–13 demonstrates that exactly such a relationship as just seen for specific gravity exists between parotid

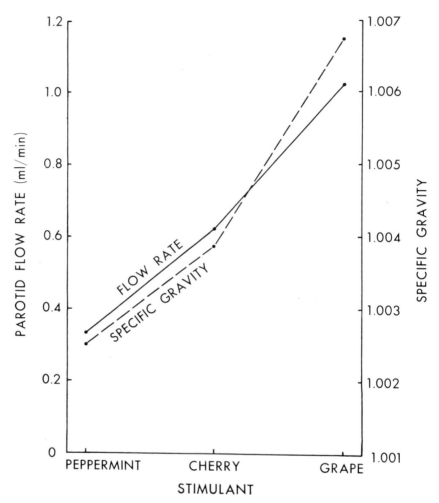

Fig. 12–12.   Effect of flow rate on parotid fluid specific gravity (314 subjects).

flow rate and total protein concentration.   Again, there is a highly significant positive correlation between flow and protein concentration in stimulated saliva, but when unstimulated collections are made, a negative correlation at this level of gland function between these two variables becomes evident.

Let us look at a variable in stimulated saliva that is not correlated with flow.   There is exactly such a correlation between the sialic acid values and flow rate when samples are collected with peppermint, cherry, and grape candy drops.   At the nonstimulated rate of flow, a negative correlation exists between sialic acid and flow rate.   That is, as flow rate is decreased there is a tremendous increase in sialic acid concentration.   We have seen that, if the variable is positively correlated with flow in stimulated saliva, or if it is devoid of correlation with flow rate in stimulated flow, there is still, for each

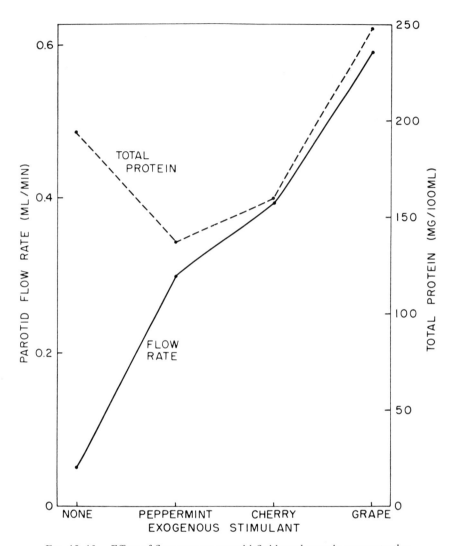

Fig. 12–13.   Effect of flow rate on parotid fluid total protein concentration.

of these two situations, a negative correlation between flow and concentration at the unstimulated level.

Figure 12–14 points out that in stimulated saliva (gum A, gum B, and gum C) there is a negative correlation between flow rate and secretory IgA concentration.   That is, as flow rate is increased in stimulated saliva, salivary IgA concentration decreases significantly.   When we direct our attention to the unstimulated collections, on the far left of Figure 12–14, we see that the same situation exists for IgA and flow rate, a highly significant negative correlation that we saw for specific gravity, for total protein, and

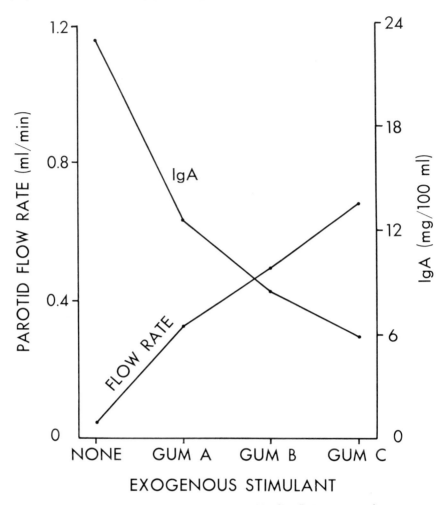

FIG. 12–14.   Effect of flow rate on parotid saliva IgA concentration.

for sialic acid.   All these variables of saliva, although differing significantly in their response to stimulation, demonstrate the same response in unstimulated fluid.

Let us now make a quick reference to osmolality, one of the measurements in a body fluid that is most meaningful when mechanisms of management are considered.   Figure 12–15 shows the highly significant positive correlation that exists in stimulated parotid saliva between flow rate and mOsm/kg. Although it is frequently stated that saliva is invariably hypotonic, it is not generally appreciated just how hypotonic the oral fluids actually are. Notice on the right side of the chart in Figure 12–15 that when flow rate is at its highest level, approximately 1.0 ml/min per parotid gland, the osmolality value is only 127 mOsm/kg.   This is far less than one-half of the osmo-

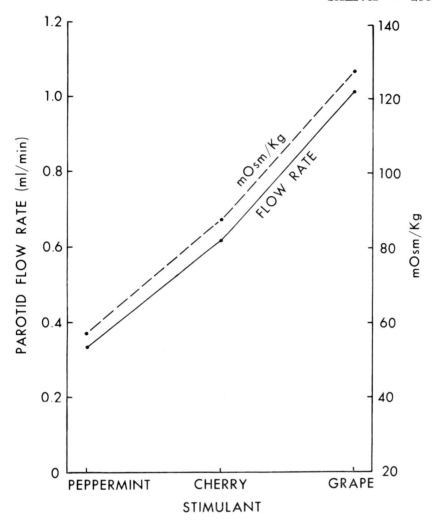

Fɪɢ. 12–15. Effect of flow rate on parotid fluid osmolality (314 subjects).

lality of plasma. As will be pointed out later in this discussion, regardless of the method employed to collect parotid saliva—extreme stimulation, no stimulation at all, and even drug-depressed unstimulated flow—this low osmolality ratio between parotid saliva and plasma persists.

In another study of osmolality, a group of 11 subjects was selected on the basis of high parotid flow rates. A total of 1,100 stimulated samples was collected from these subjects over a 4-week period. The subject with the highest flow rate mean for 100 samples, 2.25 ml/min, also had the highest osmolality mean, 180.4 mOsm/kg. Even at these high rates of flow it is impossible to obtain a parotid saliva that in any manner approaches plasma in osmolality.

Although it is not shown in Figure 12–15, the osmolality response in unstimulated parotid fluid is exactly that which we have seen in earlier parts of this presentation. That is, although a highly significant positive correlation exists between flow rate and osmolality in stimulated saliva, a highly significant negative correlation exists between these two variables in the unstimulated rate of flow.

To this point, the saliva discussed had been collected with exogenous stimulants, and the results compared one stimulant with another. Statements were also made concerning the means for a large group of individuals from whom unstimulated saliva had been collected. Unfortunately, it is not possible when collecting nonstimulated saliva to direct glandular activity to the point where one can study rate of flow at more than one level in each individual. There is, however, another way that this situation can be viewed. Figure 12–16 presents osmolality means for subjects who have furnished unstimulated parotid fluid samples. These 503 subjects were divided into five groups based upon the unstimulated rate of flow. The longest bar, on the far left, denoting the highest osmolality, is for the sub-

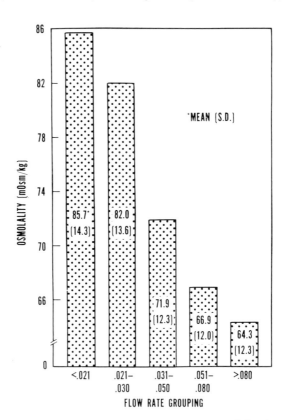

Fig. 12–16. Effect of flow rate on parotid fluid osmolality (503 subjects).

jects with unstimulated rates of flow at 0.020 ml/min or less. The shortest bar, on the far right, represents the subjects whose unstimulated rate of flow was more than 0.080 ml/min. This figure may be looked upon as representing an extension of the negative correlation between osmolality and flow rate that we saw exhibited when we compared peppermint-stimulated saliva to nonstimulated saliva for the entire group of subjects. The implication in this figure is clear—the longer the low flowing parotid saliva lies in the ductal apparatus of the gland, the more concentrated it becomes. Virtually all the constituents of parotid saliva give a result that is similar to that seen in this osmolality figure. This suggests the possibility of what might be classified as an "apparent" increase in the various constituents, and that all of these increases, as flow rate is decreased, may be related to removal of water from the luminal fluid.

There is one exception to this pattern of increase in concentration at the lower rates of flow. That exception is sodium and, if we printed a figure of sodium values for these 503 subjects divided into these five flow rate groups, there would be no significant differences between the means for the five groups. This is a peculiarity of sodium that will become more important as we pursue this discussion further. Please let the point be made once more that, at the nonstimulated rate of flow, the physiological rate of flow if you will, the lower the rate of flow the more concentrated the saliva becomes, and this is highly suggestive of water resorption from the luminal fluid.

A study was conducted on the effect of rate of flow on glucose concentration in 507 subjects who provided unstimulated parotid saliva samples. Again, a highly significant negative correlation between flow and the variable under study was seen.

Armed with the foregoing information on glandular management, studies were made on the unstimulated flow at an even lower level. Figure 12–17 gives flow rate and osmolality for a group of 20 subjects before and after the administration of atropine sulfate. Before administration of atropine the unstimulated salivary flow rate mean for these 20 subjects was 0.053 ml/min (S.D. = 0.031) and after atropine dosage this mean decreased significantly (P = 0.01) to 0.023 ml/min (S.D. = 0.014). Along with this highly significant decrease in rate of flow induced by atropine administration, the osmolality mean increased significantly (P = 0.01) from 48.6 mOsm/kg (S.D. = 15.76) to 83.5 mOsm/kg (S.D. = 35.81). Thus, the negative correlation between osmolality and flow rate within a group of subjects providing unstimulated samples is manifest even more when the unstimulated rate of flow is depressed significantly by the administration of this anticholinergic agent.

A large number of other variables were studied by the atropine approach. Figure 12–18 demonstrates the type of change that took place with some of these variables. The solid lines below the horizontal midpoint of this figure represent the percentage decrease in rates of flow for the different groups of

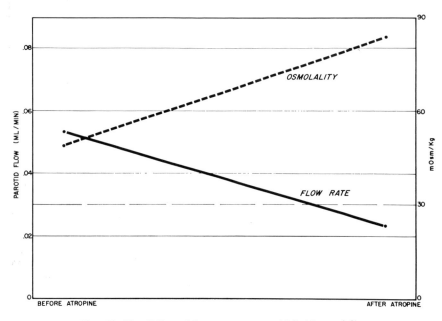

FIG. 12–17. Effect of flow rate on parotid fluid osmolality.

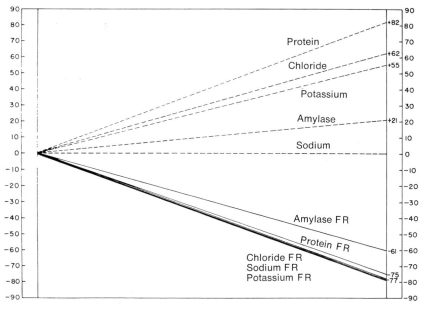

FIG. 12–18. Per cent changes in flow rate (solid line) and concentrations (broken lines) after administration of atropine.

subjects employed to study each variable. The broken lines above the mid-point of the figure represent the percentage increases in the various variables represented here. These include protein, chloride, potassium, and amylase, all of which increased significantly with decreases in flow rate brought about by administration of atropine. The significant point in this figure, and the fact to be emphasized particularly, is that the concentration of sodium did not change at all following the administration of atropine. The unbroken flow rate line demonstrates a significant decrease in flow associated with administration of atropine to the sodium group but the horizontal broken line shows that the sodium concentration did not change.

The actual means for flow rate and sodium concentration before and after the administration of atropine follow. Flow rate was depressed from 0.052 ml/min (S.D. = 0.028) to 0.012 ml/min (S.D. = 0.006). Along with this highly significant decrease in flow rate, the sodium mean for the unstimulated samples was 2.0 mEq/L (S.D. = 1.38) and after administration of atropine the sodium level remained at exactly this 2.0 mEq/L (S.D. = 1.30) level.

Recalling our observations on the effect of light and light deprivation on parotid flow rate, we designed an experiment to determine whether light deprivation could be substituted for administration of atropine and, in this drug-free state, the biochemical observations could be duplicated. Blindfolding brought about a significant (P = 0.01) decrease in unstimulated parotid flow from 0.056 ml/min (S.D. = 0.025) to 0.026 ml/min (S.D. = 0.015). With this significant decrease in gland function, the potassium concentration increased from 29.9 mEq/L (S.D. = 0.91) to 38.3 mEq/L (S.D. = 3.71) and chloride increased from 19.3 mEq/L (S.D. = 0.96) to 24.9 mEq/L (S.D. = 2.02). Each of these changes in concentration was highly significant. The means for all four variables are presented in Figure 12–19. The upper left section of the graph shows the significant decrease in flow rate, the lower left shows a significant increase in potassium concentration, the lower right shows a significant increase in chloride concentration, and the upper right portion demonstrates the point that the difference between the sodium means before and after blindfolding was not significant. The mean for sodium concentration under routine lighting was 5.82 mEq/L (S.D. = 3.18); with the blindfold in position it was 6.00 mEq/L (S.D. = 3.57). The chemical changes that took place under atropine were identical to those in the blindfolded patients.

The lack of effect of flow rate on sodium concentration at the low ranges of flow rate in this discussion probably results from a balanced outward diffusion of water from the luminal fluid caused by sodium resorption. Thus, at these low rates of flow, sodium appears to be the trigger ion. Resorption of sodium from the luminal fluid produces a gradient down which water flows. This resorption of water in proportion to the amount of sodium removed from the fluid maintains the sodium level in the luminal fluid in

SELECTED REFERENCES

BARYLKO-PIKIELNA, N., DANGBORN, R. M., and SHANNON, I. L.: Effect of cigarette smoking on parotid secretion. Arch. Environ. Health, *17*, 731, 1968.

BURGEN, A. S. V., and EMMELIN, N. G.: *Physiology of the Salivary Glands.* Baltimore, Williams & Wilkins, 1961.

ENFORS, B.: The parotid and submandibular secretion in man. Acta Otolaryngol., (Suppl.) *172*, 1, 1962.

KERR, A. C.: *The Physiological Regulation of Salivary Secretions in Man.* New York, Pergamon Press, 1961.

KORCHIN, B., and WINSOR, A. L.: Glandular dominance in humans. J. Exp. Psychol., *27*, 184, 1940.

LASHLEY, K. S.: Reflex secretion of the human parotid gland. J. Exp. Psychol., *1*, 461, 1916.

SCHEYER, L. H., and LEVIN, L. K.: Rate of secretion by individual salivary gland pairs of man under condition of reduced exogenous stimulation. J. Dent. Res., *34*, 725, 1955 (Abstract).

SCHNEYER, L. H., and SCHNEYER, C. A.: *Secretory Mechanisms of Salivary Glands.* New York, Academic Press, 1967.

SHANNON, I. L.: Effect of mental exercise on parotid flow rate in the human. Texas Dent. J., *87*, 10, 1969.

SHANNON, I. L., and FELLER, R. P.: Effects of lights of specific spectral characteristics on human resting parotid gland function. Arch. Oral Biol., *19*, 1077–1078, 1974.

SHANNON, I. L., SUDDICK, R. P., and DOWD, F. J., JR.: *Saliva: Composition and Secretion.* New York, Karger Press, 1974.

SHANNON, I. L., SUDDICK, R. P., and EDMONDS, E. J.: Effect of rate of gland function of parotid saliva fluoride concentration in the human. Caries Res., 7, 1, 1973.

SREEBNY, L. M., and MEYER, J.: *Salivary Glands and Their Secretions.* New York, Macmillan, 1964.

SUDDICK, R. P., and DOWD, F. J., JR.: The microvascular architecture of the rat submaxillary gland: Possible relationship to secretory mechanisms. Arch. Oral Biol., *14*, 567–576, 1969.

WINSOR, A. L.: Conditions affecting human parotid secretion. J. Exp. Psychol., *11*, 355, 1928.

Chapter **13**

The Acquired Enamel Integuments: Pellicle, Plaque and Calculus

ROBERT R. WHITE, Ph.D.

Several renewable organic films develop on the enamel surface after eruption of the tooth. These films, called the acquired enamel integuments, may be removed by brushing or abrasion, but they reappear repeatedly. Numerous names appear in the literature describing these films but a standard nomenclature has been suggested (Table 13–1). The acquired pellicle, dental plaque, and dental calculus are of especial interest not only from a biological viewpoint but also as a result of their roles in the pathologic changes in the dentition and periodontium.

ACQUIRED PELLICLE

The acquired pellicle is the acellular and bacteria-free organic film primarily composed of salivary glycoproteins lying immediately over the enamel. If the surface of a tooth is cleaned with an abrasive to remove all of the material covering the enamel, or if cleaned enamel slabs or mylar strips are placed in the oral cavity where they may be bathed with saliva, an organic film, the acquired pellicle, will form rapidly (Figs. 13–1 and 13–2). The deposition of pellicle begins within minutes after exposure to saliva and the initial layers are essentially complete within 90 minutes. This "short-term" pellicle may continue to grow slowly by additional deposition of salivary glycoproteins or bacteria may adsorb to its surface initiating formation of plaque.

The pellicle is found on the dentition throughout the oral cavity. Its thickness is determined by the abrasive forces of mastication and the formation of the overlying integument, dental plaque. It can be differentiated from plaque by the relative absence of bacteria and by the fact that, unlike dental plaque, it cannot be removed by toothbrushing. Application of an

Table 13–1. Nomenclature of the Acquired Integuments of the Teeth

Name	Description	Previous Names
Acquired pellicle	a. A cuticle acquired after eruption	1. Mucin plaque 2. Acquired cuticle 3. Plaque and film 4. Dental cuticle 5. Enamel cuticle 6. Brown pellicle 7. Acquired enamel cuticle 8. Dental plaque 9. Posteruption cuticle
Food debris	b. Food debris	1. Materia alba 2. Sordes 3. Food debris
Dental plaque	c. A dense bacterial layer	1. Plaque 2. Materia alba 3. Muco-bacterial film
Calculus	d. Calcified material	1. Calculus 2. Tartar

From Dawes, C., Jenkins, G. N., and Tonge, C. H.: The nomenclature of the integuments of the enamel surface of the teeth, Brit. Dent. J., *115*, 65–68, 1963.

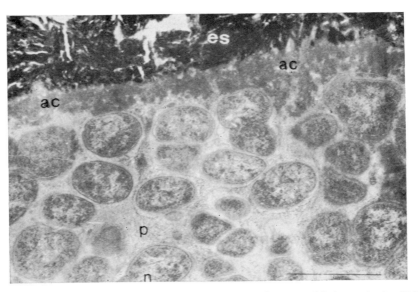

FIG. 13–1. Electron micrograph of tooth section showing enamel (es), acquired pellicle (AC), and plaque (P). ×30,000. (From Frank, R. M., and Houver, G.: An ultrastructural study of human supragingival dental plaque formation. In *Dental Plaque*. W. D. McHugh (Ed.). Edinburgh, E. & S. Livingstone Ltd., 1970, pp. 85–108.)

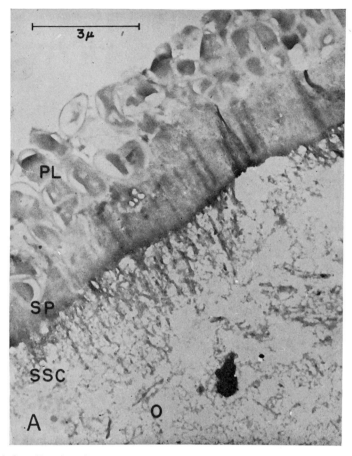

FIG. 13–2a. Demineralized cross section of tooth's surface showing structures described by Meckel, including plaque (PL), stained pellicle (SP), and subsurface cuticle (SSC). O is the organic residue of enamel. (From Meckel, A. H.: The formation and properties of organic films on teeth, Arch. Oral Biol., *10*, 585–597, 1965.)

abrasive such as pumice is necessary for removal of the pellicle from the enamel surface.

Although the acquired pellicle is usually referred to as a single structure, Meckel subdivided the acquired pellicle into three layers based on electron microscopic observations. These are the subsurface cuticle, the surface cuticle, and the stained pellicle (Fig. 13–2a and b). These "cuticles" should not be confused with the primary enamel cuticle, a product of the embryological development of the tooth. The subsurface cuticle is a network of fibrils extending into the enamel. Apparently it is pellicle material that has penetrated through defects in the enamel surface. The subsurface cuticle ranges from 1 to 3 μm in depth and is present on enamel surfaces damaged by previous injury or demineralization. The surface cuticle is a

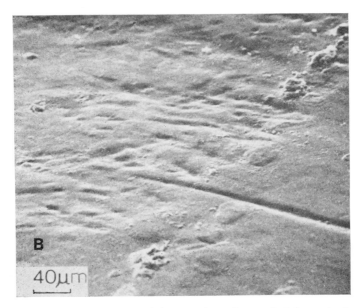

Fɪɢ. 13–2b. The formation of pellicle on a cleaned enamel surface. A piece of tape protected the upper left half of a cleaned tooth from saliva. After 1 hr. the tape was removed. The layer of organic film masks the scratches in the enamel surface on the lower right half. ×225. (Courtesy of C. A. Saxton, Unilever Research, from Scanning electron microscope study of the formation of dental plaque, Caries Res., 7, 102–119, 1973.)

layer of amorphous material immediately covering the enamel. Meckel reported that the surface cuticle was approximately 0.2 μm thick. However, it has been demonstrated that this cuticle may be 5 μm or more in thickness. The outermost part of the acquired pellicle, the stained pellicle, is a smooth brownish layer ranging in depth from 1 to 10 μm. Although Meckel differentiated the stained pellicle from the surface cuticle, it may be simply a part of the cuticle that has taken up stain. It is also possible that it may be the result of bacterial infiltration and metabolism within the pellicle. All teeth do not necessarily possess a demonstrable pellicle, nor are all three layers discernible when a pellicle is present.

Chemical Composition

Correlation of different chemical analyses of pellicles is complicated due to differences in the pellicle preparations analyzed. Mature pellicle and pellicle recently formed on cleaned enamel or mylar strips placed in the mouth (short-term pellicle) have been used for analyses. Pellicle has been harvested by scraping the enamel surface and removing the scrapings with a pipette or by acid demineralization of the surface of extracted teeth. Studies of the pellicle removed by demineralization have also varied with respect to the material analyzed; some have used only the acid-insoluble portion of pellicle, whereas others have combined both soluble and insoluble portions, the "total" pellicle.

Assays of hydrolyzed plaque indicate that 45 to 50% of the acquired pellicle is composed of amino acids. Amino acid analyses of different pellicle preparations are shown in Table 13–2. In all samples there are high concentrations of acidic amino acids and low concentrations of sulfur-containing amino acids. The acidic amino acids are expected because of their known tendency to adsorb to hydroxyapatite. There are some variations in the preparations, especially with regard to serine, tyrosine, glycine, and

Table 13–2. Amino Acid Composition of Pellicles, Plaque, and Saliva (residues per 1000 residues)

	Pellicle Samples				*Subman-dibular-Parotid Saliva Mixture‡*
	Scraped Short Term*	*Mature Insoluble Acid Extract†*	*Mature Total Acid Extract‡*	*24-Hr Plaque Matrix†*	
ASP	74	70	89.0	76.8	73
THR	36	37	47.4	10.7	45
SER	100	57	147.1	50.0	43
GLU	128	147	132.7	185.5	209
PRO	23	64	61.9	270.3	88
GLY	160	128	151.7	169.9	99
ALA	75	125	79.9	23.6	186
VAL	42	53	36.7	21.3	54
MET	—	—	6.1	1.5	—
ILEU	30	32	26.5	15.5	27
LEU	62	59	56.1	25.6	55
TYR	19	34	28.2	19.2	22
PHE	30	38	30.5	16.6	25
LYS	68	58	37.6	46.3	44
HIS	42	35	28.1	18.8	13
ARG	40	63	28.9	43.8	13
MET S			Tr	Tr	
DAP	—	—	Tr	0	
CYS	10		8.4	0.9	
CYS 2			3.7	4.1	

* Estimated from Sonju, T., and Rolla, G.: Caries Res., 7, 30–38, 1973.
† Leach, S. A., Critchley, P., Kolendo, A. P., and Saxton, C.: Caries Res., 1, 104–111, 1967.
‡ Mayhall, C. W.: Arch. Oral Biol., 15, 1327–1341, 1970.

alanine. These large variations reflect the variations in the times and methods of sampling.

The carbohydrate content of different pellicle preparations also varies. Armstrong reported that the pellicle contained 10 to 15% carbohydrates, whereas Mayhall reported an average of 5.6 mg of carbohydrate per 100 mg of ash-free sample. Glucose, fucose, mannose, galactose, glucosamine, and galactosamine are present in the pellicle. Glucose makes up over 60% of the carbohydrates in short-term pellicle. Since salivary proteins are considered to be the source of pellicle material, the absence of sialic acid, a carbohydrate unique to such glycoproteins, is unusual. However, its absence has been attributed to enzymatic degradation by oral bacteria.

Despite the definition "bacterial-free" it is apparent that there is some bacterial invasion of mature pellicle samples. The extent of this bacterial invasion varies with the age and location of the pellicle. Detection of muramic acid, diaminopimelic acid, and rhamnose, all bacterial markers, in pellicle analyses indicates that bacteria are present. The concentrations of these compounds range from none to minimal, or trace, contaminants in short-term pellicle to much greater concentrations in older pellicle. Armstrong reported that as much as 40% of his sample could have been of bacterial composition. However, since pellicles form in germ-free animals, it is apparent that bacteria are not necessary for their formation.

The chemical composition of pellicle resembles that of glycoproteins, and its formation is primarily the result of salivary glycoprotein deposition. However, the amino acid compositions of pellicle preparations vary from that of saliva (Table 13–2). This variation probably results from selective adsorption of salivary proteins. Indirect evidence of this selectivity is suggested by the high degree of similarity in amino acid analyses of short-term pellicles collected in different areas of the mouth. Nonspecific adsorption of salivary proteins would be expected to result in variable analyses, reflecting the composition of the saliva bathing the particular area.

The selective adsorption of specific salivary proteins to enamel or hydroxyapatite has been reported by several investigators. Hay isolated several proteins from parotid saliva that have much higher affinity for hydroxyapatite than do other salivary proteins. These included two small acidic proteins and four proline-rich proteins. A high molecular weight protein capable of aggregating bacteria and of adsorbing to tooth enamel also has been described. This protein may be involved not only in pellicle formation but also in plaque formation.

Specific identification of some of the proteins present in the pellicle has been accomplished through immunofluorescence. Short-term pellicles formed on enamel slabs placed in the mouth have been analyzed with specific immune sera. Thirteen different proteins were detected in the pellicle, including albumin, immunoglobulins, complement components, amylase, lactoferrin, fibrinogen, and lysozyme. The specific mechanisms by which these particular proteins are incorporated into the pellicle are unknown.

Formation

Formation of the pellicle is probably a result of several different mechanisms. The initial molecular layers of the short-term pellicle are probably composed of the proteins described by Hay and others—those that selectively adsorb directly to the enamel. Once this layer has completely coated the enamel, other mechanisms probably predominate. Two that have been suggested and for which there is evidence are precipitation of salivary glycoproteins following bacterial degradation and precipitation of these proteins as a result of increased salivary pH.

Undenatured salivary glycoproteins are soluble at pH 7.0. However, if the sialic acid moiety is cleaved from these proteins, the normal molecular configuration of these proteins is disrupted, there is a shift in the isoelectric point, and the proteins become insoluble at a pH near neutrality. Thus, they precipitate out of saliva and can adsorb to the teeth. Oral bacteria are known to possess the enzyme neuraminidase which hydrolyzes the sialic acid from glycoproteins. Incubation of fresh saliva with oral bacteria *in vitro* results in loss of the sialic acid and formation of glycoprotein precipitates. This theory of protein deposition to form pellicle is substantiated by the absence of sialic acid from the pellicle.

Another mechanism of deposition of pellicle material has been proposed by Kleinberg. As the saliva enters the oral cavity it loses carbon dioxide with a subsequent increase in pH. This rise in pH is within the range demonstrated by Kleinberg to cause precipitation of salivary glycoproteins through formation of a protein-carbohydrate-calcium phosphate complex. As the saliva passes over the tooth's surface these complexes could adsorb to enamel or the previously deposited layers.

The properties of the acquired pellicle vary as it matures. Pellicle removed from teeth within hours after formation is much more susceptible to acid solubilization than that removed several days later. This may result from denaturation, either surface or bacterial, of the glycoproteins. The laminar appearance of pellicle, which has been described by several investigators, is also indicative of changes in pellicle during maturation. The lamination may result from periodic deposition of different materials or alteration of the outermost surfaces at different times with subsequent overlayering of new materials.

Function

Both protective and harmful functions have been attributed to the acquired pellicle. The pellicle can act as the initial matrix to which oral bacteria adhere to initiate formation of plaque with its subsequent injurious effect. Electron micrographs demonstrate the colonization of the pellicle by oral bacteria. However, bacteria can initiate plaque formation in the absence of the acquired pellicle.

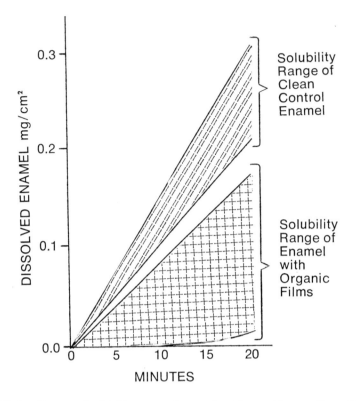

Fig. 13–3. Ranges of solubility rates of enamel, with or without salivary films, immersed in 0.1 N lactic acid, pH 4.0. (Modified from Meckel, A. H.: The nature and importance of organic deposits on dental enamel, Caries Res., 2, 104–114 1968.)

On the other hand, it has been demonstrated experimentally that the acquired pellicle has definite protective properties in the retardation of enamel demineralization (Fig. 13–3). This protective effect has been attributed to two possible mechanisms. The pellicle may act as a barrier to diffusion of acids from plaque to the enamel surface; a phenomenon that would tend to retard the demineralization of the enamel by decreasing the concentration of the demineralizing agent. The second mechanism proposed is enhancement of the remineralization process. The presence of the pellicle retards diffusion of the calcium and phosphate ions from the area of demineralization and the entrapped minerals may increase the efficiency of the remineralization process. The dissolution of enamel is not inhibited, rather the repair process is enhanced by the elevated levels of necessary minerals. Both processes may occur, and the possible significance of each under natural conditions has yet to be determined.

DENTAL PLAQUE

Dental plaque is the organic film, usually overlying the acquired pellicle, composed of bacteria and their products, and constituents derived from saliva and gingival fluid. Plaque is a complex and dynamic ecological system. As it develops on a newly cleansed tooth surface, its cellular and intercellular components are in a state of flux in response to the endogenous contributions of the host, the exogenous contributions of diet, and the ever-changing interrelationships of the bacterial populations within it. It is apparent that plaque varies from mouth to mouth, from tooth to tooth in the same mouth, and even from surface to surface on the same tooth. On a cleansed tooth, plaque may be seen to build up from the gingival margin and spread over the tooth's surface. In the absence of oral hygiene, it can cover the gingival areas of the tooth within days. The thickness of plaque is limited by the abrasive effects of the masticatory movements of teeth and the movements of tongue and cheeks. Plaque is thickest in protected areas such as the gingival crevice, the interproximal spaces, pits and fissures, and areas of slight imperfections of the teeth. If the normal occlusive forces are absent, plaque will form over normally plaque-free surfaces.

Plaque is divided into two major types: supragingival and subgingival. Of these, the former has received the most study, and information on it far outweighs that which is known concerning subgingival plaque. This emphasis on supragingival plaque reflects the relative ease with which it can be obtained for study. Supragingival plaque receives contributions of bacterial nutrients and matrix components from saliva and ingested foods. There is a small contribution from gingival fluid. Subgingival plaque probably receives its major contributions from gingival fluid, with smaller contributions from diet and saliva. Although differences in nutrients can influence the composition of plaque, an even more important factor is the differences in oxygen potential. This is the principal determinant of the bacterial flora. Because of its sequestered location, subgingival plaque supports a larger population of anaerobic bacteria than supragingival plaque.

Bacterial Composition

Bacteria are the major constituents of plaque (Fig. 13–4). Total microscopic counts of bacteria (viable and nonviable cells) are reported to be as high as 2.5×10^{11} cells per gram of supragingival plaque. Viable counts of aerobic and anaerobic bacteria were 2.5 and 4.6×10^{10}, respectively. Gingival debris adjacent to subgingival plaque has been reported to contain 2×10^{11} bacterial cells per gram of debris. Since a preparation of centrifuge-packed bacterial cells has a similar density, this indicates that these plaques were composed almost entirely of bacteria. However, the number of cells per unit of plaque is subject to variation, because the diet of the individual influences the volume of the extracellular matrix. For example, plaque

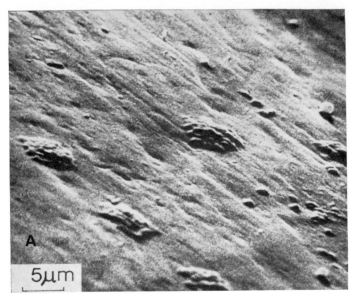

Fig. 13–4a. Formation of plaque on cleansed enamel surface at 24 hr. ×2,000. (Courtesy of C. A. Saxton, Unilever Research, from Scanning electron microscope study of the formation of dental plaque, Caries Res., 7, 102–119, 1973.)

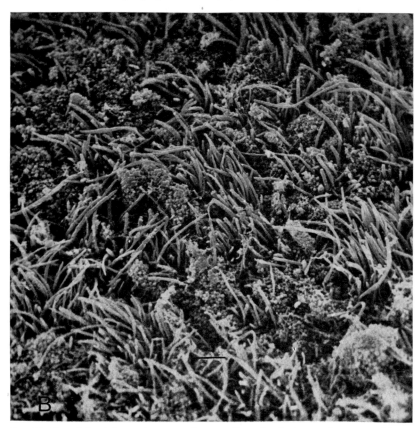

Fig. 13–4b. Mixed flora of mature plaque. Coccal colonies are interspersed between groups of filaments. Field width is 100 μm. (From Jones, S. J.: The tooth surface in periodontal disease, Dent. Pract., 22, 462–473, 1972.)

formed in the presence of a high sucrose diet can contain as much as 30% extracellular polysaccharides based on wet weights.

At least 27 different types of bacteria have been reported to be present in plaque. This figure probably errs on the low side as a result of inadequate methods of cultivating all of the species of bacteria in plaque. The bacterial flora in plaque varies depending on the age and location of the plaque and the diet of the individual from whom it is obtained.

Ritz followed the bacterial populations in supragingival plaque developing on cleaned tooth surfaces for 9 days (Fig. 13–5). Initially, high levels of aerobic bacteria were present. These declined with time, and there was a concomitant increase in numbers of anaerobic bacteria as the plaque increased in weight. The predominant bacteria throughout the study were facultative (either aerobic or anaerobic) streptococci. Their total numbers were highest initially and declined only slightly over the 9-day period. Studies on the distribution of the three types in plaque established that the aerobes were present in the outer layers, the anaerobes were in the deepest areas of plaque, and the facultative organisms could be found throughout the plaque.

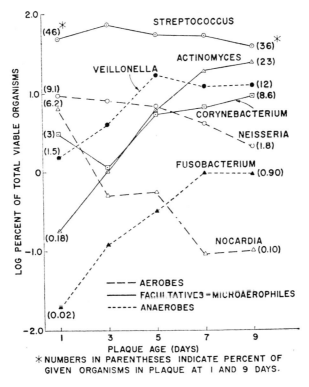

Fig. 13–5. Relative proportions of selected organisms in developing plaque. (From Ritz, H. L.: Microbial population shifts in developing human dental plaque, Arch. Oral Biol., *12*, 1561–1568, 1967.)

As plaque grows, there is also a change in the morphological types of bacteria present. Initially, the bacterial flora consists of gram-positive cocci and rods. This gradually changes to a complex population containing gram-positive cocci and rods, gram-negative cocci and rods, filaments, and spiral forms. The changes in bacterial composition in developing plaque are due, in large part, to the thickening of the plaque layer, resulting in anaerobiosis in the plaque nearer the tooth's surface. The oxygen that permeates the outer layer of plaque is consumed by the aerobes at the surface, rendering the inner layers anaerobic. That the increasing complexity of the bacterial flora is a result of the increasing anaerobiosis is reflected in subgingival plaque; in this sequestered area the bacterial flora at 2 days resembles that of 1- to 2-week-old supragingival plaque.

The large amount of dialyzable material found in plaque indicates plaque has diffusion-limiting properties. The structure of plaque varies from a gel to a floc depending on the dietary status of the individual. Fasting plaque

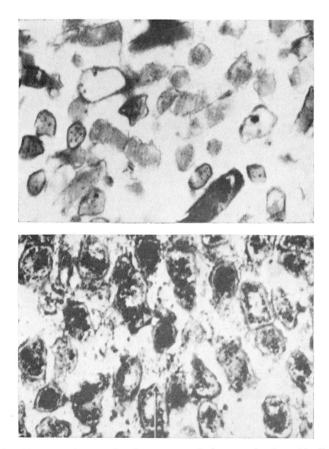

Fig. 13–6. Electron micrographs of sugar-starved plaque stained specifically for carbohydrates before (top) and 6 min after (bottom) rinsing the mouth with sucrose solution. (From Leach, S. A.: Plaque chemistry and caries, Ala. J. Med. Sci., *5*, 247–255, 1968.)

is probably a floc with spaces between the aggregated bacterial cells. The floc structure allows exchange of dietary, salivary, and bacterial constituents. After meals, accumulations of bacterial by-products within the intercellular spaces convert the plaque to a less permeable gel (Fig. 13–6). During subsequent fasting periods the plaque reverts to a floc as a result of bacterial utilization of the extracellular matrix.

Chemical Composition

Plaque consists of approximately 80% water, most of which is found within bacterial cells. The remainder is in the acellular portion of the plaque either bound to other components such as proteins or free within the matrix. Krembel and co-workers separated mature dental plaque into its cellular and acellular components and analyzed it (Table 13–3). Lipids and carbohydrates predominate in the acellular or matrix fraction, whereas proteins and nucleotide-like materials predominate in the cellular or bacterial portion. About 25 to 30% of the acellular matrix is dialyzable.

It is assumed that the protein found in the matrix of plaque is primarily of salivary origin, since the amino acid composition of water-extractable plaque protein is similar to that of salivary glycoproteins (Table 13–2). Thus, the protein of the extracellular plaque matrix and that of the acquired pellicle are derived from the same source and probably deposited by some of the same mechanisms.

Silverman and Kleinberg subjected the solubilized acellular matrix of plaque to column chromatography and found 11 different protein-containing fractions, all having molecular weights greater than 100,000. Most of the fractions contained both calcium and phosphate bound to the large molecular weight components.

Specific identification of some of the proteins of the plaque matrix has been carried out using immunological methods. Material from the plaque adjacent to the gingival tissue has been shown to contain immunoglobulin G, immunoglobulin A, and the enzyme amylase. The significance of these particular proteins with regard to plaque mass is unknown. Further analysis by

Table 13–3. Composition of Mature Human Dental Plaques in Per Cent of Dry Weight

	Ash	Free Lipids	Proteins	Carbohydrates	Ultraviolet-Absorbing Substances
Total plaques	10	10–14	40–50	13–17	10–15
Acellular fraction	15	26–30	6.7–7	31–41	2–6
Cellular fraction	11	1.3–5	40–70	7–14	10–15

From Krembel, J., Frank, R. M., and Deluzarche, A.: Fractionation of human dental plaques, Arch. Oral Biol., *14*, 563–565, 1969.

disc electrophoresis demonstrated the presence of components homologous with saliva and serum (*i.e.*, gingival fluid), and some that resemble neither and are probably of bacterial origin.

Other matrix proteins that are probably of minor significance structurally but may be of major importance with regard to the pathological potential of plaque are the enzymes in dental plaque. Most of these are of bacterial origin and include proteases, hyaluronidases, chondroitinsulfatases, and glycosyltransferases, among others.

Hotz and colleagues extracted plaque by several methods and determined its carbohydrate content by gas chromatography. Glucose was the predominant carbohydrate. Glycerol, arabinose, ribose, mannose, galactose, maltose, and isomaltose were also present. Other investigators have reported the presence of rhamnose, fructose, methylpentose, glucosamine, and galactosamine. Sialic acid is not found in plaque, and several reports indicate that fucose, another moiety of salivary glycoproteins, is absent from the matrix. These two carbohydrates are probably removed from the proteins and metabolized by bacteria either before or after deposition in the plaque matrix.

A major part of the matrix is composed of bacterial polysaccharides including glucans, fructans, and heteroglycans. The glucans, which can comprise as much as 10% of the dry weight of plaque, were initially identified as dextrans, and are often referred to as such. However, these glucans include polymers in which the predominant linkage is $\alpha1-3$, whereas true dextrans are linked by $\alpha1-6$ bonds. The term "mutan" has been proposed for the $\alpha1-3$ polyglucans most of which are synthesized by *Streptococcus mutans*. The glucans, dextran and mutan, are relatively resistant to degradation by most plaque bacteria and play roles as adhesive and structural components in plaque.

The fructans or levans, composed of fructose molecules, are the other major extracellular polysaccharides found in the plaque matrix. They may comprise as much as 1% of the dry weight of plaque. Levans play a role as energy storage compounds in plaque, because in the absence of other carbohydrates they are rapidly metabolized by plaque bacteria.

It has become evident that the polysaccharides, mutan, dextran, and levan, are of major significance in the formation and metabolism of dental plaque. Of the various dietary carbohydrates, sucrose is the major precursor for these polysaccharides in plaque. Intracellular polysaccharide synthesis involves phosphorylated intermediates built up within the cell. However, as a result of the extracellular synthesis of these plaque polysaccharides, the energy necessary for polymerization must be present in the components involved, and when released, must be conserved for later use. The link between the fructose and glucose molecules in sucrose is a dihemiacetal bond containing a high energy of hydrolysis. None of the other common dietary carbohydrates possesses this bond. Several oral bacteria, especially streptococci, produce extracellular enzymes capable of hydrolyzing the bond, conserving the energy released, and using it to transfer the glucose or fructose monomers to polymers. These enzymes are commonly called dextransucrase, mutansucrase, or levansucrase, but are better described as glucosyltransferases or fructosyltransferases. These have been isolated from oral streptococci, and have been shown to be capable of *in vitro* synthesis of polysaccharides similar to those of dental plaque.

The heteroglycans found in the plaque matrix have received little study. The plaque of subjects on a glucose diet has been found to contain a heteroglycan composed of glucose, galactose, hexosamine, and other unidentified sugars. Although these polymers were demonstrated under special circumstances, they probably are at least minor components of natural plaque matrix. The means by which these polymers are synthesized is unknown. The possibility that secreted phosphorylated intermediates may be involved in their synthesis has been suggested.

The major intracellular polysaccharides are the glucose polymers of the glycogen–amylopectin type. These glucans act as carbohydrate storage compounds for use in the absence of exogenous carbohydrate. They are rapidly formed in the presence of excess dietary carbohydrates and used as an energy source during periods of fasting.

The carbohydrate content of plaque is extremely variable because many factors can affect it. For example, plaque taken within minutes after eating has a much higher carbohydrate content than that collected following a period of fasting, because the polysaccharides used as energy storage compounds, especially amylopectins and levans, are consumed during the fasting period. This is easily visualized in sections of plaque taken before and after fasting and stained with carbohydrate disclosing stains (Fig. 13–6).

An individual's diet can also determine the carbohydrate composition of plaque. Plaque taken from subjects on a high sucrose diet has been shown to have a carbohydrate/nitrogen ratio five times higher than plaque of subjects on a high glucose diet. In the former there is a preponderance of dextrans and levans, whereas in the latter, the previously described heteroglycans are formed.

Although there is a high lipid content in plaque, little work has been done in plaque lipid research. Krembel and colleagues reported that the free lipids of the acellular fraction of plaque comprised about 20 to 26% of the dry weight of plaque. The lipid fraction contained saturated even carbon chain acids from C_{12} to C_{20} and the unsaturated acids $C_{16:1}$, $C_{16:2}$, and $C_{18:1}$. They did not determine if these were of salivary or bacterial origin.

Table 13–4 lists the levels of the major inorganic components of plaque. The possible extreme variability in the chemical composition of different samples of plaque is apparent in these analyses. The higher levels were derived from the plaque of heavy calculus formers in areas of dentition on which heavy accumulations of plaque commonly occur. The lower levels represent the other extreme, plaque from light calculus formers on areas of light plaque formation. The major source of these inorganic constituents is saliva. Plaque selectively accumulates calcium, phosphate, and mag-

Table 13-4. Inorganic Components of Three-Day-Old Plaque
(% of lyophilized weight)

	Maxillary Plaque*	Lingual Lower Anterior Plaque†
Calcium	1.6	9.0
Phosphorus		
Unhydrolyzed	.5	5.0
Hydrolyzed	1.2	6.6
Sodium	.3	.2
Potassium	1.8	.6
Magnesium	.2	.4

* Three-day-old plaque of light calculus former.
† Three-day-old plaque of heavy calculus former.
From Mandel, I. D.: Biochemical aspects of calculus formation, J. Periodont. Res., 9, 10–17, 1974.

nesium, therefore levels of these minerals are much higher in plaque than in saliva.

Kleinberg and his colleagues measured calcium and phosphorus levels in plaque 1, 2, and 4 days after cleaning the tooth's surface. Relative concentrations of these two minerals declined after the first day and remained relatively constant through day four. The investigators attributed the presence of the calcium and phosphorus to formation of a calcium phosphate-carbohydrate-protein complex on the tooth's surface. Initial deposition of these complexes (probably acquired pellicle) results in a high calcium- and phosphorus-to-dry-weight ratio. After initial deposition, the ratio changes as the proteins to which the calcium is bound are metabolized by plaque bacteria and as the mechanisms of plaque deposition change.

Concentrations of calcium and phosphorus in plaque are influenced by the age of the subject, age of the plaque, pH of the plaque, location of plaque on the dentition, and the tendency of the individual to form calculus. Adolescents have less calcium in their plaque than adults. This is due in part to the lower levels of salivary calcium in children. The fact that mandibular plaque has a higher calcium content than maxillary plaque has been attributed to several factors. One factor is the higher calcium levels in the submaxillary saliva bathing the mandibular dentition. Another factor which may be responsible is the higher pH in the mandibular areas. This may increase the precipitation of calcium and phosphorus in these regions. Older plaque usually has a higher calcium phosphate level as a result of calculus formation within the plaque.

Levels of fluoride, like those of calcium and phosphorus, also are much higher in plaque than in saliva. Reported average concentrations of fluoride in plaque range as high as 67 ppm. The sources for the plaque fluoride are saliva, drinking water, and the diet. The enamel surface also contributes some fluoride to the plaque overlying it, because it has been demonstrated that plaque produced on mylar foils contains less fluoride than plaque formed on enamel surfaces in the same mouth. However, the levels of fluoride normally found in plaque can be supplied easily by the fluoride in saliva and water. The fluoride in drinking water can be the determinant of plaque fluoride concentrations. Fluoride levels were nearly twice as high in plaque obtained from children in an area in which the water had a high fluoride content as those in plaque obtained from children in a low fluoride-containing area.

Since there is a concentration difference between plaque fluoride and the saliva bathing it, the fluoride must be bound within the plaque. The method or location of this binding is unknown. Previously, it was proposed that fluoride was within bacterial cells or that it could be bound to proteins. However, it has been demonstrated that there are small molecular weight dialyzable components in saliva that can bind the fluoride. Complexes with these components within plaque could be the means by which the fluoride is bound within plaque. In addition, x-ray diffraction patterns obtained with early calculus suggests that fluorapatite formation may be a mechanism of fluoride binding in plaque.

Formation

There are numerous theories concerning the mechanisms of plaque formation. These center around the three major plaque components: saliva, bacteria, and bacterial products. Varying degrees of evidence in support of these different theories have been presented and it is probable that all may be involved in the formation of plaque.

The deposition of salivary glycoproteins responsible for the acquired pellicle probably continues by the same mechanisms during plaque formation. Hydrolysis of the carbohydrate moieties of the glycoproteins by bacterial enzymes continues, causing precipitation of these proteins on the plaque surface. The protein deposition resulting from increases in salivary pH as a result of the loss of carbon dioxide may also occur.

Kleinberg has reported another pH-dependent mechanism of protein precipitation that may be involved in plaque formation. At acidic pHs, within the range of those that can occur in the oral cavity, there is another aggregative effect on salivary proteins. The complex formed at an acidic pH varies from that formed at an alkaline pH because the calcium and phosphorus content is much lower in the acid than in the alkaline precipitate. The decrease of salivary pH to levels capable of aggregating proteins could result from the acidity of saliva in individuals with slow salivary flow rates. In addition, acid formation by bacteria populating the surrounding soft tissues or those already present in the plaque would decrease the pH. Precipitation of salivary proteins passing over these areas also could contribute to the plaque mass.

Reports in the literature indicate that the development of the bacterial populations in plaque involves a predictable transition from a simple to a complex flora. When variations of diet, dentition, and salivary flow are considered, the members and numbers of these populations are fairly reproducible. Their presence is the result of two factors: adsorption of the bacteria to the acquired pellicle or previous layers of plaque, and multiplication of the adsorbed bacteria to increase their numbers in plaque. Neither of these is a haphazard phenomenon; both appear to be selective mechanisms.

The specificity of adsorption is readily apparent when comparing the initial populations of bacteria adsorbed to the acquired pellicle with the populations found in the saliva bathing the tooth's surface. The numbers of each species in each population have been found to be disproportionate. In addition, tests with pure cultures of different oral bacteria reveal differences in their efficiency of adsorption to enamel coated with salivary proteins. It is obvious that the presence of bacteria in plaque is not simply a matter of entrapment in the precipitated salivary proteins, but that there is a selectivity of adsorption.

Several mechanisms by which bacteria can adsorb to pellicle, to other bacteria, or to previously formed plaque have been described (Fig. 13–7). Ordinarily the negative charge on bacteria and glycoproteins at oral pH would tend to discourage complexing between these components. However, calcium ions present in saliva can neutralize the charge and act as a bridge between bacteria or bacteria and glycoproteins. Thus, bacteria-calcium-bacteria aggregates or bacteria-calcium-protein complexes could form. The

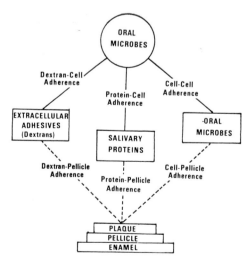

Fig. 13–7. Adhesive interactions involved in the formation of dental plaque. (Modified from Schachtele, C. S.: Recent developments in the microbiology of dental plaque formation, Northwest Dent., *51*, 108–113, 1972.)

protein could be free in saliva and induce further aggregation and precipitation, or it could be pellicle or plaque protein and act as the adsorption site on the tooth surface.

It has been demonstrated that specific bacteria, including those adsorbed in largest numbers on pellicle, have a tendency to aggregate in the presence of saliva. A large molecular weight protein that in the presence of calcium causes bacterial cells to aggregate has been isolated from saliva. Similarly acting proteins have been demonstrated in plaque. Some of these molecules not only aggregate bacteria but also adsorb to apatite.

Aggregating mechanisms with bacterial products replacing the salivary component have been demonstrated. Certain species of streptococci will agglutinate when high molecular weight dextrans are added to suspensions of these bacteria. These same streptococci are the major dextran-producing species in plaque. In addition, these dextran-coated bacteria also adsorb much more readily to enamel and hydroxyapatite than other bacteria. Thus, they synthesize their own adhesive substance which can act to attach them to each other and to the tooth. Other species of bacteria produce similarly acting but not identical substances.

Selective interspecies aggregation also has been demonstrated with plaque bacteria. Adsorption of cocci to filamentous bacteria in plaque has been demonstrated with the scanning electron microscope. This is a specific reaction because specific bacteria are involved. The mechanism by which this interspecies attachment occurs is unknown; specific receptor sites, the synthesis of an adhesive polymer such as dextran, or both are possible.

Another source of the bacteria populating plaque is bacteria retained on the enamel surface after prophylaxis. Meckel reported that, despite a thorough cleaning of the tooth, bacteria still remained in wedge-shaped defects in the enamel surface. Although this supplies some of the bacteria, the extent of its contribution to the total plaque population has not been determined.

After establishment of the initial layers of plaque on the enamel surface, plaque continues to grow in mass. The rate of growth is rapid initially and levels off within days. It has been demonstrated that 90% of the plaque mass in 32-day-old plaque was already present by the eighth day of growth. The increase is the result of additional deposition of components, bacterial and salivary, on the surface, and by reproduction of bacteria and production of bacterial products, especially polysaccharides, within the plaque. Plaque continues to grow until it reaches the limits determined by abrasive forces within the oral cavity.

The relative volume of cellular and extracellular components in plaque varies. Among the bacterial products comprising the matrix of plaque, glucans play the most significant role in plaque mass. The extent of their involvement is determined by the diet of the individual. This is especially a function of the dietary carbohydrates. In the presence of large amounts of sucrose a larger proportion of the plaque is composed of extracellular polysaccharides, and the plaque is of a heavy gelatinous nature. The numbers of bacteria and the levels of salivary glycoproteins are reduced proportionally. In tube-fed subjects or those fed carbohydrate-free diets, the plaque is much thinner and there is a higher density of bacteria and a larger proportion of nitrogenous substances than in other subjects.

Plaque and Caries

Although protective functions have been suggested for plaque, the harmful effects of this film on the teeth or the gingiva are such that they easily override any possible benefit. Plaque is the major etiological agent for caries and periodontal disease. The cariogenicity of plaque is predominantly the result of the acidogenic metabolism of plaque bacteria. Although it has been definitely established that plaque is involved in periodontal disease, its role is more complex and many different factors have been implicated.

The chemicoparasitic theory of caries formation is based on the acidogenic nature of plaque. The carious lesion results from the demineralization of enamel during exposure to the acid produced by plaque bacteria. The critical

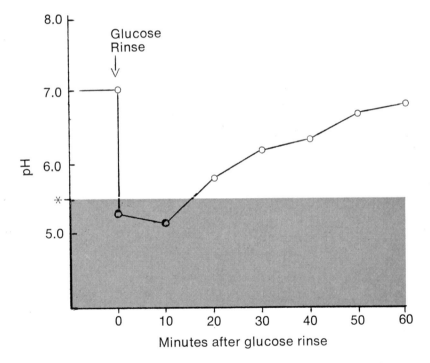

*approximate decalcification point of enamel.

Fig. 13–8.   pH curve in dental plaque *in situ* following application of glucose rinse. (Modified from Stephan, R. M.: Intra-oral hydrogen-ion concentrations associated with dental caries activity, J. Dent. Res., *23*, 257–266, 1944.)

point for demineralization of dental enamel is around pH 5.6. When presented with suitable substrates, plaque bacteria can easily produce such an acid environment while undertaking their normal metabolic activities.

Stephan used antimony electrodes *in vivo* to measure acid production by plaque exposed to carbohydrate rinses. He demonstrated that the plaque pH dropped to levels well below the decalcification point of enamel within minutes after application of carbohydrates (Fig. 13–8). After a short period the pH slowly returned to the original levels. This phenomenon, known as a "Stephan curve," occurs repeatedly upon application of fermentable carbohydrates to plaque.

Proof that the production of acid is a function of plaque and not of the tooth surface alone can be demonstrated by measuring acid production *in vivo* before and after removal of plaque (Fig. 13–9). In the presence of plaque the Stephan curve occurs on application of glucose. However, following removal of plaque from the same tooth's surface, there is no drop in pH when the tooth again is exposed to glucose.

Further evidence of the relationship of plaque acidogenesis to caries may be gained by comparison of caries activity and plaque pH in different individuals or in different areas of the dentition. Stephan noted that the fasting pH and the extent and duration of acid production by plaque after a carbohydrate rinse were directly related to the caries activity of the particular individual (Fig. 13–10). Others have measured plaque pH in different areas

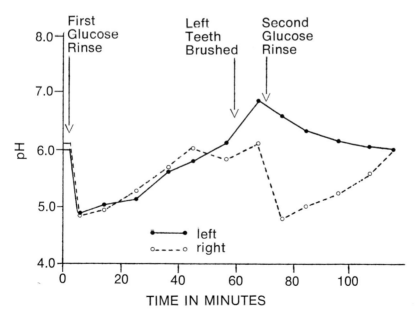

FIG. 13–9. pH curves following application of glucose rinses. Left teeth were brushed following initial rinse with glucose. (Modified from Stephan, R. M. and Miller, B. F.: A quantitative method for evaluating physical and chemical agents which modify production of acids in bacterial plaques on human teeth, J. Dent. Res., *22*, 45–51, 1943.)

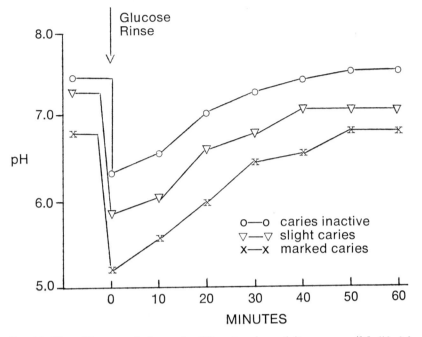

Fɪɢ. 13–10. pH curves of plaques in different caries activity groups. (Modified from Stephan, R. M.: Intra-oral hydrogen-ion concentrations associated with dental caries activity, J. Dent. Res., *23*, 257–266, 1944.)

of the dentition and found that regions with the lowest plaque pH correlate with areas of increased caries activity.

The acids responsible for the demineralization are those resulting from normal metabolic activities of the plaque bacteria. Several organic acids including lactic, acetic, propionic, formic, and butyric acid are produced in plaque exposed to carbohydrates. Of these, lactic acid apparently contributes most to the drop in pH, for the rate of lactic acid formation by plaque corresponds to the initial rapid decrease in pH demonstrated in Stephan's curve.

The diffusion-limiting nature of plaque potentiates the effects of the acids because it retards their movement out of plaque. This results in the accumulation of acids in close proximity to the enamel surface, enhancing the demineralization process.

Stephan-type curves also occur following carbohydrate-containing meals. However, the reversion to fasting pH levels is usually slower. Kleinberg and Jenkins reported that the pH rose only to 70 to 80% of fasting levels $3\frac{1}{2}$ hours after initial exposure to the carbohydrate. The delay is the result of retention of foods in the oral cavity and/or production of polysaccharides by the plaque bacteria. The retention properties of different foods have been demonstrated to affect the pH curves produced by plaque; the longer the clearance time, the longer the duration of acid production. In addition, many oral bacteria produce either or both intracellular and extracellular polysaccharides in the presence of excess fermentable carbohydrates. These are utilized after other carbohydrates are consumed, and this delayed fermentation retards the return to fasting pH levels.

The return to fasting pH levels is the result of neutralization or removal of the acids by the combined actions of plaque, bacteria, and saliva. Diffusion of saliva into the plaque and of bacterial products out of the plaque dilutes the acids. The efficiency of this action varies with the structure of the plaque matrix, the more open the matrix the faster the exchange of saliva and plaque fluids.

The buffering capacity of saliva also neutralizes the acidic environment. These buffering effects are mediated primarily by bicarbonate. In addition, saliva contains compounds that serve as precursors for base production by plaque bacteria.

Within plaque itself are several factors that reverse the pH. Plaque possesses an even greater buffering capacity, mediated by proteins and calcium phosphate, than that of saliva. Members of the bacterial flora within plaque also metabolize the lactic acid to less acidic compounds such as acetic or propionic acids. Finally, plaque metabolism of salivary constituents can lead to formation of basic products that neutralize the previously formed acids.

Kleinberg and his associates have carried out extensive investigations into the metabolism of plaque, especially with regard to plaque pH. Kleinberg and Jenkins measured the pH of plaque in different areas of the dentition, and noted a correlation between pH and plaque location. Maxillary plaque pH was found to be lower than mandibular in corresponding areas. The pH of maxillary posterior plaque was higher than maxillary anterior, but mandibular anterior was higher than mandibular posterior. Finally, the lingual plaque pH was higher than both labial and buccal plaque pH in corresponding areas. From these results, Kleinberg and his co-workers concluded that plaque in areas of the dentition having more access to saliva had higher pHs both during fasting and following the ingestion of carbohydrates. This, coupled with the fact that individuals with faster resting salivary flow rates had higher plaque pHs than those with slower rates, indicated that saliva must play a major role in determining plaque pH.

Of the various components in saliva the only one capable of serving as a ready source of alkali is urea. Plaque metabolism of urea to form ammonium ion is even more rapid than glycolysis. Although other nitrogenous compounds such as proteins and amino acids can serve as a source for acid neutralization, bacterial metabolism of these is too slow. Thus, salivary urea is a key factor in the maintenance of plaque pH, especially during fasting periods.

The pH of plaque primarily is a result of the effects of alkali production from salivary urea and acid production from glycolysis. At any given time the sum of these two determines the pH of the plaque at that time. Thus, during a period of fasting, alkali production from salivary urea will render the plaque pH basic. In the presence of dietary carbohydrates during meals, or extracellular bacterial polysaccharides after meals, there is a decrease in plaque pH as a result of glycolysis.

During either feeding or fasting, the pH of plaque varies from that of the saliva bathing it. Again, this results from the metabolism of carbohydrates and urea, both of which are delivered to the plaque bacteria by the saliva. Depending on the substrate, either acid or base is produced more rapidly by the plaque than it can be neutralized by saliva. During and following meals plaque will be more acidic than saliva as a result of fermentation of dietary carbohydrates; during fasting, plaque will be more alkaline than saliva as a result of the metabolism of salivary urea.

Of the common dietary carbohydrates, sucrose is one of the most cariogenic, for metabolism of the sugar by plaque bacteria results in a number of processes that enhance the demineralization process. At low carbohydrate levels bacteria readily utilize sucrose as an energy source and produce abundant amounts of acid from it. In the presence of higher levels of carbohydrates, plaque bacteria, especially streptococci, synthesize the polymers, dextran, mutan, and levan, from sucrose. These polysaccharides play multiple roles in the demineralization process. They are synthesized in the extracellular spaces of plaque and change its structure from that of a relatively open floc to a gel structure with a resultant decrease in diffusibility of soluble compounds. Since this occurs at the time when there is excess carbohydrate available to the plaque, this is also a period of high acid production, and the decreased diffusion through plaque increases the duration of the acidic environment, extending the period of demineralization. Finally, as the levels of ingested carbohydrates fall off, these polysaccharides, especially levan, are metabolized and this, again, tends to extend the time of exposure to acid.

Plaque and Periodontal Disease

Loe and Theilade and associates demonstrated the importance of plaque in gingival inflammation by scoring the development of plaque and gingivitis in subjects who had suspended all oral hygiene procedures. The accumulation of plaque was closely correlated with the development of gingivitis (Fig. 13–11). During this period there was a change in the bacterial population from a simple one containing cocci and rods to a complex population of cocci, rods, filaments, and spirals. The diagnosis of mild gingivitis, which occurred within 9 to 21 days, coincided with the establishment of the complex bacterial flora in each individual. Reinstitution of oral hygiene resulted in a reversion to normal healthy gingiva with the original simple bacterial flora. Similar studies have repeatedly demonstrated this correlation of gingivitis with accumulations of plaque.

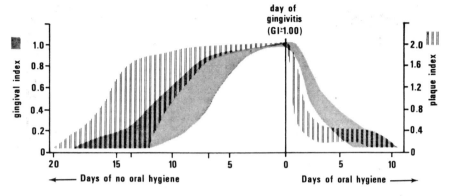

FIG. 13–11. Summation of gingival and plaque indices of a group of 11 individuals during periods without oral hygiene and subsequent periods of oral hygiene. (Modified from Theilade, E., et al.: Experimental gingivitis in man, J. Periodont. Res., 1, 1–13, 1966.)

The mechanisms by which plaque induces periodontal disease have not been definitely established. Many different products of plaque bacteria have been suggested as agents for gingivitis and periodontal disease, including toxins, enzymes, proteins, and polysaccharides which can act as antigens in immune reactions and tissue-irritating metabolites. All these factors are present in plaque, and all have been demonstrated to induce injury in tissues under experimental conditions. There is also ample clinical evidence that some of these play a role in the natural disease process. However, it has not yet been determined which of these factors, if any, plays the major role in periodontal disease and what the roles of the remaining components might be.

CALCULUS

Shortly after pellicle and plaque form on the tooth's surface, the process of mineralization resulting in the formation of calculus begins (Fig. 13–12). The presence of crystalline foci may be demonstrated within hours after the deposition of the initial plaque layers. Although it may occur within bacterial cells, crystallization usually begins in the extracellular matrix of plaque. As it grows, the area of mineralization encompasses plaque bacteria and they become mineralized. Calcification can also occur in the pellicle, especially in the lingual areas.

Calculus is formed both subgingivally and supragingivally. Although supragingival calculus may be found throughout the dentition, it is heaviest in areas where the salivary glands empty into the oral cavity. Thus, supragingival calculus is most abundant on lingual surfaces of the mandibular anterior teeth and the buccal surfaces of maxillary molars. This difference in distribution is also present with subgingival plaque.

Subgingival calculus is harder and denser than supragingival calculus and is often pigmented. Supragingival calculus is usually yellowish white,

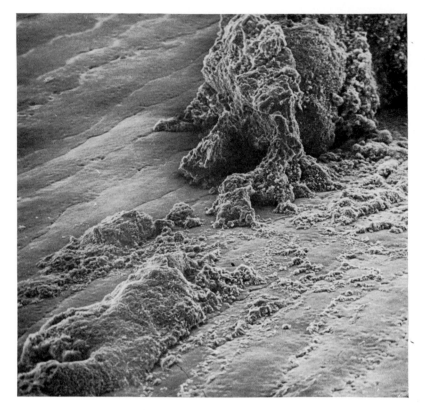

Fig. 13–12. Accretion of calculus on enamel. The organic matrix has been removed by treatment with sodium hypochlorite. Field width is 200 μm. (From Jones, S. J.: The tooth surface in periodontal disease, Dent. Pract., 22, 462–473, 1972.)

whereas subgingival calculus may be brown, greenish, or black. The differences in composition are dependent primarily on the relative contributions of saliva and gingival fluid and variations in the bacterial populations in the areas in which each is formed.

The bacterial population of calculus resembles that of mature plaque. A study of the cultivable organisms in calculus plaques indicated that streptococci were predominant up to 4 weeks. In older calculus filamentous forms predominated. The large populations of filamentous bacteria in calculus have led to the theory that they may be directly involved in the mechanisms of calculus formation.

Chemical Composition

Mature calculus, by definition, is composed of approximately 80% mineralized materials and 20% water and organic constituents. Table 13–5 illustrates the results reported by Little and colleagues. They noted that the

Table 13–5. Chemical Content of Calculus in
Per Cent of Dry Weight

	Calculus	*Matrix*
Ash (%)	73.0	2.10
Recoverable matrix (%)	13.15	–·
Ca: P (wt.)	1.75	1.21
Nitrogen	1.51	9.05
Protein		
(N × 6.25)	8.10	56.0
Saccharide (%)	4.06	21.4
Lipid (%)*	3.13	24.7
Nucleic acid	–	2.3%

* Much lower lipid values have been reported by others.

From Little, M. F., Bowman, L., Casciani, C. A., and Rowley, J.: The composition of dental calculus, Arch. Oral Biol., *11*, 385–396, 1966.

nitrogen content and amino acid composition of calculus from different areas of the dentition varied, whereas the carbohydrate content was relatively constant. From comparisons of the amino acid and carbohydrate composition of the calculus matrix, they decided that the calculus matrix reflects the composition of dental plaque in general and is not derived from any specific source such as salivary glycoproteins.

The crystalline material is primarily calcium phosphate containing around 30 to 35% calcium and 15 to 18% phosphorus. The Ca: P ratio is between 1.75 and 2.0 depending on the age and location of the calculus. Little and Hazen compared deep subgingival calculus, marginal calculus, and supragingival calculus. The subgingival calculus had a slightly higher calcium content than the others but there was no difference in the phosphorus content. The marginal calculus varied from one location to another. The calcium-to-phosphorus ratio of deep subgingival calculus was 2.04 and that of supragingival calculus was 1.75. The ratio for marginal calculus fell in between these figures at 1.89.

Rowles and others have studied the calcium phosphate crystals in calculus and identified apatite, whitlockite, octacalcium phosphate, and brushite. As illustrated in Table 13–6, the relative proportions of these varied with the age of the calculus and the area of the dentition from which it was obtained. Subgingival calculus contains higher concentrations of whitlockite than supragingival calculus. This probably results from the higher levels of magnesium present in crevicular fluid. Whitlockite is also less often present in calculus under six-months' duration, indicating that it is a product of mature calculus.

Table 13–6. Incidence, Abundance, Areas of Prevalence, and Age Changes of Calcium Phosphate Crystals in Calculus

Component	Incidence (%)	Abundance (%)	Area of Prevalence	Change with Age
Apatite	99.5	55.3	throughout	no change
Whitlockite	80.7	24.2	posterior	increase
Octacalcium phosphate	94.8	20.0	upper anterior	no change
Brushite	43.6	8.9	lower anterior	decrease

From Rowles, S. L.: The Inorganic Composition of Dental Calculus, In *Proceedings of the First European Bone and Tooth Symposium*, H. J. J. Blackwood (Ed.). Oxford, Pergamon Press, 1964, pp. 175–183.

Fluoride levels are also elevated in calculus, the concentration being severalfold that of plaque and saliva. The fluoride concentration ranges from 200 to 300 ppm but it can rise two- or threefold following topical application of fluoride. Magnesium is also sequestered by calculus, and levels as high as 0.9% have been reported. Many other elements have been reported to be present in minute concentrations in calculus.

Formation

X-ray diffraction studies indicate that crystallization of the calcium phosphate in plaque may be initiated within hours after deposition of the plaque on a cleaned tooth surface. Two forms of calcium phosphate crystals, brushite and apatite, were present. This early calculus had a poorly defined crystalline structure but as time progressed it became more crystalline. The time it takes for plaque to attain an inorganic content of 75 to 80% is called the "calculus formation time." In heavy calculus formers the calculus formation time may be only 12 days. However, although the inorganic content may reach this level rapidly, the crystalline composition may not resemble that of mature calculus for months or years.

Two types of crystals have been identified in the areas of initiation of mineralization (Fig. 13–13). A-foci are fine needle-like or platelet-shaped crystals of apatite. These appear mainly in the extracellular matrix of plaque, but they may be found within bacterial cells. B-foci are rod-like crystals which are aggregates of brushite. They are found extracellularly. Whereas A-type mineralization centers may be intermixed with some organic material, the crystals of B-centers have no organic material associated with them.

The mechanism by which calculus formation is initiated is unknown. Several theories have been advanced, but none has been proved. The possibility that bacteria or their products are responsible for calculus formation was once considered but is now known to be incorrect, because gnotobiotic animals, which have no bacteria, form calculus. In addition, as has

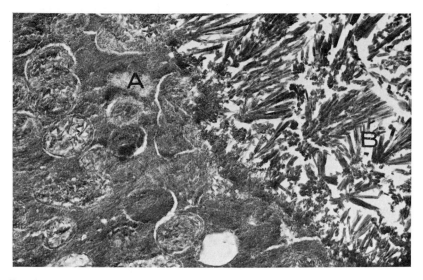

Fig. 13–13. A- and B-centers of mineralization in supragingival plaque. A-centers consist of densely packed needle-shaped or platelet-shaped crystals. B-centers consist of hexagonal crystals. ×30,000. (From Schroeder, H. E.: *Formation and Inhibition of Dental Calculus*, Berne, H. Huber, 1969.)

been described previously, calculus formation usually begins in the matrix rather than in the bacterial cells. However, it is probable that bacteria or their products influence the formation of calculus under natural conditions.

Saliva is saturated with calcium and phosphate, and this has led to theories based on the precipitation of calcium phosphate from saliva as a result of increases in salivary pH. These changes could result from loss of CO_2 from saliva as it enters the oral cavity or from alkali production during bacterial metabolism of salivary urea.

The possibility that localized increases of calcium and phosphate within plaque could initiate crystallization also has been considered. This could be caused by release of protein-bound calcium from bacterial metabolism or by release of phosphate by phosphatases in plaque.

Despite the aforementioned possibilities, the most accepted concept at this time is that of an epitactic mechanism in which formation is initiated with the help of another compound. It is presumed that the organic matrix of plaque contains compounds that provide sites for deposition and alignment of calcium and phosphate in a configuration corresponding to that of the crystal. This initial crystal then acts as a seed or a nucleus for the mineralization to proceed by continued precipitation of calcium and phosphate.

There is a great deal of variation in the rate of calculus formation in different individuals and many investigations have been carried out to determine the reason for this difference. The possibility that salivary calcium and phosphorus levels might be involved has been studied several times with contradictory results. One report indicated that calculus formers had higher levels of these minerals in their saliva; others found no significant differences.

Rapid calculus formers have significantly higher salivary protein levels than do calculus nonformers. It has been suggested that this may reflect a qualitative rather than a quantitative difference; calculus formers may possess an additional protein that enhances the formation of calculus. Calculus formers have higher salivary urea levels than do calculus nonformers. This salivary urea could serve as a source of base, resulting in a higher plaque pH which would enhance deposition of calcium phosphate and possibly crystallization. Significantly higher levels of salivary esterase, pyrophosphatase, and acid phosphatase have been found in rapid calculus formers. Salivary viscosity has also been implicated, because saliva of calculus formers is less viscous than that of calculus nonformers.

On the other hand, the possibility exists that the difference in rate of formation is not the result of an added factor in the rapid formers, but rather the absence of a constituent in saliva. It has been reported that nonformers of calculus have higher levels of pyrophosphate in their saliva. This compound has been shown to be an inhibitor of calculus formation. Thus, the difference could be a matter of inhibition of calculus formation in calculus nonformers rather than enhancement in calculus formers. Despite these possibilities, an explanation of the differences in the rate of calculus formation has yet to be found.

The possible role of calculus in periodontal disease has led to much speculation. However, since it has been demonstrated that calculus is usually covered with plaque, and that mechanical injury is not as significant in the cause of the disease as was previously thought, it is apparent that calculus is not a primary cause of periodontal disease. It can potentiate the harmful effects of plaque, because it has been shown that plaque and calculus combined appear to be more inflammatory than plaque alone.

SELECTED REFERENCES

ARMSTRONG, W. G.: Origin and nature of the aquired pellicle, Proc. R. Soc. Med., *61*, 923–930, 1968.

GIBBONS, R. J., and VON HOUTE, J.: On the formation of dental plaque, J. Periodontol., *44*, 347–360, 1973.

HAY, D. I.: The interaction of human parotid salivary proteins with hydroxyapatite, Arch. Oral Biol., *18*, 1517–1529, 1973.

HOTZ, P., GUGGENHEIM, B., and SCHMID, R.: Carbohydrates in pooled dental plaque, Caries Res., *6*, 103–121, 1972.

KLEINBERG, I.: Biochemistry of the dental plaque, Adv. Oral Biol., *4*, 44–90, 1970.

KLEINBERG, I.: The role of dental plaque in caries and inflammatory periodontal disease, J. Can. Dent. Assoc., *40*, 56–66, 1974.

MANDEL, I. D.: Biochemical aspects of calculus formation, J. Periodont. Res., *9*, 10–17, 1974.

MANDEL, I. D.: Relation of saliva and plaque to caries, J. Dent. Res., *53*, 246–266, 1974.

McHUGH, W. D. (Ed.): *Dental Plaque*, Edinburgh, E. & S. Livingstone Ltd., 1970.

ORSTAVIK, D., and KRAUS, F. W.: The acquired pellicle: Immunfluorescent demonstration of specific proteins, J. Oral Pathol., *2*, 68–76, 1973.

ROWE, N. H. (Ed.): *Proceedings of Symposium on Dental Plaque: Interfaces*, Ann Arbor, Mich., University of Michigan, School of Dentistry, 1973.

SCHROEDER, H. E.: *Formation and Inhibition of Dental Calculus.* Berne, Hans Huber, 1969.

SONJU, T., and ROLLA, G.: Chemical analysis of the acquired pellicle formed in two hours on cleaned human teeth in vivo, Caries Res., *7*, 30–38, 1973.

Chapter 14

Mechanisms of Dental Caries

SAMUEL DREIZEN, D.D.S., M.D.

Enamel, the primary site of the carious lesion, is the hardest of all human tissues. When fully formed it is acellular, avascular, aneural, and completely devoid of biologic powers of self-repair.

Dental caries is an anatomically specific and biochemically controversial disease of the calcified tissues of the teeth. Pathologically, caries begins as a subsurface demineralization of the enamel which progresses along the radial course of the enamel prisms to the dentino-enamel junction. At the junction, caries spreads laterally and centrally into the underlying dentine assuming a conical configuration with the apex toward the pulp. The dentinal tubules become infiltrated with bacteria and dilate at the expense of the intervening matrix. Liquefaction foci are formed by the coalescence and destruction of adjacent tubules. Softening of the dentine precedes disorganization and discoloration culminating in the formation of a cheese-like or leathery mass. Further disintegration undermines the cusps and sound tissue causing secondary fractures and enlargement of the cavity. If unchecked, caries will eventually involve the pulp and destroy the vitality of the tooth.

THEORIES OF CARIES FORMATION

Numerous theories have been advanced to explain the mechanism of dental caries. All are tailored to fit the form created by the chemical and physical properties of enamel and dentine. Some maintain that caries arises from within the tooth; others that it originates from without. Some ascribe caries to structural or biochemical defects in the tooth; others to a propitious local environment. Some incriminate the organic matrix as the initial point of attack; others the inorganic prisms or rods. Some have gained wide acceptance; others are relegated to their avid and persistent progenitors. The most prominent are the chemicoparasitic, proteolytic and proteolysis-chelation concepts. The endogenous, glycogen, organotropic, and biophysical theories represent some of the currently held minority views.

The Chemicoparasitic Theory

This theory was formulated by Miller, who in 1882 proclaimed that, "Dental decay is a chemico-parasitical disease consisting of two distinctly marked stages; decalcification or softening of the tissue and dissolution of the softened residue. In the case of enamel, however, the second stage is practically wanting, decalcification of the enamel practically signifying its total destruction." The cause was attributed to ". . . all microorganisms of the human mouth which possess the power of exciting an acid fermentation of foods may and do take part in producing the first stage of dental caries . . . all possessing a peptonizing or digestive action upon albuminous substances may take part in the second stage."

Fosdick and Hutchinson have updated the theory that the initiation and progress of a carious lesion require the fermentation of sugars in or under a dental plaque and the production *in situ* of lactic acid and other weak acids. Caries was equated with a specialized series of reactions based on the diffusion of substances through the enamel. Caries penetration was attributed to changes in the physical and chemical characteristics of enamel during the life of the tooth and to the semipermeable nature of enamel in the living tooth.

Direction and rate of migration of substances through tooth structure appear to be influenced by the diffusion pressure. For uncharged particles, diffusion pressure depends mainly on molecular size and molecular concentration differential. The lines of diffusion are principally through the rod sheaths and inter-rod substance comprised of apatite crystals with comparatively little organic matter. Lines of Retzius and incremental lines may also serve as pathways for diffusion. During ionic migration from the saliva to enamel, apatite crystals either react with or capture ions from the diffusant. Reaction or capture most probably occurs in the inter-rod substance through which the diffusant passes. The affected crystals become more or less stable and more or less soluble depending on the ions involved. Capture of calcium and phosphate ions tends to plug the diffusion pathways. Substitution of fluoride ions for hydroxyl ions in the apatite crystal forms a more stable and less soluble compound. Capture of hydrogen ions from acid diffusants, with the formation of water and soluble phosphates, destroys the enamel membrane (Eq. 14–1).

$$Ca_{10}(PO_4)_6(OH)_2 + 8H^+ \rightleftharpoons 10Ca^{2+} + 6HPO_4^{2-} + 2H_2O \qquad \text{Eq. 14–1}$$

If the surface of the tooth has been exposed to the oral environment long enough for maturation to occur, the diffusion pathways at or near the enamel surface contain salts which are more resistant to acids. When this layer of posteruptive maturation forms and is not too dense and impermeable it

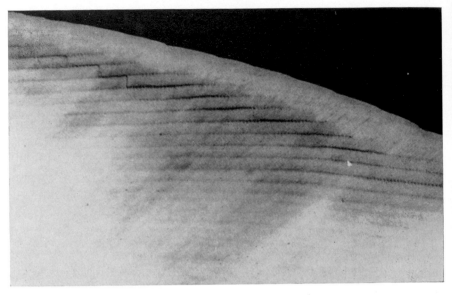

Fig. 14–1. Microradiograph of thin section of carious lesion showing parallel rods, inter-rod substance, lines of Retzius, Darling layer, and incremental growth lines. (Fosdick and Hutchinson, courtesy of Ann. New York Acad. Sci., *131*, 758–770, 1965.)

results in a "Darling layer," if a lesion develops. Acids then have to penetrate to a considerable depth before encountering apatite crystals susceptible to dissolution. The surface may thus remain intact, while the deeper layers become water soluble producing the subsurface demineralization characteristic of initial enamel caries (Fig. 14–1). Figure 14–2 shows the same structures as Figure 14–1 with a more advanced carious lesion. Note that the Darling layer has suffered serious dissolution.

Electron microscopic studies of early enamel caries confirm the presence of at least four different layers created by the acid decalcification process. These consist of (1) a relatively intact layer at the surface comprised of mineral of low acid solubility resulting from the presence of fluoride in the crystals and from the reprecipitation of salts liberated by solubilization from the depths of the lesion, (2) a partially demineralized layer beneath the surface enamel composed of mineral residues from which most of the more soluble fractions have been dissolved, (3) a reaction zone where the more soluble components are being actively lost by dissolution, and (4) sound enamel of low permeability deep to the lesion which can temporarily withstand the demineralization process. According to Brown, the physicochemical factors controlling events in the body of the lesion and in the reaction zone are thermodynamic in nature (variable solubility), whereas those dominating events in the intact layer and in the plaque are kinetic in nature (restricted diffusion).

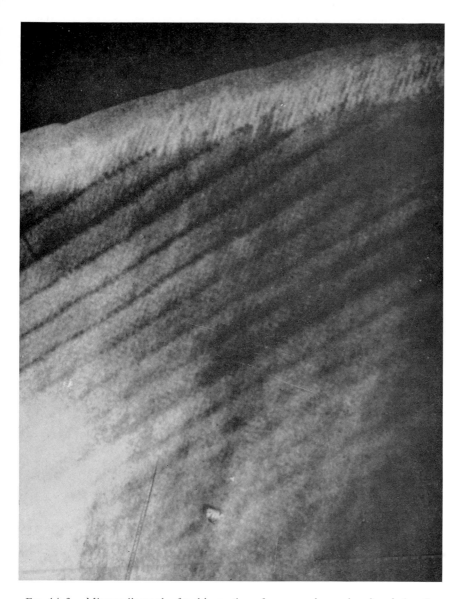

FIG. 14–2. Microradiograph of a thin section of a more advanced carious lesion than that shown in Figure 14–1. Note the parallel rods, inter-rod substance, lines of Retzius, partially dissolved Darling layer and incremental growth lines.

Some of the histological features of enamel caries have been attributed to mineral redeposition during the caries attack. Before porosity can become evident, the mineral dissolved from the interior enamel must be transported out of the tooth by a process of slow diffusion during which some of the mineral may reprecipitate. Weatherell maintains that mineral redeposition in the surface enamel would account, in part, for the seemingly intact surface zone, because this zone is not perfectly intact, does have spaces, and does contain altered enamel.

The Proteolytic Theory

Proponents of the proteolytic theory and its various modifications regard the enamel matrix as the key to the initiation and penetration of dental caries. The mechanism is attributed to protein-splitting microorganisms which invade and destroy the organic elements of enamel and dentine. The digestion of the organic matter is followed by a physical and/or acid dissolution of the inorganic salts.

Gottlieb maintained that caries begins in those enamel lamellae or uncalcified prism sheaths which lack a protective cuticular covering at the surface. The caries process spreads along these structural defects as the proteins are destroyed by enzymes liberated by the invading organisms. In time the calcified prisms are attacked and necrotized. The destruction is characterized by the elaboration of a yellow pigment which appears from the time the tooth structure is first involved. The pigment is presumed to be a metabolic product of the proteolytic organisms. In most instances the protein degradation is accompanied by limited acid production. In rare cases proteolysis alone may cause caries. Only yellow pigmentation, with or without acid formation, denotes "true caries"; acid action alone produces "chalky enamel" and not true caries. Acids not only fail to produce caries but are responsible for erecting a barrier against the spread of caries by contributing to the development of transparent enamel. Transparent enamel results from an internal shift of calcium salts. The salts at the site of acid action are dissolved with some going to the surface where they are washed out and some penetrating into the deeper layers where they are precipitated to form hypercalcified transparent enamel. The microbial invasion roads are obstructed by the increased calcification and further bacterial penetration is prevented. Fluoridation, whether by topical application or by ingestion of fluoridated water, protects the teeth against caries by fluoridizing the noncalcified organic pathways. This presumably attracts calcium from the adjacent prisms and obstructs the invasion roads.

Frisbie interpreted the microscopic phase of caries which occurs prior to a visible break in the enamel surface continuity as a process entailing a progressive alteration of the organic matrix and a projection of microorganisms into the tooth substance. The caries mechanism is identified as a depolymerization of the organic matrix of enamel and dentine by enzymes released by proteolytic bacteria. Both acid formed during the hydrolysis of dental proteins and mechanical trauma contribute to the loss of the calcified component and to the enlargement of the cavity.

Pincus related caries activity to the action of sulfatase-producing bacteria on the mucoproteins of enamel and dentine. The polysaccharide portion of these mucoproteins contains sulfate ester groups. Following hydrolytic release of the polysaccharides, sulfatase liberates the bound sulfate as sulfuric acid. The acid dissolves enamel and then combines with calcium to form calcium sulfate. In this concept the teeth themselves contain the substances necessary for acid production by bacteria. An external source of carbohydrate is not required. The changes in the organic structure are primary; those in the mineral phase secondary.

The main support for the proteolytic theory is derived from histopathological demonstrations that some regions of the enamel are relatively rich in protein and may serve as avenues for the spread of caries. The theory does not account for such clinical characteristics of dental caries as localization to specific tooth sites, relation to food habits, and dietary prevention. It does not explain the production of caries in experimental animals by high carbohydrate diets nor the prevention of experimental caries by glycolytic inhibitors. No mechanism has been demonstrated to show how proteolysis can destroy calcified tissue except through the formation of acid end products. It has been calculated that the total amount of acid potentially available from enamel protein is capable of dissolving only a small fraction of the total calcium salt content of enamel. Furthermore, there is no chemical evidence that there is an early loss of organic material in enamel caries nor have proteolytic forms been consistently isolated from early enamel lesions. In contrast, it has been found that before tooth protein in general and glycoproteins in particular can be depolymerized and hydrolyzed, demineralization is necessary to expose the protein linkages bonded to the inorganic fraction. Electron microscope examinations demonstrate a filamentous organic framework interspersed in enamel mineral between and within the enamel prisms. The fibrils are about 50 millimicrons in thickness. Unless the adjacent inorganic substance is first demineralized, the spacing would hardly be sufficient for bacterial penetration.

The Proteolysis-Chelation Theory

Schatz and co-workers extended the proteolytic theory to include chelation as an explanation for the concomitant destruction of enamel mineral and matrix. The proteolysis-chelation theory affixes the etiology of caries to two interrelated and simultaneously occurring reactions; microbial destruction of the largely proteinaceous organic matrix and loss of apatite through dissolution by organic chelators, some of which originate as matrix breakdown products.

10

The bacterial attack is initiated by keratinolytic microorganisms which decompose protein and other organic substances in the enamel. Enzymatic degradation of the protein and carbohydrate elements yields substances that chelate calcium and dissolve the insoluble calcium phosphate. Chelation can sometimes cause solubilization and transport of ordinarily insoluble mineral matter. It is accomplished through the formation of coordinate covalent bonds and electrostatic interactions between the metal and the chelating agent.

$$M^{++} + H_4EDTA \rightleftharpoons H_2MEDTA + 2H^+ \qquad \text{Eq. 14-2}$$

Calcium chelators including acid anions, amines, peptides, polyphosphates, and carbohydrates are present in food, saliva, and plaque material and may conceivably contribute to the caries process.

The theory also holds that, since proteolytic organisms are generally more active in an alkaline environment, tooth destruction can take place at a neutral or alkaline pH. The acid-producing oral microflora, instead of causing caries, actually protects the teeth by controlling and inhibiting the proteolytic forms. The chelating properties of organic compounds are sometimes altered by fluorine which can form covalent bonds with some metals. Fluorides may thus affect the linkages between enamel organic and mineral matter in a manner which confers resistance to caries.

There are serious questions as to the validity of some of the basic premises of the proteolysis-chelation theory. Although the solubilizing effect of chelating and complexing agents on insoluble calcium salts is well documented, it has not been shown that a similar phenomenon occurs in enamel *in vivo*. Recent scanning electron microscope studies of enamel caries have shown that the pattern resembles that of acid attack much more closely than that of chelation by EDTA. Keratinolytic organisms are not part of the oral flora except as occasional transients. Enamel protein is extremely resistant to microbial degradation. Bacteria that attack keratins have not been shown to destroy enamel organic matrix. A survey of the biochemical characteristics of 250 oral proteolytic bacteria uncovered none that could attack unaltered enamel. Jenkins maintains that the proportion of organic matter in enamel is so small that even if all was suddenly converted into active chelating agents, these products would not be capable of dissolving more than a tiny fraction of the enamel apatite. Also, there is no convincing evidence that plaque bacteria can, in the natural environment which is presumably saturated with calcium phosphate, attack the organic matter of enamel before decalcification has occurred. In contrast, Jenkins' data suggest that the chelators in plaque, far from causing decalcification of the tooth, may actually hold a reservoir of calcium which is released in ionic form under acid conditions to maintain saturation of calcium phosphate over a wide pH range. Like the proteolytic theory, the proteolysis-chelation theory fails to explain the relationship between diet and dental caries either in man or in experimental animals.

The Endogenous Theory

The endogenous theory was promulgated by Csernyei, who claimed that caries results from a biochemical derangement beginning in the pulp and manifested clinically in the enamel and dentine. It is precipitated by an elective localized influence of the central nervous system or some of its nuclei on magnesium and fluorine metabolism of individual teeth. This accounts for caries affecting some teeth and sparing others. The caries process is pulpogenous in nature and emanates from a disturbance in the physiological balance between phosphatase activators (magnesium) and phosphatase inhibitors (fluorine) in the pulp. At equilibrium, pulp phosphatase acts on glycerophosphates and hexosephosphates to build calcium phosphate. When the equilibrium is disrupted, pulp phosphatase promotes the formation of phosphoric acid which dissolves the calcified tissues.

Eggers-Lura agreed that caries is caused by a disturbance of phosphorus metabolism and by an accumulation of phosphatase in the affected tissue but disagreed as to the source and mechanism of action of phosphatase. Since caries attacks teeth with either living or dead pulps, the origin of the enzyme must come not from within the pulp but from without the tooth, that is, the saliva or oral flora. Phosphatase dissolves tooth enamel by splitting the phosphate salts and not by acid decalcification. According to its proponents, the phosphatase hypothesis explains the individuality of caries and the caries-inhibiting effects of fluorides and phosphates. The relationship between phosphatase and dental caries activity has not, however, been confirmed experimentally.

The Glycogen Theory

Egyedi maintained that susceptibility to caries is related to a high carbohydrate intake during the period of tooth development which results in the deposition of excess glycogen and glycoprotein in tooth structure. The two substances are immobilized in the apatite of the enamel and dentine during the maturation of the matrix, thus increasing the vulnerability of the teeth to bacterial attack after eruption. Plaque acids convert the glycogen and glycoprotein into glucose and glucosamine. Caries begins when the plaque bacteria invade the organic tracts of the enamel and degrade the glucose and glucosamine into demineralizing acids. This theory has been criticized as being highly speculative and unsubstantiated.

The Organotropic Theory

The organotropic theory of Leimgruber holds that caries is not a local destruction of the dental tissues, but a disease of the entire dental organ. The tooth is considered part of a biological system composed of pulp, hard tissues, and saliva. The hard tissues act as a membrane between the blood and saliva. Direction of exchange between the two depends on the biochemical and biophysical properties of the media and on the active or passive role of the membrane. Saliva contains a "maturation factor" which unites the submicroscopic protein and mineral constituents of the tooth and maintains a state of biodynamic equilibrium. At equilibrium the mineral and matrix of enamel and dentine are joined by homopolar valent linkages. Any agent capable of destroying the polar or valency linkages will disrupt the equilibrium and cause caries. These are to be distinguished from substances which destroy tooth structure once the linkages have been ruptured. The active molecules forming the linkages are water or the "saliva maturation factor" identified tentatively as 2-thio-S-imidazolon-5. This compound is biologically active in an acid medium and fluorine acts as a catalyst in its formation. Supportive evidence for the Leimgruber theory is extremely meager.

The Biophysical Theory

Neumann and DiSalvo developed the load theory of caries immunity based on the response of fibrous proteins to compression stress. They postulate that high chewing loads produce a sclerosing effect on the teeth divorced from either attrition or detergent action. The sclerotic changes are presumably mediated through a steady loss of the water content of the teeth possibly connected with an uncoiling of polypeptide chains or a closer packing of fibrillary crystallites. The structural changes produced by compression are alleged to increase tooth resistance to the destructive agents in the mouth. The validity of this theory has not yet been proven due to technical difficulties which have prevented testing the concept of stress-sclerosis in human enamel.

SOLUBILITY OF TOOTH ENAMEL

All of the foregoing theories of caries formation agree that the disease involves a dissolution of tooth enamel. The points of contention are the initial site and the method involved. Mechanisms have been proposed to explain the dissolution of enamel under acid, neutral, and alkaline conditions. Evidence derived from carefully controlled morphological, biophysical, and biochemical studies overwhelmingly supports the conclusion that in developing caries, enamel mineral is solubilized before the matrix is lost. Direct pH measurements indicate that carious dissolution takes place in an acid environment. Acid is present in detectable quantities in all stages and at all depths of the carious lesion. When measured *in situ* in the resting state with an antimony microelectrode, the pH averages 5.5. There is a return to the acid condition in the lesion even after repeated buffering. Either acid is formed continuously or there is a large reservoir of acid in the depths of the lesion which constantly diffuses to the surface.

Brudevold lists the evidence which suggests that enamel caries is primarily a process of demineralization as: (1) The morphological changes characteristic of the initial lesions can be reproduced in sound enamel by etching with weak acids. (2) Bacterial degradation of the organic matrix in intact enamel has not been demonstrated. (3) The matrix of demineralized enamel is so fragile that it is easily destroyed by slight mechanical trauma obviating the necessity of postulating degradation of the matrix.

The chemistry of tooth enamel solubility in acid solutions is complicated by changes in apatite composition induced by the interchange of ions between the crystal and liquid phases. Accordingly, enamel apatite does not have a constant solubility product. The solubility increases with a decrease in pH and is similar to that of secondary calcium phosphate at pH 6 and to that of primary calcium phosphate at pH 4. Carbonate tends to increase and fluorides to decrease the solubility of enamel apatite. In acid solutions, the solubility of enamel apatite is also affected by the concentration and viscosity of available buffers, the volume ratio between mineral and buffer, and the interionic action occurring during the dissolution process.

Chemical kinetic studies show that the diffusion of hydrogen ions and molecules of undissociated acid into the enamel and the rate of reaction between acid and mineral are of utmost importance in controlling the speed and extent of acid attack. Diffusion barriers on the tooth surface or in the outer enamel layer reduce the rate of acid dissolution and retard surface demineralization. Once past the protected surface layer, the acidic ions and molecules are free to react with and to dissolve the tooth structure. As soon as local concentrations of dissolved calcium and phosphate become appreciable, the acid attack stops. It resumes again when the acids have diffused further into the enamel structure or when the released calcium and phosphate ions have passed out of the involved area. Cyclic repetition of these diffusion-controlled processes leads to the ultimate decalcification of tooth structure in depth.

Microradiographical and electron microscope probes provide confirmatory evidence that demineralization antedates disintegration of the organic matrix in both enamel and dentinal caries. Zones of varying radiolucency manifested as alternating light and dark bands indicative of differences in mineral content are visible microradiographically in early enamel caries. Crystallites isolated from advanced lesions show perforations and surface erosions when examined under the electron microscope. Within the lesions, islands of organic matrix remain between the invading bacterial columns which contributed to the loss of rod substance. In dentinal caries, the collagenous fibers are remarkably intact even in regions of extensive demineralization.

The morphological changes are accompanied by alterations in the chemical composition of the affected tissues (see Chapter 1). Carious enamel and carious dentine contain more water, more organic matter and less mineral, when measured on a weight basis, than corresponding sound tissue in the same tooth. In the inorganic fraction, the most pronounced caries-associated changes are a diminution in carbonate and magnesium and an elevation in fluoride content. Decrease in total ash reflects the degree of tissue demineralization; changes in the inorganic component represent alterations in the remaining crystallites. The higher fluoride values connote that some fluorapatite remains in the lesion after the more soluble crystals have been dissolved. The increase in organic matter may be relative and/or absolute. A relative increase is associated with tissue demineralization without proteolysis; an absolute increase, with an influx of organic molecules from the salivary fluid and bacterial invasion of the involved tissues. The change in moisture content represents a replacement of the destroyed tissue elements by water.

The basic premise of the chemicoparasitic theory that the acids responsible for enamel demineralization are bacterial in origin is supported by an impressive array of experimental and clinical data. Proof that microorganisms are essential to the caries process is found in demonstrations that "germ-free" animals do not develop decay when fed a caries-promoting diet under sterile conditions. Bacteriological analyses of the dental plaques covering the sites of enamel caries invariably show a predominance of acidogenic and aciduric organisms. In the presence of a suitable substrate, these organisms produce acids in amounts which penetrate the enamel and dissolve the mineral element. The dissolution is initially confined to the subsurface enamel as the outermost layer is protected by a high fluoride content and by an organic surface film derived from the saliva. Eventually, sufficiently large spaces are created in the surface enamel to permit invasion by bacteria. Inward progression of the lesion is followed by a gradual pulpward migration of the microorganisms.

A wealth of clinical data accords with the proposition that caries is caused by acids formed from the bacterial fermentation of foods retained in the oral cavity. In man, caries invariably begins at those anatomical sites on the tooth which are sheltered from the cleansing action of mastication and where food debris and plaque are most likely to accumulate. The plaque is comprised of a matrix incorporating finely divided food particles, residues of mucin and desquamated epithelial cells and various microorganisms and their metabolites. Plaque is permeable to glucose and sucrose but relatively impermeable to starch. It contains the enzyme systems required for the conversion of fermentable carbohydrates into acid end products. Direct intraoral determinations of human plaque pH reveal that plaque acidity reaches levels capable of dissolving tooth structure within 4 minutes after oral introduction of a glucose-containing test solution. The demineralizing plaque pH is maintained for approximately 30 to 45 minutes before returning to the pretest values. The temporal sequence of acid production in the plaque corresponds closely to the oral glucose clearance time. These studies indicate that acid formation in the plaque is a discontinuous process with periods of activity directly related to the frequency with which fermentable carbohydrates are introduced into the oral cavity.

Numerous surveys show that the dental caries incidence in susceptible individuals exists in direct proportion to the quantity, form, and frequency of ingestion of fermentable carbohydrates. The carbohydrates are dietary in origin, since freshly secreted human saliva contains only negligible amounts of carbohydrate regardless of the blood sugar level. The salivary carbohydrates are bound to proteins chiefly as the glycoproteins sialomucin and fucomucin, which are resistant to degradation by the oral acidogens. Dietary regulation of carbohydrate intake, when carefully controlled and faithfully adhered to, has been reported effective in inhibition of caries formation.

Variations in caries susceptibility of teeth in different regions of the mouth have been explained, in part, by local variations in the chemical composition of the plaque. Reported differences include a high calcium concentration in lower incisor plaques, a high phosphate level in lingual plaques and a high fasting plaque pH in caries resistant areas. Fasting plaque pH values often exceed the pH of the surrounding saliva signifying that alkalies are actively produced within some plaques and may contribute to caries prevention.

EFFECT ON THE ORGANIC MATRIX

As originally postulated by Miller, after caries enters the dentine, the process becomes one of both decalcification and proteolysis. Confirmation is derived from studies of the bacterial populations of carious lesions. In dentinal caries, the microbial composition differs significantly from that of enamel caries. There is a dichotomy of predominance associated with the depth of the dentinal lesion. The deepest penetration contains a preponderance of aciduric forms with a virtual absence of dentinolytic organisms. Bacteria capable of hydrolyzing the organic residues of decalcified dentine are concentrated in the superficial aspects of the lesion. The microbial distribution suggests that in dentinal caries, as in enamel caries, decalcification precedes proteolysis.

Histological studies demonstrate further that proteolysis of the insoluble organic matrix occurs only after demineralization is well established. According to Darling, lysis of the organic component does not occur until there has been a breakdown of the enamel surface. Microradiographical and polarized light studies show that there is a differential demineralization of the enamel in caries. The earliest evidence of demineralization in the surface zone is found, most often, along the striae of Retzius. The underlying enamel already shows marked salt loss. From the striae of Retzius, demineralization spreads to the interprismatic areas and thence to the prism cores. The sequence is precipitated primarily by the loss of soluble organic matter which facilitates differential demineralization. It has been duplicated experimentally by exposing teeth to the action of dilute lactic acid and to formic acid. Whether chelating agents produce a similar pattern of mineral loss remains to be determined.

Because of technical difficulties, studies of caries-associated changes in the properties and composition of the organic matrix have usually been confined to dentine. Armstrong categorized these changes as: (1) Reduction in the concentrations of arginine, histidine, hydroxylysine, proline and hydroxyproline. (2) Increase in the quantities of phenylalanine, tyrosine and methionine. (3) Modification of the basic amino acid residues in the intact matrix. (4) Acquisition of resistance to collagenase attack. (5) Formation of a characteristic brown pigmentation. (6) Apparent loss of fluorescence activity. (7) Increased amounts of bound carbohydrate, particularly in the completely collagenase-resistant fraction. These alterations are believed to result from a combination of proteolytic degradation of dentinal collagen by bacterial collagenases, formation of a dentine-carbohydrate complex between dentinal protein and carbohydrates or allied substances and contamination of the residual matrix by non-collagenous protein.

A yellow-brown discoloration is an integral part of the organic component of the lesion in advanced caries. The discoloration has been ascribed either to exogenous staining or to an endogenous pigmentation. The former denotes a physical deposition of microbial or food stains onto the involved tooth structure; the latter a chemical combination between the organic fraction of the tooth and chromogenic substances elaborated during the caries process. The pigment has been recovered from carious lesions and identified chemically as a melanoidin. There is now substantial evidence that the pigmentation represents a nonenzymatic browning reaction between exposed dental proteins and carbohydrate derivatives. Reactive carbonyl-containing fermentation products of glucose, specifically, dihydroxy-acetone and glyceric aldehyde, and chemical decomposition products of pentoses and hexoses, notably, furfural and hydroxymethylfurfural, have been found to interact with decalcified human coronal protein to yield a yellow-brown pigment. The pigment thus formed is identical in chemical and physical properties with that present in the carious lesion. Each of the 18 amino acids with a functional amino or imino group, which are common to both human enamel and dentine, brown nonenzymatically when exposed to carbonyl-containing carbohydrate degradation products under conditions of temperature and pH which prevail in the oral cavity and in the carious lesion.

EFFECT OF FLUORIDE AND OTHER IONS

It has become increasingly apparent that fluorides play a multiple and complex role in the prevention of dental caries. The effect of ingesting fluoridated water is related primarily to the fluoride deposited in enamel preeruptively and in the few years immediately following eruption. In the posteruptive state, accessible surfaces acquire fluoride to a greater extent than inaccessible areas, thus limiting the effectiveness of fluorides in the sites most susceptible to caries attack.

Ingested fluoride is deposited in enamel as fluorapatite which is more resistant to caries formation than hydroxyapatite. Fluoride also has the unique ability to induce apatite formation from solutions of calcium and phosphate. It favors the conversion of soluble acid phosphates to solid basic phosphate thereby maintaining the apatite structure even at low pH values. In the alternating process of demineralization and reprecipitation which characterizes the reaction between acid and tooth mineral, fluoride promotes the deposition of apatite. This effect is counteracted by carbonate, magnesium, and other ions that possess a tendency to disturb the apatite lattice and by agents such as pyrophosphate and other organic phosphates which alter the surface of the apatite crystal and prevent crystal growth. Since there are no detectable changes in the concentrations of other tooth components as a result of fluoride deposition, the caries-resistant effect of fluoride appears to be mediated in part through the maintenance of the integrity of the apatite crystal.

EFFECT OF AGE

Resistance of human teeth to carious attack appears to increase with age. Newly erupted teeth are considerably more susceptible to caries than are older teeth. The diminished propensity to decay has been ascribed usually to a posteruptive maturation process in the enamel. While the mechanism responsible for maturation and enhanced resistance is unknown, it is generally associated with exposure to saliva. Following eruption, teeth will undergo both physical and chemical alterations with time. Saliva contributes significantly to the change in ionic content and permeability of enamel. Thus, the bone-seeking elements, fluorine, zinc, lead, and iron, accumulate in the surface enamel in quantities related to the external environment of the tooth. With increasing age, there is also an increase in the fluoride and a decrease in the carbonate concentrations of surface enamel. In addition to affecting sound enamel, there is evidence that the organic and mineral constituents of saliva may deposit in areas of defective or demineralized enamel to decrease the rate of development of the carious lesion.

BIOCHEMISTRY OF THE SHEATH SPACES IN CARIES

Polarization microscopy and impregnation techniques which have been used to investigate the biochemistry of the sheath spaces in caries provide additional evidence that the disease is essentially an acid-induced, inorganic leaching process. The sheath spaces partially surround the enamel rods and separate them from the interprismatic substance. The spaces are completely enclosed in fully calcified enamel except in the regions of the enamel tufts. During calcification, the sheath spaces fill with crystals of the type present in the prisms and interprismatic substance. In caries, the sheath spaces reopen. The reopening has been attributed to the early dissolution of the rod crystals lining the sheath spaces. The position and greater solubility of these crystals, due to a high carbonate content, render them highly susceptible to acid action.

Electron micrographs of experimentally produced enamel caries show (1) a widening of the inter-rod spaces in the relatively sound outer enamel layer, suggestive of acid diffusion between the rods; (2) a generalized destruction of the rods deep to the outer layer, attributable to direct penetration by acids; and (3) an advancing front below the lesion with inter-rod space enlargement, denotive of a return to the original acid diffusion pathway.

In addition to penetrating between the organic matrix and enamel crystallites, acids also attack dislocation sites in the center of the enamel prisms to produce hollow cores. These dislocation sites are formed during enamel deposition and maturation when the inorganic material is deposited in an organic matrix which has a helical structure comparable to collagen.

REMINERALIZATION

Although human enamel is lacking in biological powers of regeneration, *in vitro* studies indicate that saliva has the capacity to remineralize slightly decalcified enamel surfaces. The ability varies between individuals but is fairly constant for samples obtained from the same subject. Saliva serves as a calcifying metastable solution with respect to enamel in this process. The oral fluids act as a source of minerals for the remineralization of submicroscopic spaces inaccessible to organic molecules and for nucleator organic molecules necessary for the repair of large spaces. Remineralization is accelerated in the presence of 1 ppm fluoride. The fluoride promotes nucleation of calcium phosphate and decreases the solvent power of the liquid phase. It is doubtful whether remineralization restores the continuity of the enamel surface in its entirety or is ever sufficient to produce complete healing of the carious lesion. It may be of considerable importance, however, in retarding or arresting caries.

SELECTED REFERENCES

Brown, W. E. (Ed.): Physicochemical mechanisms of dental caries, J. Dent. Res., *53*, 155–318, 1974.

Sognnaes, R. F. (Ed.): *Chemistry and Prevention of Dental Caries*, Springfield, Charles C Thomas, 1962.

Staple, P. H. (Ed.): *Advances in Oral Biology*, New York, Academic Press, Inc., vol. 1, 1964; vol. 2, 1966.

Whipple, H. E., (Ed.): Mechanisms of dental caries, Ann. New York Acad. Sci., *131*, 685–930, 1965.

Wolstenholme, G. E. W. and O'Connor, M. (Eds.): *Caries Resistant Teeth*, Boston, Little, Brown & Company, 1965.

Chapter 15

Nutritional Basis of Oral Health

KENNETH O. MADSEN, Ph.D.

Beliefs about foods and proper diets are ancient; however, nutrition and chemistry as sciences developed concurrently mostly during the 18th century emerging finally as biochemistry near the end of the 19th century. Biochemistry remained synonymous with nutrition until recently when there has been an increasing tendency to make nutritional biochemistry a separate discipline.

The nutritional aspects of biochemistry began with the study of calorimetry. It was established that carbohydrate, fat, and protein were the gross constituents of foods that, upon oxidation in the body (respiration), released characteristic equivalents of energy.* It was soon recognized, however, that protein probably played a more specific role than that of providing body heat. Today, a host of specific roles in body chemistry has been assigned to the amino acids and proteins, although the amino acid threonine was not recognized as being required in the diet until 1935.

About the same time it was realized that certain amino acids were necessary, it was also discovered that there existed other essential materials or "accessory food factors" besides the gross components of foods. That is, in addition to carbohydrate, fat, protein, and minerals, other factors were required for growth and health. The discovery of these factors, the vitamins, excited the interest of nutritional biochemists for several decades. Vitamin B_{12}, latest to be discovered, was not structurally defined in its coenzyme form until 1955. All the water-soluble vitamins have now been assigned one or more specific roles in intermediary metabolism. Understanding of the roles of ascorbic acid and the fat-soluble vitamins is still incomplete.

The need for many dietary minerals is well known. By the beginning of this century, the requirements for the major mineral elements sodium, chlorine, calcium, and phosphorus, and the trace element iron were fairly

* In this chapter, "calories" always refers to large calories, *i.e.*, kilocalories (kcal or C).

Table 15–1.   Significant Constituents of Foods and Estimates of Daily Consumption by the American Adult Male (Essential Nutrients Capitalized)

Energy Metabolism

Carbohydrates (gm)		Lipids (gm)		Proteins (Amino Acids) (gm)	
Starches, Dextrins	150	Fats & Oils*	130	8 ESSENTIAL AMINO ACIDS	30
Sucrose	110	Phospholipids*	5	10 Semi- or Non-essential	
Other Sugars	70	ESSENTIAL FREE FATTY ACIDS*	2	Amino Acids	50
(Organic Acids	2)	Cholesterol	1		
Bulk (Indigestible)	20				

Body Structure and Homeostasis

Major minerals (gm)

SODIUM	4	CHLORIDE†	5	POTASSIUM†	6
CALCIUM†	0.8	PHOSPHATE† (as P)	1.5	MAGNESIUM†	0.4

Catalysts

Micronutrient Elements (mg)

IRON	10	MANGANESE	5	SELENIUM	0.5
ZINC	10	MOLYBDENUM	0.3	CHROMIUM	0.06
COPPER	2	IODIDE	0.1	FLUORIDE	2
		COBALT	0.1	Vanadium	2
				Nickel	0.3
				Silicon	?

Vitamins (mg)

Fat-Soluble

VITAMIN A (and active CAROTENES)	6	VITAMIN E (TOCOPHEROLS)	6
VITAMIN D (CALCIFEROLS)	0.04	VITAMIN K (active forms)	2

Water-Soluble

THIAMINE (B₁)	1.5	PYRIDOXINE (B₆)	3	BIOTIN	0.2
RIBOFLAVIN (B₂)	1.8	CYANOCOBALAMINE (B₁₂)	0.01	CHOLINE	700
NIACIN	15	PANTOTHENIC ACID	10	Inositol	1000
ASCORBIC ACID	75	FOLIC ACID (FOLACIN)	1	Vitamin P Complex	25

*TOTAL ESSENTIAL FATTY ACIDS   40 gm.
† Also function as catalysts.

well recognized. The importance of other major elements such as potassium and magnesium, as well as other trace elements, was subsequently discovered. Metabolic roles for a number of trace or catalytic mineral elements are quite well known. Those nutrients remaining undiscovered are most likely to be found among the trace minerals of foods. Recently, chromium, selenium, and fluoride have been classified as nutritionally essential. Fluoride, long considered only beneficial for prevention of dental caries, may stabilize bone when ingested over a life span and also promote growth, fertility, and hematopoiesis. Vanadium, nickel, and silicon are suspected to be essential for man.

That our knowledge of man's nutritional needs is essentially complete is shown by the fact that mixtures of known chemical compounds have supported life and apparent health in young adults for several weeks.

The essential elements and compounds and other significant food constituents that must be obtained from the external environment, usually diet, are listed in Table 15–1. Despite the occurrence of thousands of different compounds in food or synthesized from food by the body, relatively few are quantitatively significant. Even the food constituents that are nutritionally essential in small amounts (micronutrients) are relatively few in number. Moreover, the significant food substances can be broadly categorized into only three groups: those necessary for energy metabolism, body structures and homeostasis, and catalysis. These categories often overlap. For example, calcium is a skeletal building block and has catalytic function. Notably, only protein, the major building block of life, defies classification. It routinely supplies calories. One-third of body protein is collagen; blood, albumin and hemoglobin are major blood homeostatic proteins. Yet, active proteins like individual enzymes and hormones demonstrate their catalytic roles at very small concentrations.

Despite the vast accumulation of data, the complete function of each nutrient is only partly understood. Even when chemical mechanisms of nutrition seem clear, the regulation of mechanisms and the relationships of mechanisms to each other and to cellular sites of action are often obscure. For example, although nutrition started with the study of energy metabolism, much about this subject is still unknown. The nutritional aspects of energy capture and transfer are still under active study at the subcellular level of the mitochondrion, and the control of energy nutrition is being studied at the whole body level as well.

The status of our current nutritional knowledge and its application to oral health may be understood best in terms of what remains unknown. Frontiers of research are listed below. It is apparent that much remains to be learned and that we can expect the new knowledge to have an ever greater significance to dental practice.

1. *Quantitative Requirements.* The most complete data have been established for average, normal young adults, yet even for these persons, the extent of individual variation has not been defined. The quantitative needs

throughout the life span, under various physiological conditions and in disease or injury situations, require further study. The best data measure only certain restricted ages during the life span, mostly under healthy non-stressful conditions. Furthermore, these requirements need to be based on more sophisticated criteria than those used in the past. For example, the importance of nutritional status to mental attitudes and performances, in addition to effects on growth or susceptibility to disease, is just now being measured.

2. *Interrelationships of Nutrients.* It is now realized that the absolute daily requirement of a nutrient may be less critical than the relative amounts of other nutrients with which it interacts. For example, more calcium for skeletal growth is required when soft tissue growth is enhanced by a diet rich in both calories and protein. Similarly, an excess of any one nutrient may produce a relative deficiency of another.

3. *Acute and Chronic Factors that Increase Requirements.* Infection, inflammation, and trauma greatly increase the demand for nutrients. For example, caloric demands may increase to 5,000 calories a day or more in extreme cases. These needs and the techniques to supply them are only now being understood. Chronically used drugs are of nutritional concern. For example, some oral contraceptives increase the demand for folic acid and perhaps for vitamin B_6.

4. *Patterns of Eating.* Currently, nutritional requirements are expressed on a daily basis, but frequency of eating throughout the day can influence minimum requirements and may determine the optimal allowances for nutrients. Frequency and size of meals affect satiety and may also influence other factors such as the effectiveness of quick-acting metabolic feedback controls. The slower adjustments of hormonal balances may also be affected by food intake habits. The pattern of eating has only recently been shown to affect oral health.

5. *Organoleptic Factors.* The effect of such physiological factors as taste, smell, and salivation on satiety is important in designing calorie-controlled diets and in the acceptability of new foods. The effect of dentures and dental materials on taste, palatability, and food selection habits has received inadequate attention. Operation may be followed by hypogeusia or dysgeusia, two unpleasant reactions to food which can be treated with zinc. Copper, vitamin A, and other nutrients have been associated with organoleptic activity, also.

6. *Inborn Errors of Metabolism.* Discovery of the genetic deficiencies affecting metabolism is making it increasingly important to devise compensating diets. Genetic error may be suspected whenever the origin of a disease is obscure and a nutritional component seems to be involved. The development of dietary regimens is expected to help those who are highly susceptible to such diseases. Psychic influences of food constituents, such as choline and catecholamine precursors, may vary among individuals.

7. *The Practice of Proper Nutrition.* As social and physiological demands change and advances are made in science and dentistry, the role of the dental profession in patient counseling and community education will change and, predictably, will increase.

Development of new foods and food enrichment programs based on a growing understanding of nutrition will help to assure optimal nutrition for population groups, but will not replace the need for nutritional guidance and education of individuals, families and communities. In fact, the correct use of new foods such as protein substitutes has not been clarified for the public. Without more training few can use the information on food labels.

The Dentist and Nutrition

The dentist may become the professional person from whom an increasing number of persons will receive nutritional advice. Since a high incidence of oral ills exist, the dentist sees a broader cross section of the population more frequently, for longer visits and under less acute conditions of illness than the physician. These factors provide opportunity not only to determine nutritional status, but also to communicate nutritional advice. Although difficult, it is especially important to detect the signs of mild nutritional deficiency. Only repeated patient contact will establish whether nervousness, fatigue and associated vague symptoms are chronic and characteristic and therefore possibly related to nutritional status. Moreover, it is noteworthy that the head and neck areas and especially the oral cavity most readily show the outward signs of nutritional deficiency. As the practice of preventive dentistry becomes increasingly possible, nutritional guidance will become a greater part of "bread and butter" dentistry.

NUTRITIONAL STANDARDS

Recommended Daily Dietary Allowances

The development of nutritional standards is the first step in the application of nutritional knowledge. In 1941, the Food and Nutrition Board of the National Research Council of the National Academy of Sciences accumulated the available data on nutritional requirements. This Board, comprised of recognized nutritional authorities, estimated average *minimum* physiological *requirements*. They then increased these requirements two to three times above the actual minimums to levels that would compensate for average variations in individual requirements and for environmental variations encountered by normal persons in the United States. These levels were called *allowances* and termed the "Recommended Daily Dietary Allowances" (RDA). They include allowances for variations due to age, sex, and reproduction. Thus far, only a small percentage of the life span has been studied as the basis for making such assessments. The best data have been

Table 15–2. Food and Nutrition Board, National Academy of Sciences-National

Designed for the maintenance of good nutrition of

	Age (yr)	Weight (kg) (lb)		Height (cm) (in)		Energy (kcal)[b]	Protein (g)	Fat-Soluble Vitamins		Vita-min D (I.U.)	Vita-min E Activity[e] (I.U.)
								Vita-min A Activity (R.E.)[c]	(I.U.)		
Infants	0.0–0.5	6	14	60	24	kg × 117	kg × 2.2	420[d]	1,400	400	4
	0.5–1.0	9	20	71	28	kg × 108	kg × 2.0	400	2,000	400	5
Children	1–3	13	28	86	34	1,300	23	400	2,000	400	7
	4–6	20	44	110	44	1,800	30	500	2,500	400	9
	7–10	30	66	135	54	2,400	36	700	3,300	400	10
Males	11–14	44	97	158	63	2,800	44	1,000	5,000	400	12
	15–18	61	134	172	69	3,000	54	1,000	5,000	400	15
	19–22	67	147	172	69	3,000	54	1,000	5,000	400	15
	23–50	70	154	172	69	2,700	56	1,000	5,000		15
	51+	70	154	172	69	2,400	56	1,000	5,000		15
Females	11–14	44	97	155	62	2,400	44	800	4,000	400	12
	15–18	54	119	162	65	2,100	48	800	4,000	400	12
	19–22	58	128	162	65	2,100	46	800	4,000	400	12
	23–50	58	128	162	65	2,000	46	800	4,000		12
	51+	58	128	162	65	1,800	46	800	4,000		12
Pregnant						+300	+30	1,000	5,000	400	15
Lactating						+500	+20	1,200	6,000	400	15

[a] The allowances are intended to provide for individual variations among most normal persons as they live in the United States under usual environmental stresses. Diets should be based on a variety of common foods in order to provide other nutrients for which human requirements have been less well defined.

[b] Kilojoules (k J) = 4.2 × kcal.

[c] Retinol equivalents.

[d] Assumed to be all as retinol in milk during the first 6 months of life. All subsequent intakes are assumed to be half as retinol and half as β-carotene when calculated from international units.

Research Council, Recommended Daily Dietary Allowances,[a] Revised 1974
practically all healthy people in the United States

	Water-Soluble Vitamins						Minerals					
Ascorbic Acid (mg)	Folacin[f] (μg)	Niacin[g] (mg)	Riboflavin (mg)	Thiamin (mg)	Vitamin B_6 (mg)	Vitamin B_{12} (μg)	Calcium (mg)	Phosphorus (mg)	Iodine (μg)	Iron (mg)	Magnesium (mg)	Zinc (mg)
35	50	5	0.4	0.3	0.3	0.3	360	240	35	10	60	3
35	50	8	0.6	0.5	0.4	0.3	540	400	45	15	70	5
40	100	9	0.8	0.7	0.6	1.0	800	800	60	15	150	10
40	200	12	1.1	0.9	0.9	1.5	800	800	80	10	200	10
40	300	16	1.2	1.2	1.2	2.0	800	800	110	10	250	10
45	400	18	1.5	1.4	1.6	3.0	1,200	1,200	130	18	350	15
45	400	20	1.8	1.5	2.0	3.0	1,200	1,200	150	18	400	15
45	400	20	1.8	1.5	2.0	3.0	800	800	140	10	350	15
45	400	18	1.6	1.4	2.0	3.0	800	800	130	10	350	15
45	400	16	1.5	1.2	2.0	3.0	800	800	110	10	350	15
45	400	16	1.3	1.2	1.6	3.0	1,200	1,200	115	18	300	15
45	400	14	1.4	1.1	2.0	3.0	1,200	1,200	115	18	300	15
45	400	14	1.4	1.1	2.0	3.0	800	800	100	18	300	15
45	400	13	1.2	1.0	2.0	3.0	800	800	100	18	300	15
45	400	12	1.1	1.0	2.0	3.0	800	800	80	10	300	15
60	800	+2	+0.3	+0.3	2.5	4.0	1,200	1,200	125	18+[h]	450	20
80	600	+4	+0.5	+0.3	2.5	4.0	1,200	1,200	150	18	150	25

As retinol equivalents, three-fourths are as retinol and one-fourth as β-carotene.

[e] Total vitamin E activity, estimated to be 80% as α-tocopherol and 20% other tocopherols.

[f] The folacin allowances refer to dietary sources as determined by *Lactobacillus casei* assay. Pure forms of folacin may be effective in doses less than one-fourth of the recommended dietary allowance.

[g] Although allowances are expressed as niacin, it is recognized that on the average 1 mg of niacin is derived from each 60 mg of dietary tryptophan.

[h] This increased requirement cannot be met by ordinary diets; therefore, the use of supplemental iron is recommended.

established with 22-year-old men and women represented in Table 15–2 as the 23- to 50-year-old groups. Much of the discussion of nutrition in this chapter will be in terms of these "standard" young adults.

Other Nutrient Standards

A variation of the RDA is the US–RDA, established recently by the Food and Drug Administration (FDA) to replace the outmoded MDR (so-called Minimum Daily Requirements) (Table 15–3). The public will become most familiar with this standard, since the FDA devised it as the legal guideline

Table 15–3.   US Recommended Daily Allowances (US-RDA) (for labeling vitamin and mineral supplements)*

Vitamins and Minerals	Unit of Measurement	Adults and Children 4 or More Years of Age	Infants and Children Under 4 Years of Age	Pregnant or Lactating Women
Vitamin A	International Units	5,000	2,500	8,000
Vitamin D	"	400†	400	400
Vitamin E	"	30	10	30
Vitamin C	Milligrams	60	40	60
Folic Acid	"	0.4	0.2	0.8
Thiamine	"	1.5	0.7	1.7
Riboflavin	"	1.7	0.8	2.0
Niacin	"	20	9.0	20
Vitamin B_6	"	2.0	0.7	2.5
Vitamin B_{12}	Micrograms	6	3	8
Biotin	Milligrams	0.3	0.15	0.3
Pantothenic Acid	"	10	5.0	10
Calcium	Grams	1.0	0.8	1.3
Phosphorus	"	1.0	0.8	1.3
Iodine	Micrograms	150	70	150
Iron	Milligrams	18	10	18
Magnesium	"	400	200	450
Copper	"	2.0	1.0	2.0
Zinc	"	15	8.0	15

* The US–RDA used for food labeling and for foods that are also vitamin and mineral supplements differ from the US–RDA in this table in the following respects: (1) they do not specify US–RDA for pregnant and lactating women; (2) the order of listing required on the label is different; and (3) protein is added at the level of 65 gm for adults and children 4 or more years of age, and 28 gm for infants and children under 4 years. If the protein efficiency ratio of protein is equal to or better than that of casein, US–RDA is 45 and 20 gm, respectively.

† Presence optional for adults and children 4 or more years of age in vitamin and mineral supplements.

Table 15–4. Suggested Guide to Interpretation of Nutrient Intake Data*
(ICNND-Values)

	Deficient	Low	Acceptable	High
Protein, gm/kg body weight	<0.5	0.5–0.9	1.0–1.4	≥1.5
Calcium, gm/day	<.3	0.30–0.39	0.4–0.7	≥0.8
Iron, mg/day	<6	6–8	9–11	≥12
Vitamin A, I.U./day	<2,000	2,000–3,499	3,500–4,999	≥5,000
Thiamine, mg/1000 Calories	<.2	0.20–0.29	0.3–0.4	≥.5
Riboflavin, mg/day	<.7	0.7–1.1	1.2–1.4	≥1.5
Niacin, mg/day	<5	5–9	10–14	≥15
Ascorbic acid, mg/day	<10	10–29	30–49	≥50
†Calories	..	..	..	..

* This guide applies to a 25-year-old physically active male of 170 cm in height and 65 kg in weight living in a temperate climate and consuming a varied diet.
† The requirement for calories is so dependent upon size, climate, age, and physical activity that no figures can be stated.

for regulating the labeling of foods and nutritional supplements. Most of the values are selected from RDA tables although they include copper and biotin, which are not listed in the RDA.

In 1951, a governmental group, the Interdepartmental Committee on Nutrition for National Defense (ICNND), established a guide which helps to interpret the numbers found in the RDA table. It describes an acceptable range of nutrient intake for a standard man slightly smaller than the average man described in the RDA table. It defines high, acceptable, low, or deficient ranges (Table 15–4).

Neither the RDA nor the ICNND standards are directly applicable to small groups or to individuals. They are based on statistical averages and some persons may have greater or less than the average requirement for one or more nutrients. Nevertheless, in lieu of biochemical data or other measurements to judge individual nutritional status, a diet can be compared to these standards for detecting probable areas of nutritional improvement.

Table 15–5. Daily Food Guide—A Revised and Amplified Version

Food Group and Recommended Minimum Daily Servings (MDS)	Serving Sizes and Descriptions	Further Recommendations
Milk and Milk Equivalents Children (Over 8) 3 Teens 4 Adults 2 Pregnancy 4 Lactation 6	8 oz. (1 cup) whole, skim, low fat, or 2% milk or reconstituted powder 1½ oz. (1½ slices) American or cheddar cheese 1½ cups cottage cheese 8 oz. yogurt or buttermilk 2 cups ice cream	1. Read labels and select products fortified with vitamins A and D when possible. 2. For weight control, choose low fat milks, cottage cheese, or plain yogurt; avoid ice cream, malts, and dairy desserts. 3. Liquid milk is not essential. Recognize and count servings of dairy products used in cooking.
Meat and Meat Equivalents 2 for everyone	2–3 oz. lean cooked meat without bone or fat (beef, veal, pork, lamb, poultry, fish, shellfish, liver, heart, kidney) 2 eggs 4 tablespoons peanut butter 1 cup cooked dry beans or peas 3 small packages or ½ cup nuts 4 slices luncheon meat 2 wieners	1. For weight control: a. Avoid fried, deep-fat fried, breaded, gravied or ground meat preparations. b. Select low fat meats and remove fat by trimming, broiling or blotting. c. Distribute meat items sparingly throughout the day; their fat content satisfies appetite. The same is true for eggs and nuts.

Food Group / Servings	Serving Sizes	Guidelines
Vegetable and Fruits 4 for everyone Include one good source of vitamin A and one of vitamin C each day	½ cup fruit, vegetable, "greens" ½ cup citrus, tomato, or "C" enriched juices 1 cup tossed salad 1 small orange, carrot, sweet potato, red pepper 1 medium-sized apple, banana, potato, tomato, lemon ½ medium-sized grapefruit; ¼ cantaloupe ¼ cup raisins 4 tablespoons catsup	1. Select a variety of fruits and vegetables. Avoid added sugar. Emphasize raw items. 2. Select items rich in: *Vitamins A and C.* All leafy "greens"; tomatoes; watermelon; red peppers; sweet potatoes; cantaloupe; broccoli. *Vitamin A.* Carrots; squash; pumpkin; apricots, and other dark yellow vegetables. *Vitamin C.* All citrus fruits; cauliflower; okra; *green* peas, beans, limas and peppers; pineapple; brussels sprouts; turnips; cabbage; strawberries; potatoes.
Breads and Cereals 4 for everyone	1 slice bread or equivalent amount of pancake, tortilla, bun, etc. ½ cup cooked cereal or grits ½ cup macaroni, spaghetti, noodles, rice 1 oz. (3/2 cup) dry cereal 6 2" × 2" saltine crackers 2" cube cornbread 2 cups popcorn	1. Whenever possible, select products that are: a. Made from whole grain or from flours and meals enriched with iron and B-vitamins. b. Less sweet—not pre-sweetened. c. Low in calories—not used as snacks or desserts. 2. Restrict selection of baked goods not listed; these are usually rich in sugar and fat and poor in nutritional content.

Table 15–5. (Continued)

Food Group and Recommended Minimum Daily Servings (MDS)	Serving Sizes and Descriptions	Further Recommendations
Typical Non-food Group Items	Alcoholic beverages, soft drinks, all creams, coffee creamers, margarine, butter, bacon, chips, dips, salad dressing, gravies, spices, Jell-O, sugar, candy, jelly, honey, syrup, many baked goods, pickles, olives. *Most of these are "empty-calorie" foods, i.e., high in calories and low in nutrients.*	1. Select remaining calories from both food group and non-food group items. 2. To give interest and added flavor to meals, include non-food group items. To control body weight, limit these rather than food group items.
Further Guidelines	1. The MDS from the Four Food Groups provides *only* about 1200 calories. 2. The MDS from a *variety* of foods provides the protein, vitamins and minerals normally needed without using further supplements, special foods or pharmaceuticals. 3. Balanced meals achieved by selecting one item from each food group at each meal are best. Snacks, also, should be selected from the Four Food Groups. 4. To complete good nutrition: (a) select *iodized* salt and use sparingly, and (b) choose one or more rich iron sources (liver, beef, lamb, shellfish, eggs, leafy green vegetables, dried beans and fruits, enriched or whole grain cereals) and use often.

Food Standards

For general public use and for the professional person giving nutritional guidance, it is desirable to have a standard based on foods rather than nutrients. First, the United States Department of Agriculture classified foods into seven groups in 1946. This was then simplified to a daily guide in which only four food groups were defined—milk, meat, vegetable-fruit and bread-cereal (Table 15–5). The minimum number of servings each food group should provide on a daily basis are 2, 2, 4 and 4, respectively. With a few exceptions in the meat group, two of the groups contain animal foods and two contain plant foods. A prime purpose of this chapter will be to describe the sound scientific basis for this food guide and to demonstrate its usefulness in the practice of dentistry.

COMPOSITION OF THE DAILY DIET

Nature and Sources of Nutrients

Although most foods contain a wide variety of nutrients, their relative importance in a daily diet usually depends upon their containing significant concentrations of one or more nutrients. On the other hand, even low concentrations of nutrients in a food item become important when that food is eaten in large quantities or when the nutrients in it are of superior quality. For example, the low protein concentration in potatoes becomes significant when potatoes are eaten in large amounts. In addition, the potato protein has a higher biological value than most plant proteins. Another exception obtains when a low total nutrient content is biologically available, that is, easily digested, absorbed, or utilized. The total iron or calcium content of some foods may be impressive, but when these elements are minimally available, foods of lower but more available content are superior sources.

Dry Matter Composition

Understanding of the gross contents of the usual diet may readily be obtained by drying and weighing the several pounds of daily food. The dry matter in the usual adult diet will weigh about 1 to $1\frac{1}{2}$ lb or about 500 to 700 gm. Carbohydrate, fat, and protein contribute most of the weight (Table 15–6).

Carbohydrate

Calories. Two-thirds of the daily dry matter eaten, that is, the weight of the diet exclusive of water, is one nutrient, carbohydrate. Assuming 4 calories per gram as a practical value for the energy level of carbohydrates, 405 gm of carbohydrate would supply the suggested 60% of 2700 kilocalories that are allowed for the standard man according to RDA values. This alone would supply nearly the entire 1800 calorie basal metabolism require-

Table 15-6. Typical Estimates of Calories and Caloric Nutrients Provided by Minimum Number of Servings from the Daily Food Guide for Adults with Estimated Minimal Requirements and Suggested Allowances

Food Group	Amount per day	Calories per Serving	Total Calories	Total Grams per Day[1]		
				Carbohydrate	Fat	Protein
Milk	2 cups	170	340	24	20	16
Meat	2 servings (3 oz. each)	220	440	—	30	42
Vegetable-Fruit	4 servings[2]	25	100	25	—	—
Bread-Cereal	4 servings	70	280	60	—	8
Total			1160	109	50	66
Estimated Minimal Requirements[3]						
23-year-old man			1800[4]	100	30	20
23-year-old woman			1200[4]	100	30	20
Suggested Allowances[3]						
23-year-old man			2700	405	90	68
23-year-old woman			2000	300	67	50

[1] Estimates exclude amounts less than 1 gram.

[2] Assumes equal selections from: (1) vegetables providing essentially no calories, (2) vegetables providing 36 calories per serving, and (3) a typical estimate of 40 calories for fruit servings.

[3] See text for rationale upon which these requirements and allowances are based.

[4] Based on a BMR of 1.85 and 1.35 kilocalories/square meter of body surface/hr for standard man and woman, respectively.

ment for the standard man. This large intake of just one nutrient has important consequences to be discussed later in terms of vitamin requirements, body weight control, metabolism and oral health, especially with respect to dental caries.

Starches. More than 90% of the dietary carbohydrate is provided by plants and about half of it is in polysaccharide form as plant starches largely from cereal grains. These are classified primarily in the bread-cereal food group. Processing and cooking may release sticky forms of starch and protein which increase oral retention and are detrimental to good oral health. Thus residues from breads, cereals and pastas such as macaroni and spaghetti are readily retained in the mouth. Newer commercial products attempt to limit sticky forms which are often the least acceptable from the standpoint of taste and texture. Further processing, toasting, and baking cause drying and hardening with subsequent reduction of stickiness. Partial hydrolysis also occurs, but the dextrins produced are probably no more soluble or fermentable than starches but less sticky so that the overall effect is beneficial. Starchy foods may increase in retention time in the following order: potatoes, pastas, whole wheat bread or toasted white bread, and white bread.

Starches and Caries. The effect of starchy foods on caries production has not been established. Such items should be eaten only during meals when saliva and other foods are available to aid in oral clearance and be avoided between meals when they enhance retention of sugars. Sugars are cariogenic and often are eaten between meals. Sugar-coated cereals, especially, and regular dry cereals normally made with addition of some sugar should be restricted to the mealtime experience. Similarly, caramel-coated popcorn should be avoided between meals, but popcorn is not retentive and would seem to be ideal as a between-meal snack from the caries preventive standpoint. Unfortunately, reliable rankings for food cariogenicities do not yet exist so caution is necessary when recommending between meal items.

Sugars and Caries. The remaining half of the daily carbohydrate intake is made up of sugars of which one-half, or about 80 to 120 gm, is sucrose. Sucrose, being readily fermented by oral microorganisms, is highly cariogenic. Sucrose more than other sugars promotes the type of dental caries associated with thick plaque deposits. These plaques, containing insoluble, highly-adhesive dextrans, which differ from food starches, are alpha-1,6 linked chains with various branching configurations. They are produced extracellularly by certain strains of oral streptococci.

Oral enzymes offer possibilities for the control of oral carbohydrates, especially since food-borne enzymes after oral clearance would be digested as any other food protein. The normally occurring enzyme salivary amylase does not demonstrably affect orally retained starchy foods; however, dextranase, a bacterial enzyme that hydrolyzes bacterial dextrans, inhibits caries production when placed in the diet or drinking water of hamsters. Caries may occur readily without dextran or copious plaque residues and all sugars, even slowly fermenting milk sugar, lactose, are cariogenic when tested in animal caries studies. The sweet sugar alcohols, sorbitol and mannitol, contained in some sugarless gums and pharmaceuticals are so slowly metabolized that they are considered noncariogenic. Therefore, these gums and some brands of "chewable" vitamins are not caries threats.

The consensus is that lactose consumed in milk, cheese, and other items of the milk food group is not cariogenic and can be consumed between meals. However, milk is retained on the oral mucosa so that, from the standpoint of caries prevention, it would be better to avoid sucrose-sweetened milk items such as malts, chocolate milk and ice cream between meals.

Lactose comprises only 5 to 10% of the dietary carbohydrate and is the only common animal food source of carbohydrate. Glycogen, animal starch, is rapidly lost during meat processing and is ingested as such only through such pleasures as raw shellfish.

The remaining sugars are glucose and fructose from honey and vegetable-fruit food group items. This group also provides starches in the form of parenchymatous fruits and legumes, as do dry beans and peas which, however, are classified in the meat food group. The carbohydrates in most of these foods are usually not highly retentive.

Carbohydrates of Vegetable-Fruit Food Group and Dental Health. Carbohydrate is the only quantitatively important constituent provided by the vegetable-fruit group and these carbohydrates are not usually present in an orally fermentable physical form. In fact, if foods such as apples, carrots, celery or even potatoes or cauliflower are only gently processed to retain their firm texture or eaten raw, then they require chewing, stimulate salivation, and serve to promote oral clearance of food debris. Accordingly, such foods are termed "detergent" foods. It is unlikely that they aid in removal of much bacterial plaque; however, they ordinarily facilitate the oral clearance of sugar-containing food debris and thereby reduce caries. Preliminary studies suggest that the frequent presence of foods requiring chewing and elimination of the carbohydrate retention factor may promote periodontal health. Raw items are ideal in lunches as well as between meals. Care must be taken to assure acceptance of these foods by preserving crispness and freshness with appropriate hydrating, wrapping, and refrigeration.

Vegetable items are best if only blanched during cooking or cooked in minimum water until tender—a skill of Chinese cooking. This not only preserves their detergent qualities, but also prevents the extraction and loss of soluble vitamins and minerals. The destruction of heat- and oxygen-labile vitamins, especially thiamine by heat and ascorbic acid by oxygen, is also minimized. The flavor and color are also retained making these foods more attractive to many who otherwise may miss their nutritional benefits.

Since the effect of very sweet fruit on caries is largely unknown, oranges, pineapple, peaches, and sweet juices, although not highly retentive, probably should be used infrequently between meals. Citrus fruits can sufficiently stimulate salivation so as to be essentially noncariogenic. A beneficial effect was reported in a preliminary experiment where malic acid from apples was incorporated with sorbitol in a noncariogenic candy mint designed to stimulate salivation between meals as an anticaries measure. Dried fruits such as raisins are unquestionably retentive, contain sugar, and are to be avoided.

Table 15–6 summarizes the carbohydrate contributions from each food group when the recommended minimum number of servings per day is consumed. Commonly, much more than 60 grams of starches from the bread-cereal group are in the daily diet. Note that honey and sucrose items such as syrups, jellies, candies, and sugar are high in caloric value and contain essentially no other nutrients. They are not included in any food group and are often termed "empty-calorie" foods.

In summary, refined, processed starchy foods present the problem of oral retention. They may be cariogenic, *per se*, or, under certain conditions and in the presence of sugars in particular, caries-promoting. The clinical evidence relating to the cariogenicity of sucrose-containing items will be discussed in connection with the control of dental caries.

Indigestible Bulk

All of the carbohydrates mentioned thus far are completely digestible by the adult. The indigestible material is termed "bulk" and comprises 3 to 5% of the daily intake of dry matter. It is mostly "crude fiber" or plant polysaccharides such as celluloses, pectins or gums. A small portion of the bulk represents fibrous proteins such as skin keratin. The bulk materials bind water and stimulate intestinal movements promoting proper fecal elimination. In excess they can cause diarrhea.

Formerly, many persons were overly worried about constipation and used cereal brans and cathartic fruits and vegetables excessively. Today, the reduced fiber level of most diets has become a matter of concern, and there is need to reemphasize the use of dietary fiber such as raw and less processed foods from the vegetable-fruit and bread-cereal groups by persons of all ages. Good peristalsis is maintained by assuring good nutrition for healthy gastrointestinal tract musculature and a reasonable amount of exercise.

Fat

Caloric Considerations. If the dry matter from an ideal diet were extracted with a fat solvent, 90 grams of fat equivalent to 30% of the total caloric intake would be obtained (Table 15–6). This is based on the 2700 calorie allowance for the standard man and a caloric equivalent of 9 kilocalories per gram for most food fats and oils.

The average person is aware of only about one-fourth of this fat, the so-called "visible" fat as butter, margarine, salad dressings, and fried foods. Another one-fourth includes, in addition, the shortenings and oils used in cooking which are hidden, except from the cook. Except for butter and lard, these fats are largely derived from plant sources and are rich in unsaturated fats. Note in Table 15–6 that plant foods included in the four food groups for their nutritional value do not contain appreciable fat. Therefore, plant fats and oils as well as butter and lard are regarded primarily for their caloric contribution. Although they contain some fat-soluble vitamins and essential fatty acids, they are often considered as "empty-calorie" foods.

Avocadoes and olives which are rich in fat content are among the noticeable exceptions in the vegetable-fruit food group. Nuts, which range in fat content from 48% in peanut butter to 73% in pecans, are listed in the meat food group.

Although the meat food group is commonly thought of in terms of its protein content, this group provides a rich source of fat (Table 15–6). For example, most meat items and eggs which are in this food group will contribute even more calories from fat than from protein because of their high fat content and the high caloric equivalent of fat. The same is true of whole milk or ordinary cheese in the milk food group. Skim milk and low-fat milks are often fortified with 5000 and 400 units of vitamins A and D respectively to be equivalent, except in fat calories, to a quart of fortified whole milk. They are excellent substitutes for those concerned with control of caloric intake but labels should be checked to be sure of both caloric and vitamin contents. Note, however, that even the 2 cups of *whole* milk suggested by the food group guide need not be inconsistent with a calorie-controlled regimen.

Metabolic Considerations. Both the carbohydrate and fat portions of the diet are primarily important for their caloric contributions. Although there are no nutritionally essential carbohydrate molecules, there are qualitative requirements for either di-, tri-, or tetra- (poly) unsaturated fatty acids. These essential fatty acids are linoleic, linolenic and arachidonic acids respectively. The word "essential" is commonly used in nutrition to describe compounds or chemical elements that cannot be synthesized by the body and must be provided by an outside source—usually the diet. The essential fatty acids are most abundant in plant oils, but even the 50 grams of animal fat provided in the recommended servings from the four food groups (Table 15–5) are sufficient to meet the essential fatty acid needs. When all food fats in the average mixed diet are considered, 30 grams or about 1 ounce is sufficient to provide essential fatty acids equivalent to the 3 to 9 grams of linoleic acid estimated to meet the daily adult need. Obviously, these fatty acids are of little caloric significance.

Food fats also contain vitamins A, D, E and K which, like fat, accumulate and are stored in plant and animal foods. However, the vegetable-fruit food group which contributes negligible dietary fat provides important amounts of vitamins E, K and also carotenes, which the body can convert into vitamin A. Many meat food group items, especially organ meats and eggs, are rich in another fat-soluble but non-essential nutrient, cholesterol.

About 5% of the fat intake may be non-essential phospholipids some of which, lecithins, contain choline. Choline enhances fat mobilization by the liver. Even more important perhaps to fat mobilization and transport and metabolism is the level of unsaturated fatty acids—not because they are essential but for their more emulsifiable nature. This physical property may yet prove important in determining the oral effects of different food fats and oils.

Fat and Caries. To date, it appears that at a certain concentration of fat, cariogenicity is lessened. For this reason, it appears that high fat, non-sweetened, starchy foods such as potato chips or corn, rice and other cereal grain snacks, peanuts and even peanut butter may be acceptable between meals. However, they probably would not overcome the effect of sugar when combined with them in items like candy-coated peanuts or peanut butter and jelly sandwiches.

Protein

Comparison of Animal and Plant Sources. The remaining large portion of the daily dry matter is protein. The ICNND and older RDA rule of 1 gram of protein per kilogram of body weight states the standard man should receive 65 to 70 grams of protein per day or about 10% of his total calories. The new 1974 RDA states 0.8 gram per kilogram body weight or 8% of calories. This recommendation includes the provision that about 40% of the recommended value be animal proteins. These are usually a rich source of the 8 essential amino acids: lysine, tryptophan, methionine, valine, phenylalanine, leucine, isoleucine, and threonine. Gelatin, a protein gel prepared from collagen, composed to a greater extent of non-essential amino acids, is a notable exception to the generality that all animal proteins are rich in essential amino acids. In general, proteins provided by the milk and meat food groups are rich in essential amino acids and are termed variously as "complete," or of "high biological value" or "balanced" or of "high quality."*

Animal protein is expensive and not easily available to many populations throughout the world or to lower income groups in this country. These populations depend on plant proteins which contain lower protein concentrations than do animal foods. Cereal grains are made into breads, cereals, pastas, biscuits, grits, and tortillas. Note the low amount of protein provided by the recommended minimum number of four servings from the bread-cereal food group (Table 15-5). Such foods must be eaten in large quantities to meet protein requirements when animal foods are not readily available. Dry beans, peas, and nuts, although plant foods, are placed in the meat food group because they are rich in protein, compared to other plant foods, and are often eaten in large amounts. They are also rich in iron, as are most other foods in this group.

SUMMARY OF GROSS DIETARY CONSTITUENTS

Calories

Ideally, the standard man will eat 405 grams of carbohydrate, 90 grams of fat, and 68 grams of protein per day. This diet will give about · 60, 30 and 10%, respectively, of the 2700 calorie daily requirement.† Comparison

---

* They may also be called "high ranking." It is convenient to use the mnemonic Lt. M. V. Plit (lysine, tryptophan, methionine, valine, phenylalanine, leucine, isoleucine, threonine) to remember the essential amino acids. The first two primarily are often low in vegetable proteins thus giving animal proteins higher rank. The last "t" is threonine, the last of the essential amino acids to be discovered.

† Since the RDA of 56 grams of protein is adequate, even 10% of calories from protein, 68 grams, is higher than necessary. The use of 56 grams as the ideal for protein allows carbohydrate to be increased by 12 grams to a total of 417 grams. For the female the corresponding ideal suggested allowances for protein and carbohydrate would be 46 and 304 grams, respectively. Note that there are no RDA guidelines for carbohydrate and fat intake.

with the diet that would be provided by the recommended number of servings from the four food groups is shown in Table 15–6. It is apparent that the food group plan of eating provides a low calorie basal diet because of low amounts of carbohydrate and fat. It thus serves as a base for upward adjustment to the caloric levels and food choices that meet individual needs. With this basal plan an adequate supply of high quality protein is assured. Both essential amino and fatty acid requirements would be met. Since other essential nutrients are also assured by this eating plan (Table 15–6), it provides the average person with a variety of calorically wise and nutritionally adequate diets. Food group items would be the foods of choice used to meet most caloric needs as long as excessive calories from the fat in the animal food groups is avoided. The nonfood group items, especially "visible" fat and "empty calorie" carbohydrates, may be added to enhance palatability and enjoyment of other food items. Caution is necessary, however, since only 2 tablespoons of fat on salad or bread, or 5 tablespoons of sugar would add 200–250 calories.

Minerals

Besides carbohydrate, fat and protein, the only other grossly significant portion of the daily intake of dry matter is the major minerals. An ashing procedure would reveal 10 to 20 grams of total inorganic matter. This amount would be highly variable because the salt component, NaCl, may vary from 5 to 15 grams in ordinary diets; only a few grams are required.

The pH of the ash predicts the urinary pH since the body also oxidizes and essentially ashes the daily diet and excretes excesses of minerals. Na^+, K^+, Ca^{2+} and Mg^{2+} predominate if the diet is higher in milk and vegetable-fruit food group items than in acidic ash foods from the meat and bread-cereal food group where the ions of HPO_4^{2-}, SO_4^{2-} and Cl^- predominate. A diet based on the four food group plan will provide a reasonable balance of metals and non-metals and a urinary pH near neutrality.

NUTRITIONAL BALANCE

The word "balance" is very useful in the nutritional context. Because it was introduced in the discussion of ash balance, it should be defined in the two senses in which it is used. First, a balanced meal implies ideal proportions of various foods so that the nutrients will be in proper proportion to each other. Three such meals provide a balanced diet. Our knowledge of what constitutes proper balance is incomplete. Relative nutrient needs appear to vary for different tissues as well as for the body as a whole. In either case they are related to age, physiological and pathological status as well as to nutritional habits such as frequency of eating. The four food group concept is emphasized repeatedly since for this nation these food groupings and intake levels seem to be the most practical means of preparing balanced meals.

The idea of balance may also refer to foods such as milk which approaches nutritional balance in itself or to a single nutrient such as protein that contains a good distribution of amino acids, especially the essential ones. Balance also means the body's balance or balance within a body system. In this context then, good ash balance promotes acid-base balance in the body. In the case of protein, if the nitrogen (protein) intake equals nitrogen output, the body is in nitrogen balance. While useful, the determination and meaning of the state of balance is very difficult. Ideally, balanced nutrition may also depend upon many other factors besides total daily food intake. The habit of eating meals, the effects of meal size, the frequency of eating, and the influences of frequent unbalanced snacks all present questions that are only now being studied.

DIETARY CATALYSTS

Although catalysts are not quantitatively important, they serve critical roles in facilitating the body chemistry. Accordingly, they are ideally provided in foods containing gross nutrients whose utilization they catalyze. Table 15–7 shows the distribution among the food groups of a number of these catalysts including the major mineral element calcium which serves both a catalytic and a structural role. Many essential nutrients are not in the table either because their quantitative requirement is still poorly defined or because of the thought behind the establishment of the list. The philosophy used in formulating the four food groups was to provide food patterns to meet the RDA standards with the assumption that adequate amounts of other nutrients would automatically be assured. This assumption seems well founded to date. A corollary is that excessive deviation from the four food group concept such as the development of food idiosyncrasies due to allergies, poor health, excessive dieting, or food faddism could exclude nutrients whose presence is normally assured. By choosing a variety of foods primarily to meet the needs for calcium, iron, vitamin A, ascorbic acid, B-vitamins (thiamine, riboflavin and niacin), and protein, other catalytic nutrient requirements will almost necessarily be adequate.

Vegetable-Fruit Food Group and Total Health Needs

The prime reason for listing the vegetable-fruit food group becomes apparent from Table 15–7. Although these foods make only a minor caloric contribution, they supply 20% of the iron, thiamine, and niacin, more than 50% of the vitamin A and more than 90% of ascorbic acid in the United States diet. In fact, it is nearly impossible to meet the RDA of the latter without this food group. Especially important are potatoes, tomatoes, other vegetables, and citrus fruits each supplying in the United States diet about 20% of the RDA for ascorbic acid. This food group is important to periodontal patients beyond the local or physical advantages noted during the discussion of carbohydrates since oral tissues are especially sensitive to ascorbic acid deficiency.

Vegetable-fruit foods may be more necessary than expected in some diets from high income groups where the intake of enriched bread-cereal is low. In low income families the enriched bread-cereal foods contribute a large portion of iron and the B-vitamins (Table 15–7). Lower income families must emphasize the vegetable-fruit group to provide vitamin A, riboflavin and calcium, whereas in higher income groups most of these nutrients are contributed by the more expensive milk and meat food group items. Thus, in lower income situations vegetable-fruit foods and the low cost enriched bread-cereal foods are especially important for healthy oral soft tissues. In fact, in such populations the symptoms of pellagra, ariboflavinosis, and other nutritional deficiency diseases were associated first of all with the head and neck area and especially with oral disease. Nutritional requirements for good general health are also required for good oral health. Deficiency symptoms, *e.g.* simple anemia from iron deficiency, which occur elsewhere than the oral cavity, would eventually affect especially anoxia-susceptible periodontal tissues. *It is academic and unnecessary to attempt to associate foods and their nutrients specifically with oral health effects in order to justify relevance when the health of the total individual is the real issue.*

Other Food Groups

Both high and low income groups may use the four food group guide for oral health. Low income groups need economic counseling for wise food purchasing but both groups require education and guidance in food selection.

On the basis of only the low calorie basal diet provided by the four food group guide, it is apparent from Table 15–7 that all of the nutrients except niacin either approach or exceed the RDA values. Actually niacin is better supplied than indicated since the high quality protein from the animal food groups contains tryptophan from which the body can obtain 1 mg of niacin from each 60 mg of this essential amino acid.

It is obviously difficult to supply the calcium allowance without liquid milk or its use in foods. In US diets, dairy foods supply 75% of the calcium, about one-half the riboflavin and an important portion of vitamin A even without vitamin A enrichment of milk. This otherwise nutrient-rich food group is noticeably lacking in significant concentrations of iron and ascorbic acid.

The meat food group, like milk, provides a good balance of nutrients. Presently, in the average US diet it supplies 50% of the protein and niacin, more than 40% of the iron, and about 25% each of vitamin A, thiamine, and riboflavin.

Since most foods are incomplete in their nutritional balance and since some nutrients are found in relatively few food sources, the value of a variety of foods in the diet is apparent. Variety may provide balanced meals if as

Table 15–7. Average Quantity of Nutrients Provided by Minimum Number of Servings Specified from Each Food Group of the Daily Food Guide and Recommended Daily Allowances of These Nutrients for Young Adults

Food Group	Amount	Calcium	Iron	Vitamin A Value	Thiamine	Riboflavin	Niacin	Ascorbic Acid
		mg	mg	I.U.	mg	mg	mg	mg
Milk and Milk Equivalents.	2 cups	514	0.3	870	0.13	0.69	0.4	Trace
Meat and Meat Equivalents.	6 ounces	70	6.9	1400	0.50	0.60	9.0	0
Vegetables and fruits								
Dark-green and deep-yellow vegetables	$\frac{1}{4}$ cup	23	0.6	2,590	0.04	0.04	0.3	13
Citrus fruits	$\frac{1}{2}$ cup	27	0.4	140	0.08	0.03	0.3	53
Other vegetables	$\frac{1}{2}$ cup	22	0.8	80	0.07	0.05	0.9	13
Other fruits	$\frac{1}{2}$ cup	16	0.7	560	0.04	0.05	0.4	7
Subtotal		(88)	(2.5)	(3370)	(0.23)	(0.17)	(1.9)	(86)
Breads and cereals Whole grain, enriched, restored	4 servings	55	2.1	30	0.30	0.16	2.5	0
Total		730	12.0	5700	1.2	1.6	14.0	86
Recommended Dietary Allowances								
23-year-old man		800	10.0	5,000	1.4	1.6	18.0	45
23-year-old woman		800	18.0	4,000	1.0	1.2	13.0	45

11

far as possible one item from each food group is selected for each meal. This allows the foods to complement each other.

FOODS AND NUTRIENTS IN METABOLISM

Biochemical Basis of Energy Nutrition

The best ratios of carbohydrate, fat and protein calories are generally unknown and may even differ with respect to age and sex. Total caloric requirements are based on the basal requirement with an additional portion of energy based on an estimate of activity. The basal requirement can be measured by the usual BMR measurement which determines the overall rate of oxygen consumption. This value is highest at birth and decreases rapidly. After the "growth spurts" of adolescence, it begins to stabilize and nearly plateaus at about age 23 or when growth ceases. Actually, it decreases slightly throughout adult life as does activity.

By age 45 the caloric need is about 5% less than at 23 and by age 65 it is reduced another 5 to 6% less than at 23. (Actually, these decreases would be about 10% and 20% if the current decreased activity with age persists. However, it is recognized that it is better for health to maintain activity rather than to further decrease the caloric allowance.) The greatest allowances are 3000 calories for 15- to 22-year-old males and 2400 for children and 11- to 14-year-old girls who mature earlier than boys. At maturity these allowances are only 2700 and 2000, respectively. For the standard man 1800 calories is the basal requirement. The remaining 900 calories represents the "activity" factor which is equal to 50% of the basal requirement as an estimate of normal activity. The basal caloric requirement is dependent upon body surface area as well as the age and sex of the individual.

Energy Release from Foods. It is not an accident of scientific discovery that the glycolysis scheme, the tricarboxylic acid cycle, and the capture of high energy phosphate occupy a central role in biology. Despite the great morphological and functional diversities manifested in living forms these strikingly similar metabolic schemes, at least in principle, represent an underlying biochemical simplicity and unity. In every living cell the *quantitatively* important metabolic pathways are those associated with the release and capture of energy. Most of our daily intake of dry matter consists of the energy-providing (caloric) nutrients. In fact, most non-caloric nutrients are needed too in direct proportion to the total amount of energy metabolism, *i.e.,* in proportion to the caloric intake or demand. This is especially true for many vitamins and trace minerals which catalyze energy release. A review of food energy will serve to describe the biochemical basis for many of our nutritional requirements.

All the energy obtained from foods was originally captured from the sun by plants during photosynthesis as shown in the familiar equation:

$$6 \ CO_2 + 6 \ H_2O + Light \rightarrow C_6 H_{12} O_6 + 6 \ O_2$$

Plants and animals that consume plants and/or other animals utilize this stored energy by a process of oxidation. Photosynthesis is the reduction of carbon dioxide by hydrogen, and to the extent the oxygen is replaced, more and more energy is stored. The caloric equivalents of carbohydrate, fat and protein are understandable in these terms. Fats contain very long hydrocarbon chains, alcohol is a slightly oxidized hydrocarbon, carbohydrates have a yet lower H to C ratio and organic acids are even less reduced. These generalities and the associated energy levels are summarized in Figure 15–1.

Catalytic Nutrients and Energy Metabolism. The overall metabolic pathways related to these energy transitions are summarized in Figure 15–2 with emphasis on the catalytic nutrients involved. Coenzymes containing vitamins are essential to nearly every aspect of the energy pathways. Oxidation is accompanied by the release of hydrogen. Niacin as niacinamide adenine dinucleotide (NAD) or its phosphate (NADP) captures this hydrogen and holds it at a high energy level as NADH or NADPH, respectively. This occurs once in glycolysis, four times in the citric acid cycle and twice in the hexose monophosphate pathway (HMP).

These hydrogens may then be used to reduce acetyl coenzyme A to cholesterol or to fatty acids. In the latter case, along with its use for glyceraldehyde reduction to glycerol, hydrogen facilitates energy storage as triglycerides (fats and oils). In oral microorganisms, it serves to reduce pyruvic acid, a ketone, to lactic acid, an alcohol. In both the formation of lactic acid in microorganisms and cholesterol in man, these reduced energy stores are lost since the products are excreted. The hydrogen stored in fats, however, may reenter energy metabolism. In fat oxidation, hydrogen is removed with the formation, again, of the reduced coenzyme NADH and the reduced riboflavin coenzyme flavin adenine dinucleotide (FADH$_2$).

Cells are limited in their ability to utilize hydrogen directly in synthesis especially since metabolites other than those possible from the direct transfer of hydrogen must be produced. Therefore, the reduced coenzymes enter a

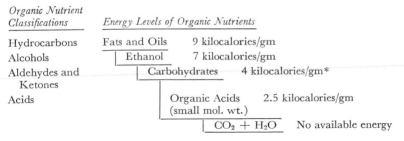

Organic Nutrient Classifications	Energy Levels of Organic Nutrients		
Hydrocarbons	Fats and Oils	9 kilocalories/gm	
Alcohols	Ethanol	7 kilocalories/gm	
Aldehydes and Ketones	Carbohydrates	4 kilocalories/gm*	
Acids	Organic Acids (small mol. wt.)	2.5 kilocalories/gm	
	CO$_2$ + H$_2$O	No available energy	

Fig. 15–1. Approximate caloric energies available from organic food constituents during bodily oxidation.

* Proteins average out at 4 kilocalories/gm—their amino acids being composed of hydrocarbons, alcohols, and acids which are oxidizable and amino groups which are not.

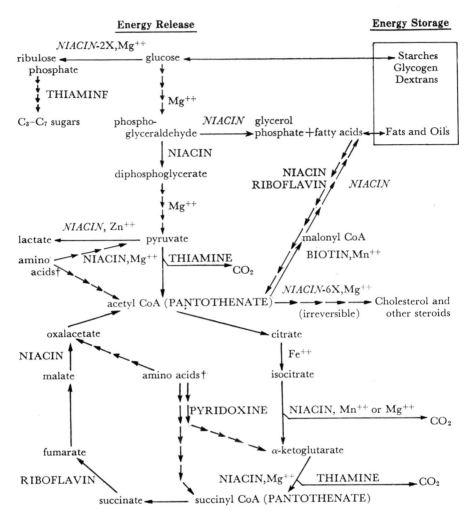

Fig. 15–2. Nutrient catalysts in energy metabolism.*

* All vitamins react in their coenzyme forms. NIACIN = NAD⁺, *NIACIN* = NADP⁺.
† Amino acid degradations require many nutritionally essential cofactors. Their conversion to carbohydrate (gluconeogenesis and glycogen storage) is not shown.

hydrogen transport scheme conveniently located in the mitochondria along with the citric acid cycle that produces the greatest amount of reduced coenzymes. In the transport sequence, hydrogen or its electron is progressively lowered in its energy level. The energy lost is captured by adenosine diphosphate and inorganic phosphate to form the high energy compound adenosine triphosphate (ATP) which the cell can use in a universal sense. ATP provides usable energy for synthesis, muscular work, active transport, and a host of other tasks. This scheme is diagrammed in Figure 15–3 which

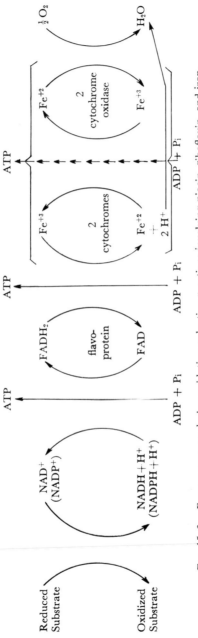

Fig. 15–3. Energy capture during oxidation-reduction reactions involving niacin, riboflavin, and iron.

shows the involvement of several nutrients. From the coupled mechanisms, termed "oxidative phosphorylation," the body obtains 3 ATP molecules for every oxygen activated as the final receptor of the hydrogen, or if an $FADH_2$ is oxidized 2 ATPs are produced. Occasionally, oxidative phosphorylation is bypassed and ATP is made directly in conjunction with substrate dephosphorylation and termed "substrate level phosphorylation."

Energy–Nutrient Demands

It is easy to be sidetracked by details in the energy pathways and miss their overall significance. We eat, first of all, to meet energy or caloric demands. More than 90% of the dry weight of the diet is processed by energy pathways. Next, we breathe mainly to supply the oxygen required to release food energy. Ninety-five per cent of the respiratory oxygen is utilized by the mitochondria in the cytochrome oxidase reaction. The net result of all cellular oxidations can be calculated, assuming a 40% efficiency of energy capture, to be a weight of ATP made and utilized each day equivalent to the body weight! Obviously, the catalytic nutrients involved in this huge biochemical expenditure must be present in adequate amounts. The great demand for these particular catalysts accounts for the fact that well-known nutritional deficiency diseases are associated with them.

B-Vitamins, Iron and Iodine. Niacin and riboflavin play key roles in energy transfer as hydrogen acceptors as does iron as an electron acceptor. Moreover, another B-vitamin, thiamine, is required for decarboxylation in energy metabolism. The advantage of enriching the starchy glucose-providing foods of the bread-cereal group with these four nutrients to aid in glucose metabolism is obvious and assures a degree of nutritional balance for these foods.

Although the B-vitamins are utilized elsewhere, their quantitative requirement is related to the degree of oxidative metabolism, *i.e.*, caloric intake. The thiamine, riboflavin, and niacin requirements are 0.5, 0.6 and 6.6 mg, respectively, per 1000 calories of food. In fact, the thiamine requirement is especially related to non-fat calories as expected since it permits glucose into the citric acid pathway as pyruvate, and is needed for pentose shunt reactions. High shunt metabolism is required for growth or wherever protein synthesis is demanded.

Growth. Higher RDA values for caloric and B-vitamin requirements have been suggested for persons during growth especially in adolescence and also during pregnancy. Iron deficiency anemia is easily incurred at these times since growth entails increased hemoglobin formation for oxygen transport. Iron is necessary also to meet the additional demands for energy metabolism via the cytochrome system. The high metabolic demands of growth require the provision of adequate iodine for thyroxine synthesis necessary for a proper basal metabolic rate, that is, a proper rate of oxygen utilization. Since the BMR decreases with age so does the RDA for iodine.

Because the need for calories continually decreases with age the RDA values for the B-vitamins, thiamine, riboflavin, and niacin have been decreased accordingly (Table 15–2). On the other hand most other requirements are less directly related to caloric intake and the RDA values recommended for the young adult should be maintained throughout the life span. For example, the vitamin A requirement is related to the body weight, and if the adult weight ideally remains relatively constant, the vitamin A requirement remains constant. The decreased RDA for iron for the post-menopausal female is noteworthy.

Other Energy-related Nutrients. Mention of other nutrients, some of which are not in the RDA tabulation, will further illustrate how the energy pathways set the demands. They include phosphorus for processing sugars as their phosphate esters, magnesium for reactions involving ATP, and pantothenic acid which is part of the coenzyme A molecule, playing a key role in energy metabolism as acetyl coenzyme A and as succinyl coenzyme A in Krebs cycle. Succinyl coenzyme A is also utilized for hemoglobin synthesis. The transportation and elimination of carbon dioxide as an end product of oxidation depend upon the zinc-containing enzyme carbonic anhydrase. The neutralization of carbonic acid and organic acids produced during metabolism is due to potassium intracellularly and sodium extracellularly with chloride as an important anion for maintaining electroneutrality.

Besides iron, each of the following nutrients prevents one of the nutritional anemias and assures adequate hematopoiesis for oxygen utilization: copper, folacin, pantothenic acid and vitamins B_6, B_{12} and C along with adequate protein, calories and the nutrient catalysts of energy metabolism.

Most amino acids from food proteins are oxidized in the body by entering the common energy pathways at various points to yield about 4 calories per gram. The transaminations of aspartic and glutamic acid requiring vitamin B_6 as pyridoxal phosphate coenzyme are quantitatively important. These two amino acids together comprise about 25% of the protein in the usual diet and enter the citric acid cycle as the alpha-keto acids oxalacetic and alpha-keto glutaric acids, respectively. Thus, the RDA for vitamin B_6 is closely related to the RDA for protein.

Although all of the nutrients mentioned in this brief review are involved elsewhere in the body chemistry, the amounts involved are determined primarily by the level of energy metabolism. Unless the energy needs are met no other metabolism is possible.

Carbohydrate Functions

Metabolic. Although there are no nutritionally essential compounds, there is a minimal daily carbohydrate need for about 100 grams or about 400 to 500 calories. This amount assures functional carbohydrate metabolism so that the acetyl coenzyme A produced by fat oxidation can enter efficiently into an operative citric acid cycle. Otherwise, ketone bodies accumulate as in diabetes in which glucose metabolism is insufficient to allow the ready oxidation of fat. These ketone bodies are acidic so that ketosis is followed by an acidosis leading to the excessive excretion of base, or sodium, and water.

An active carbohydrate metabolism also conserves the electrolyte potassium as well as sodium, both of which are necessary to neutralize organic acids. The introduction of a low carbohydrate diet is followed by a decrease in body weight due to the loss of water caused by a decrease in organic acids from carbohydrate metabolism and their accompanying electrolytes that maintain normal osmotic pressure by holding water.

Without the minimal level of 100 grams of carbohydrate to maintain the minimum of 1800 calories of adult glycogen stores, an excessive catabolism of body protein occurs to meet energy needs and for the obligatory maintenance of glycogen stores by the reversal of glycolytic pathways (glyconeogenesis). The minimum amount of carbohydrate is readily supplied by the servings specified in the four food group guide (Table 15–6).

Physiologic. Of more practical significance, a certain carbohydrate level decreases the need for calories from fat. Too high fat diets are currently highly suspect as factors in vascular and heart disease.

Some investigators argue that a sweet (cariogenic) snack, containing highly soluble and readily absorbed sugar calories, can decrease fatigue and provide a "carbohydrate lift." However, such snacks not only endanger oral health and appetite, but, when habitual and of high sugar content, also promote hypoglycemia and diabetes. Moreover, when a meal does not follow soon the appetite returns and another, perhaps harmful, snack is likely. Even meals that provide primarily sugar calories produce similar hazards.

Fat Functions

About 30 grams of fat from mixed food sources assure the proper amount of essential fatty acids and fat-soluble vitamins, but fat also has practical value. Fat satisfies the appetite due to a slower rate of digestion and absorption and a higher caloric value than carbohydrate. It also decreases gastric motility which is associated with hunger. This high satiety value paradoxically makes it an ideal constituent of each meal of a *reducing* diet. The recommended servings in the four food group guide provide less than 1200 calories of which 40% is from fat (Table 15–6). This is certainly sufficiently low for weight reduction, and if this 50 grams of fat were distributed into each of three meals, it would aid greatly in satisfying appetite.

Fat is highly palatable since many food flavors are fat soluble. Persons choosing a low calorie diet often fail to take advantage of the appetite- and taste-satisfying values of fat. They further add to their appetite problem by eliminating breakfast which should be emphasized and should contain some fat. It has been suggested that on a regular diet all the advantages of dietary fat could be supplied by 30% of the daily calories as discussed previously. This provides about 900 calories or 100 grams and is much lower than that currently eaten by the average person.

Biochemical Basis of Protein (Amino Acid) Nutrition

Functions. Proteins play central roles in living processes. They function as enzymes and hormones, in blood clotting and immune reactions, in muscular, connective and skin tissues and in calcifying matrices. They permit the transport and storage of materials and contribute to the maintenance of the proper osmotic pressure and pH. They even serve to meet energy needs. Apparently, about 100 calories, 20 to 30 grams, *must* be oxidized each day; the remainder is either oxidized or converted to fat or glycogen and stored.

Amino Acid Pool. The origin of the body proteins that perform these myriad functions is, of course, the food proteins. The nutritional aspects of protein metabolism are shown in Figure 15–4. Food proteins must first be hydrolyzed to amino acids before being reassembled into proteins characteristic of the host. The real requirement, therefore, is not for protein as such but for a balance of amino acids. Food protein contributes to the so-called amino acid pool which is defined as the total free amino acids distributed throughout the body at any one time. This pool contains the 20 or so common amino acids found in food and body proteins and weighs about 250 grams. The pool is fed by the digestion of proteins in the digestive secretions themselves (60 to 260 grams per day) as well as protein from desquamated cells (about 90 grams) sloughed into the GI tract. In addition, each day some body protein is degraded or catabolized by intracellular, lysosomal digestion and these amino acids are contributed to the pool. Enzymes have a high turnover rate so each day about half of the protein synthesis is of enzymes, one-third of which are digestive enzymes.

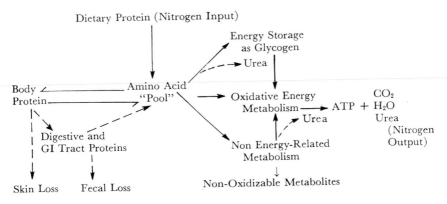

Fig. 15–4. Summary of amino acid and protein metabolism.

Continual Need for Amino Acids. All body constituents are maintained by a dynamic equilibrium which involves their continual synthesis and degradation or turnover. This balance of anabolism and catabolism and the associated maintenance of correct osmotic pressure, pH, temperature, etc., are all part of the condition termed "homeostasis" that characterizes all living things. Protein promotes and is itself maintained by homeostatic conditions. Such interdependence unites the body so that the body functions providing oral health are inseparable from those needed for total health.

As one criterion for the determination of dietary adequacy to maintain homeostasis, a balance study may be done. Nitrogen balance is used to measure the adequacy of protein nutrition by comparing nitrogen intake from food with nitrogen output as urinary urea. The usual situation for healthy adults eating adequate protein is a condition where nitrogen input and output are equal. For children, who are accumulating rather than merely maintaining existent body protein in dynamic equilibrium, the nitrogen input is greater than the output, and the balance is termed positive. To meet requirements for new tissue synthesis in pregnancy, nitrogen balance is also positive as it is during recovery from any illness or injury associated with protein losses such as the fever of acute periodontitis or tissue loss from dental surgery.

For an individual to maintain nitrogen balance, a fixed quantity of protein is not necessarily involved in the dynamic equilibrium that maintains homeostasis. In fact, the body can adapt to a low protein intake and eventually drift into nitrogen balance, and it is very difficult to determine the point at which the adapted state becomes bad for health. Usually the intake low enough to produce negative nitrogen balance over a short time period is undesirable. The readily produced negative balance is undoubtedly due to the constant demands on the amino acid pool, not only for protein synthesis, but also for such purposes as glutamine for brain metabolism, maintenance of the urea cycle, synthesis of epinephrine, and formation of the amino sugars of ground substances as well as the nitrogen bases of DNA and RNA.

Also, amino acids are constantly being deaminated and transaminated and shunted into the energy pathways and thus lost from the pool. This occurs in the post-absorptive state when gluconeogenesis from amino acids is necessary to meet the obligatory demand for glucose by the brain and certain other tissues. Although the functional requirement is primarily to maintain the possibility for continual protein synthesis, the constant caloric loss determines the minimal protein requirement. As the caloric intake is decreased amino acids will be used and body protein catabolized to meet the need. This is analogous to burning the furniture to keep the house warm. Moreover, if carbohydrate calories are limited, protein is catabolized to maintain an energy storage of glycogen even in starvation. As a corollary of this, it has been shown that recovery from protein loss, such as in wound healing, is dependent upon adequate caloric as well as protein intake. As discussed earlier, about 100 grams of carbohydrate in the daily diet have a protein catabolism-sparing action. It allows optimal dietary protein utilization from a low calorie diet.

A conclusion is that the amino acid pool is fairly small and easily depleted by the continual demands made upon it. It is generally stated that protein, *i.e.*, amino acids, is like the water-soluble vitamins and is not appreciably stored in the body.

Simultaneous Amino Acid Needs. The labile and small size of the amino acid pool is especially noteworthy because of the mechanism of protein synthesis. Each protein molecule has a unique amino acid sequence and its own relative proportions of amino acids. If each amino acid is not available almost simultaneously and in adequate amounts, the particular sequence of amino acids cannot be assembled on the RNA template at the ribosome and the protein is not synthesized. Since the cell will not normally synthesize incomplete protein, negative nitrogen balance can result if only one amino acid is limiting.

To assure adequate protein synthesis the pool must contain all the essential amino acids in adequate amounts. The most labile of amino acids may be lost from the pool and drop to a level that inhibits protein synthesis within a matter of hours. Enough total nitrogen from either essential or non-essential amino acids must be present to provide for the synthesis of non-essential amino acids.

Provision of Adequate Protein

Sources. Because adequate protein nutrition is dictated by the continual and simultaneous need for maintaining a balanced amino acid pool and because of the lability and size of this pool, it is sound nutrition to distribute the protein in three protein-balanced meals per day. Inclusion of milk and meat food group items in each meal will maintain a balance of amino acids along with a good nitrogen supply.

Recent evidence suggests that a balanced mixture of essential and non-essential amino acids is superior to the total nitrogen equivalent provided only by essential amino acids. Moreover, a natural balanced mixture of protein is superior to an equivalent mixture of amino acids. Thus, the presence of both high quality animal proteins and lower quality plant proteins as provided by the four food group guide has merit.

The lower the daily protein intake, the more critical it becomes to eat protein-balanced meals throughout the day. A person in nitrogen balance may go into a negative balance by eating his low ration of daily protein all at one meal. Nitrogen balance has been restored in such borderline situations by adding as little as 6 grams of high quality protein, one egg, to one of the protein-poor meals; such is the delicate nature of protein nutrition.

When protein intake is low, about one-third of the protein should be provided by animal proteins to assure a good allowance of essential amino acids. Specifically, only about 20 grams of egg protein, which has the highest biological value of all food protein, is required, whereas 24 grams of the major milk protein, casein, gives an equivalent of 5 to 7 grams of essential amino acids required daily, plus total nitrogen needs.

With plant proteins such as wheat and vegetable mixtures, about 30 and 50 grams, respectively, will be required to meet essential amino acid and total nitrogen requirements. These quantities represent the minimum requirements for maintaining nitrogen balance if no other proteins are ingested.

General Needs. Compared to minimum requirements for animal and plant protein diets, the RDA of 46 to 56 grams of proteins for adults does not include a large safety factor. Even the ICNND guide (Table 15–4), which tends toward conservative allowances based on world needs where economy of expensive protein foods is a factor, suggests about 32 to 58 grams of protein from mixed food sources for a 65-kilogram standard man. Similarly, the World Health Organization (WHO) recommends 29 to 37 grams (0.4 to 0.6 grams per kilogram of body weight) of egg or milk quality of protein. The low values in these ranges would meet only minimal needs if the source was primarily from only one cereal grain protein. Even US Army emergency rations designed to meet survival needs for only 2 to 4 weeks specify a minimum allowance of 35 grams of balanced protein per day.* When the protein intake is near or above the RDA level, protein quality and its frequency of ingestion are of minor importance.

Needs under Various Conditions. On the basis of grams of protein per kilogram of desirable weight, the protein requirement, like that for calories, decreases from birth. The infant is allowed about 2.0 grams per kilogram of body weight. This value decreases to about 1.4 for prepubertal children prior to the sex-mediated growth differences occurring at age 10. Thereafter, even at the peak of adolescent growth and into adulthood, the allowance decreases to about 1.0, exclusive of reproductive demands. Actually, the progressive decrease with age is less dramatic than the figures indicate. Growth proceeds with the accumulation of an increasing percentage of body weight as skeleton and collagenous connective tissue in which protein metabolism is less active. Nevertheless, there is a progressive decrease in basal metabolic rate with age suggesting that the more vigorous cellular activities do slow. With a lower energy requirement, presumably, less protein would also be required. Lower RDA levels have not been suggested for protein intake by older persons because of the fundamental need for amino acids on a continual and simultaneous basis. The lability of the amino acid pool has been

---

* A minimum requirement of 36 grams of protein is obtained if 3.2 mg of nitrogen per basal kilocalorie is taken as a minimum requirement. This nitrogen value is obtained from measurements of nitrogen losses per basal calorie as 2 mg in urine, 0.4 mg in feces and 0.8 mg as skin loss. The calculation for protein is then as follows: 3.2 mg nitrogen per basal kilocalorie × 1800 kilocalories × 6.25. The 1800 kilocalories represents the minimal requirement based on BMR measurements. The protein factor of 6.25 is based on an average of 16% of nitrogen in most proteins.

discussed and a depleted pool becomes a more serious health threat as one grows older and the circulation and other body functions decrease in efficiency. The progressive decrease in BMR itself implies decreased mobilization rates of antibodies, leukocytes and anti-infective processes as well as less efficient wound repair. To override such factors termed "conditioning factors" the RDA for protein has been maintained at the young adult level, which has the effect of providing a continually increasing allowance for protein. Even so, for old persons, an allowance of 2 grams per kilogram of weight is often suggested but not yet recommended in the RDA.

Negative nitrogen balance is almost always undesirable. However, under conditions of extreme fasting in very obese individuals hospitalized for weight reduction, negative nitrogen balance occurs as the excess musculature developed to support the overweight body is appropriately lost. For the average overweight individual, however, a weight control diet should be adequate in protein and high enough in calories to avoid negative nitrogen balance with its threat to health and normal performance. Even dissatisfaction with the caloric restriction itself should diminish if good protein nutrition is maintained. The four food group guide assures good protein nutrition along with a low calorie basal diet.

Mineral Nutrition and Related Nonmineral Nutrients

Minerals accompany the gross constituents of foods. In the usual diet, metals and nonmetals usually balance each other to provide an excess of neutral ash when the diet is adequate in other respects. Excess minerals, if absorbed, are excreted primarily by the kidney and usually determine urinary pH. Sufficient sodium, potassium, chloride, and phosphate are retained to maintain normal pH, osmotic pressure, and membrane potentials for nerve and muscle excitability. Extracellular sodium and intracellular potassium are involved in the latter functions and seem to counterbalance each other in characteristic ratios maintained by normal hormonal and kidney function. Calcium and magnesium act similarly but in much lower concentrations.

Even in unbalanced or inadequate diets the only mineral elements of particular nutritional concern are calcium, iron, and iodine.

Calcium. Calcium is of great interest both metabolically and nutritionally. It is not only the nutrient for which the RDA is most difficult to establish, but one for which the present RDA levels are very difficult to achieve. Suggestions for daily calcium intake are described throughout the life span as follows:

	Children	*Adolescents (at Peak Growth)*	*Adults*
Calcium	0.8 gm	1.2 gm	0.8 gm
Milk	3 cups	4 cups	2 cups
(or equivalent)	(0.9 gm)	(1.2 gm)	(0.6 gm)

During pregnancy and lactation 0.4 and 0.5 gram of calcium are added, respectively. The newborn infant is largely cartilaginous but contains 20 to 30 grams of calcium which must be obtained from the mother. This allowance is about three times greater than fetal needs, but it takes into account the inefficient absorption of calcium and the decreased efficiency with greater intake.

The dynamic state of calcium metabolism is described in Figure 15–5. In the diagram the net loss of endogenous body calcium is only about 320 mg which should be the daily requirement for maintaining calcium balance. In the typical adult in whom dietary and endogenous intestinal absorption are 40 and 75%, respectively, an 800 mg RDA provides 320 mg of calcium. During pubertal growth, when the skeletal accumulation of calcium may rise as high as 400 mg per day, absorption efficiency is increased. Also, if calcium intake is decreased, the efficiency of absorption increases, and calcium balance has been observed in adults with intakes of less than 300 mg. As with protein balance, it is impossible to state the point at which adaptation to low calcium intake is undesirable so the authorities differ about minimum requirements and RDA for different age groups.

In normal adults neither as little as 300 nor as much as 2000 mg of calcium is associated with demonstrable problems. Both national and international standards range from 400 to 1000 mg per day. The reasons for the caution reflected in the generous RDA values are the many known and unknown factors which inhibit calcium absorption. Dietary factors include excessive phytates in cereals and oxalates in green vegetables that form insoluble

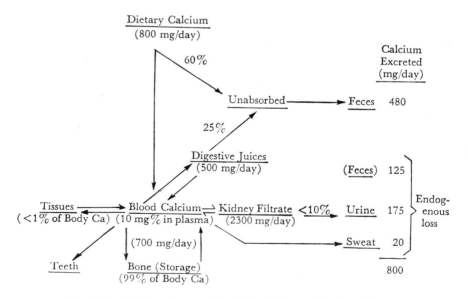

FIG. 15–5. Calcium homeostasis with typical quantitative estimates.

calcium salts. In fact some greens are so rich in oxalic acid that their calcium content is completely unavailable for absorption. Phosphate also inhibits absorption when the calcium intake and the calcium-to-phosphate ratio are too low.

The many physiological factors involved in calcium metabolism also result in cautious estimates. Bone is continually resorbed and redeposited throughout adult life, especially in facilitating growth in the young. A study of the equilibrium indicates that there exists a constant threat of calcium loss via turnover of bone salt, the gastrointestinal secretions, primarily bile, saliva and pancreatic juice, and by urine and sweat. There are data indicating that in profuse sweating and even in severe tension calcium loss may increase to 1 gram a day. Obviously, calcium needs continue throughout life after the completion of bone and tooth growth.

Milk Food Group. The major dietary source of calcium in the United States is milk. Babies who are allergic to cow's milk must resort to other natural milks or simulated milks available as formulas containing the nutrient values of milk. A notable exception is that for infants the higher ratio of calcium to phosphorus found in human milk is favored and is reflected in the current RDA values. Adults who do not care to drink milk may obtain it from milks used in cooking, from cheeses, ice cream, and other dairy foods.

Less rich but significant supplemental sources of calcium are greens, nuts, egg yolk, beans, and seafood, especially canned salmon. The eventual use of whole fish meal as human food is being seriously considered and would provide a good calcium source. Many of the virtues of milk may be reviewed within the context of calcium nutrition. Not only is the level of calcium high, but the calcium-to-phosphorus ratio is about ideal for their absorption and utilization together for bone formation. The fortification of milk with vitamin D is credited with the virtual elimination of rickets in this country. Vitamin D also facilitates calcium absorption and utilization. The high quality protein in milk contains the basic amino acids lysine and arginine which may enhance calcium absorption. The lactose of milk may also aid absorption. The relative importance and the mechanism of action of these milk factors are unknown but the preponderance of the evidence makes a strong case for milk as a calcium source.

Milk supplies calcium for the major task of bone formation and for restoring mature bone lost in its function of maintaining a constant blood calcium level. Optimal protein metabolism and ascorbic acid are required to form a normal collagen matrix for calcification. Normal bone growth also depends upon the formation of the mucopolysaccharide chondroitin sulfate which requires adequate vitamin A. Moreover, adequate protein is required for absorption of either vitamin A or the carotenes, its plant precursors. Although notably lacking in ascorbic acid, milk is rich in both protein and vitamin A. The colostrum, the first milk produced, is especially rich in vitamin A, and human milk is several times richer than cow's milk in vitamin A. This is especially important since the infant at birth is essentially deficient in vitamin A which does not cross the placental barrier.

The basis for eating protein frequently throughout the day has already been stated. Since calcium absorption is a major factor influencing calcium nutrition and since calcium like all nutrients must compete for absorption sites, it seems desirable to distribute milk, milk-containing foods or at least rich sources of protein and calcium throughout the day.

Maintenance of Teeth and Bones. It is intriguing that the teeth will calcify even when deficiencies in vitamin D or calcium are limiting bone formation or causing a net resorption of bone. Tooth formation occurs at a rapid rate and does not appear to be involved in the turnover equilibrium operative in bone. Therefore, teeth may retain within their structure a record of nutritional and other events which occurred during their formation. Someday we may be able to relate even short-term nutritional deficiency that did not influence any other part of the body to effects on teeth. Dental caries does not appear to be increased by nutritional deficiencies common to man, since the least caries occurs in some of the most nutritionally deprived situations. Conversely caries is prevalent in the United States where gross undernutrition afflicts only a minority.

Fluoride is one nutrient that does influence tooth formation and subsequent susceptibility to caries. Recent findings suggest fluoride stabilizes bones against the osteoporosis manifested during aging and in the osteomalacia of pregnancy, possibly due to an excessive rate of bone resorption. It is probable that this bone loss is not replaced because adults tend to ingest insufficient calcium. Over many years the cumulative loss may become significant although on a daily basis there may be no detectable negative calcium balance. This explanation is more likely than systemic malfunction, because high calcium retention can occur in older persons provided with high calcium diets. While adults usually obtain sufficient vitamin D, maintenance of bone including alveolar bone so important in oral health is assured only with adequate calcium and protein nutrition and perhaps fluoride.

Iron and Other "Trace" Nutrients. In many respects iron metabolism presents the same nutritional problems as calcium. About 1 mg per day is lost by the adult man, but the RDA is set at 10 mg because iron absorption is only about 10% efficient. A larger RDA of 18 mg for the adult woman replaces iron lost through menstruation. An even greater allowance on a body weight basis is provided by the 18 mg RDA for adolescents in whom the actual iron growth requirement is estimated at 0.6 mg per day. Most of this is required for hemoglobin synthesis.

As with calcification, hemoglobin synthesis also depends upon a number of nutrients, and therefore a balanced diet. It is interesting that the roles of vitamins A, D, and C and the mechanism of calcification itself are poorly understood, whereas the mode of action of the nutrients in hemoglobin synthesis are fairly well known:

$$\text{glycine} + \text{succinyl coenzyme A} \xrightarrow{\text{pyridoxal-PO}_4} \longrightarrow \longrightarrow \xrightarrow[\text{(Cu)}]{\text{Fe}} \text{heme}$$

To assure synthesis of the heme portion of hemoglobin, two vitamins, pantothenic acid in coenzyme A and vitamin B_6 as pyridoxal phosphate, are required. A pyridoxine deficiency produces a microcytic anemia. Copper is required to incorporate iron into heme. Simple iron-deficiency anemia is frequent, especially during rapid growth. Red blood cells are synthesized at the estimated rate of 2.5 million per second to replace those lost due to their limited life span. Normally, most of the iron released from old cells is stored in bone marrow, spleen and liver in the iron-containing proteins ferritin and hemosiderin.

Whenever iron stores are used or iron is lost from the body, the blood protein transferrin becomes less saturated with iron and iron absorption is stimulated. The continual involvement of iron with protein suggests that in protein deficiency iron metabolism would be hindered. Also, hemoglobin formation requires the globin or protein moiety as well as heme. A frequent supply of iron and protein such as in meat food group items would assure efficient absorption and utilization of iron.

Iodine. As discussed earlier iron is involved in cytochromes in all cellular oxidations. Another trace nutrient, iodine, is also necessary for the proper rate of cellular oxidation. Also like iron, its requirement is increased during puberty and pregnancy. Just as the iron enrichment of bread-cereal food group items has alleviated some of the iron-deficiency anemia, the fortification of table salt with iodine has lessened the simple goiter problem in the United States since it is due to iodine (thyroxine) deficiency. The use of iodized salt by everyone is to be recommended as a prophylactic measure. This is not to recommend an increased salt intake, however, since excessive salt aggravates hypertension which is a far greater problem than lack of iodine. There is no problem of receiving excess iodine in this manner even if seafood, a good source of iodine, is eaten often and if local foods and water are rich in this element. Persons on low salt diets may require iodine supplementation if they eat primarily locally grown foods and live in the so-called "goiter belt" in the central part of the United States. The possibilities for trace element deficiencies in general are much less today because foods commonly originate from many different soils. Excessive food processing may remove them, however.

Considerations for Ideal Nutrition

Ideal Eating. In summary, the ideal diet should contain three meals with each meal balanced on the following basis:

Appetite/ Body Weight Control	Nutrients Not Stored	Nutrients Difficult to Absorb
One-third of daily calories including fat and carbohydrate	One-third of daily protein including some animal protein. Also continual and simultaneous need for balanced amino acid pool. Water-soluble vitamins: B-vitamins and ascorbic acid	One-third of all calcium and iron

Not all meals can conveniently contain foods rich in all of the above nutrients nor will many persons eat three isocaloric meals; however, current nutritional knowledge indicates that such a plan is sound. The satiety value of such eating will usually decrease between-meal appetite so that the frequency of snack eating may be reduced. In fact, the value for the average healthy US citizen of eating protein, or of animal food groups, *throughout the day* is not because his amino acid pool is at risk but to satisfy appetite with the high fat content of these foods. Between-meal eating usually produces three major problems by providing (1) undesirable excessive calories, (2) "empty calorie" foods that reduce appetite for meals especially in young children, and (3) highly cariogenic items.

Occasionally, suggestions are made that "nibbling," that is eating in small amounts continually, would solve many nutritional problems. Besides the immense oral hygiene problem this would present, the probability of selecting or guiding people to select balanced diets in this manner seems very unlikely.

Adaptation. As previously stated, the body can adapt to low calcium and protein intakes and can achieve balance when output is not greater than input. This requires time, and the initiation of low intake levels results first in negative balances. At high intake levels excesses are excreted, but there may be some adaptation towards retention if high intakes are maintained. In the case of protein, the body can adapt to a higher maintenance level by developing greater muscle mass. Higher antibody levels may also result. On the other hand, to what extent do excesses unnecessarily overload body mechanisms?

Adaptation is essential to life. In fact, living organisms are first of all adaptive control systems. For each genetic and environmental situation there must be an ideal level for providing nutrition to facilitate adaptation. The question may well be, "adaptation for what?" For example, a higher muscle mass may be desirable for athletes but lower body weight may increase longevity. Animal husbandrymen can vary many characteristics of livestock by nutritional feeding procedures designed for particular objectives.

Nutritional Goals. RDA do not allow for tissue saturation with the vitamins since less than saturation supports apparent health. In the final analysis, balance studies or measurement of blood and urinary levels of nutrients must be correlated with the performance desired and this unfortunately must be tempered within the limitations of genetics, health status, and economics. Perhaps young persons wish most for optimal physical and psychological response, while older persons are concerned over longevity and response to illness. Fortunately, most aims do not seem mutually exclusive. Overnutrition and undernutrition are extremes to be avoided. They have to do more with the achievement of overall desirable health aims than the individual effects of each nutrient provided at an excess or deficient level. This means that for all recognized health aims there must be relative amounts of nutrients at which maximum adaptation can occur with a minimum of difficulty in maintaining homeostasis. *

From this discussion, it should be apparent that the prime function of optimal nutrition is to provide a maximum of freedom for the individual to express his genetic potential in response to environmental demands. Not only deficiencies, but excesses of nutrients also are threats to this freedom. If one meal or snack item is unbalanced in either quality or quantity of nutrients, the next food *may* or *may not* compensate but the body *must* compensate. The demand for some level of compensation to nutrition variables may offer a beneficial internal stimulus just as a variety of physical and mental experiences are stimulating. For example, fasting might have such stimulating benefits. This makes fine philosophy, but to date it seems that the best adaptation requires the best nutrition—a continual supply of balanced food.

MALNUTRITION

Present nutritional knowledge seems adequate for describing nutrient intake levels that will prevent gross nutritional deficiencies in populations. It is still inadequate to define the best body composition, body weight or functional levels of organs such as kidney, heart, liver, brain, etc. All these factors have been considered by nutritional scientists attempting to arrive at the compromise which best determines the total quantity of nutrients of the meal and their relative distribution or balance. Within this context, because the sources and functions of the more critical nutrients have already been defined, the nature of malnutrition may be discussed.

Overnutrition

Patterns of Caloric Intake. The major malnutritional problem in the US is probably excessive caloric intake. This includes not only too many calories,

---

* An analogy may be helpful. An ideal buffer is one that maintains the finest control of pH against both excess and deficiency of acid and is also of sufficient concentration never to be deficient and never so concentrated that it interferes with the system it is supposed to benefit.

but also the habits of eating them. Also, the nature of our carbohydrate and fat calories and their ratios have changed, and the problem may include quantitative imbalances or excesses in the use of various caloric sources. Trends in food consumption patterns during the past 50 to 60 years indicate a 10 to 20% decline in the percentage of calories supplied by carbohydrates. These are being replaced mostly by calories from fat and some protein. Fat calories may be most significant having increased from 25 to 30% to 40 to 45%.

The following comparison by food experts of the caloric distribution in the average US diet may be utilized to describe an ideal diet.

Estimated Percentage of Calories

	Present	Recommended
Carbohydrate	47	50–60
Fat	41	30
Protein	12	10–20

Surveys of dental students and hygienists at the University of Texas Dental Branch over a 5-year period suggest that the present data for the general US population are true also for those in dental school.

The changes in diet have been qualitative as well. Less starch, 50% less potatoes and 60% less bread-cereal items are eaten now, while the consumption of sugars and syrups has increased by 220% according to Department of Agriculture data. There has been about a 40% increase in unsaturated types of fat, largely vegetable oils. These qualitative changes were caused partly by food economics and partly by public preference for a host of sweets and fat-fried foods associated with convenience, availability, and taste. This is seen in the development of coffee-break snack habits and the replacement of adequate breakfast and lunch by sweet rolls, soft drinks, candy bars, french fried potatoes and pastries. These have been termed "pleasure foods" and are often empty calorie, highly unbalanced food items. Such eating habits often are associated with one overly heavy evening meal. Alternatively, the convenience of satisfying appetite, but not nutritional needs, with such eating habits eliminates any semblance of meal-eating. Frequently the lack of a meal-eating pattern is directly related to the development of both overnutrition resulting in overweight or undernutrition leading to deficiency effects. Such unfortunate eating habits were less common at the turn of the century but are readily found today in the general population.

Recent surveys among students at the University of Texas Dental Branch indicate about 44% of the daily calories are eaten at evening meals and 9%, about 260 kilocalories, are eaten between meals. Sixty per cent of these between-meal items were sugared soft drinks and pastries and 20% were candy and coffee with cream and/or sugar. These between-meals items, if in excess of caloric requirements, would cause a gain of about 2 pounds of fat per month. (One pound of fat is equivalent to 3500 calories.)

Prior to age 23 the basal caloric requirement includes caloric requirements for growth. Thereafter only maintenance requirements are included in the BMR. Aside from the body surface area, sex and age which determine the BMR, estimates must be made for activity. Typically, activity slows at about the same time as growth ceases—at least in the US population. However, one partly psychological aspect of hunger, appetite, remains. (A similar situation occurs when the large energy demands of pregnancy and lactation are suddenly decreased at the time of parturition or weaning and the mother continues to maintain the same caloric intake.)

Overweight. Recent measurements of body composition indicate that with cessation of growth a progressive decline in the percentage of body muscle and bone begins. Accordingly, about age 23 the ideal adult body weight should be achieved and either maintained or decreased with age. Often the reverse is true and the spread between ideal and actual body weight increases. This results in "middle-aged spread." Many poor nutritional habits develop during teenage years and by the early twenties result in excessive body weight and associated health problems. Excessive caloric intake early in life contributes to excessive and irreversible fat cell hyperplasia and to a lifelong problem in preventing fat cell hypertrophy whenever calories are excessive.

Ideal body weight is difficult to determine but to the extent that longevity is a goal then the population statistics favor the lean or slightly underweight. Life insurance companies in particular have found lower weights associated with longer life spans, and their actuarial tables indicate a 1% increase in death rate for every pound of body weight above these lean standards.

In recognition of the need to prevent excessive caloric intake and because average caloric expenditures are lower in our technological society, the 1958 RDA were decreased from 3200 and 2300 calories to 2800 and 2000 calories for male and female adults, respectively in 1968, and to 2700 for the male in 1974 (Table 15–2).

Statistics also show that overweight persons are more susceptible to the health complications that are the main causes of death in our country. They are diabetes, hypertension, abnormal heart size, cerebrovascular accidents or arteriosclerosis, and coronary artery disease or atherosclerosis. The blood vessel diseases are associated with increased tendencies for thrombosis and decreased fibrinolysis of those clots which do form. Although these diseases are emphasized in adults, they can also occur during the growing years. It should be mentioned that surgical complications are greater in the obese at any age. Burns, diarrhea, and other situations leading to dehydration are especially serious in obese children whose extracellular fluid volumes may be double those of lean children.

Vascular Disease. There has been an intense interest in the fat and cholesterol portion of the diet since atherosclerosis is associated with the deposition of cholesterol in the blood vessels. The elimination of high cholesterol foods such as egg yolks and organ meats is often recommended. To the degree that (poly) unsaturated oils replace saturated fat, plasma cholesterolemia is lowered by the substitution of mostly saturated animal fats with plant oils.

Recently, sucrose, whose consumption has increased so dramatically during the past 50 to 60 years, has been associated with fat metabolism. The assumption had been that starches and sugars were nearly equivalent nutritional forms of carbohydrate. Now, it appears that sucrose is converted to fat much more rapidly than an equivalent amount of starch. Perhaps the greater solubility and minimal digestive action required causes a faster absorption rate. Fat formed from carbohydrate is saturated fat so not only is the free fatty acid level of the blood elevated by the rapid entry of sucrose, but also the ratio of saturated to unsaturated fatty acids is increased. Both of these increases in blood concentrations are associated with vascular diseases.

Much debate is possible and currently extant concerning dietary regimens for controlling weight and preventing atherosclerosis and other vascular problems. Atherosclerosis may be related to hormonal status, stress, smoking, race, and heredity and like dental caries is a multifactorial disease. One rational approach may be suggested by summarizing the major dietary excesses involved in many US diets:

(1) Excessive caloric intake (either per day or per meal).
(2) Excessive fat intake.
(3) Excessive sucrose intake.
(4) High saturated : unsaturated fat intake.
(5) High cholesterol foods.

There is no mechanism to prevent absorption of excessive calories such as for iron and somewhat for calcium. Once absorbed, there is no mechanism for eliminating excess energy so it is stored as fat. The synthesis and excretion of cholesterol and bile salts may represent such an elimination. Their synthesis requires a large amount of energy, and they are not catabolized in the body to release energy. When excessive calories are contributed by fat or sucrose which is quickly convertible to fat, the cholesterol level is often elevated. Recently, ethanol (7 cal/gm) has been shown to stimulate both cholesterol and triglyceride synthesis. Normally cholesterol synthesis by the body is under feedback control and even depressed by cholesterol ingestion. The transport and metabolism of a surfeit of cholesterol and the control of its synthesis both may be more difficult under conditions where all energy pathways are flooded and the blood lipid level is high. Such conditions seem most likely whenever high levels of dietary fat and sucrose reinforce each other during any meal. Unknown factors, like stress from tension, may hamper circulation also with a resultant increase in cholesterol accumulation, thrombus formation, or vascular disease. In this way the blood levels of saturated fats and cholesterol may act more as indicators than as the cause of these health problems. Restricting saturated animal fats and food cholesterol seems warranted if the intake of fats and total calories is excessive on either a daily or a mealtime basis. On the other hand, it seems highly reasonable to suggest avoiding the overloading of the energy pathways with fats, sucrose or ethanol at anytime, but particularly at a heavy meal. Especially, total fat intake should be reduced from the present high levels so that it never represents more than 30% of the calories at any time. Heavy meals alone have been shown to promote lipogenesis and the clinically pathognomonic blood lipid values.

Conclusions for Ideal Caloric Intake. The problems associated with energy malnutrition may be solved by using the standard suggestion of eating three balanced meals a day in order to satisfy appetite and cellular needs regularly. Meals planned using the daily food guide provide about 40% of the first 1200 calories as fat. Therefore, when using the food guide to avoid overnutrition problems the calorie control recommendations in Table 15–5 should be noted. Each meal ideally would contain about one-third of the daily fat, carbohydrate, and protein. The tendency toward increased dietary protein has resulted in increased dietary fat. (A large portion of the increased fat intake in present diets exists as hidden fat in meat items.) This protein may be desirable provided the penalty is not an excessive fat intake. When the caloric nutrients are supplied by a balanced meal, not as empty calories or in overwhelming excesses, the probability of other nutrients being available for their proper utilization is increased. Ideally, a strong case can be made for replacing all non-naturally occurring sucrose with starch by using plant food groups. At least, the body is given an option for utilizing nutrients where needed rather than being forced to adapt to the stress of excessive calories alone. The fact that an overweight person gets hungry may indicate a time lag in the body control of energy metabolism during which it cannot adequately catabolize stored saturated fats. Exercise helps release fatty acids into the blood and decreases appetite.

The distribution of the proper amount of daily fat and total caloric intake into three isocaloric meals should aid in satisfying appetite without resorting to high calorie meals or to between-meal eating. These diet and exercise habits should result in a more easily controlled caloric intake and therefore a lower body weight with a good possibility of reduction in the dietary factors promoting vascular disease.

Some of the calories may be used for protein synthesis which is most efficient when the mixture of amino acids consumed is balanced. When protein and calorie nutrition are optimal, the use of the ATP and proteins in calcification, erythropoiesis, muscular work, kidney resorption, and a host of other processes requires the other nutrients to be present. The quantities must be such that no system is either overwhelmed or deficient, but has the freedom to respond as best meets bodily needs. This response includes meeting nutritional needs such as the freedom to absorb calcium and iron without the competition imposed by excessive nutrients at any one meal.

No simpler, more sound scheme for planning a balanced meal is available than the four food group guide. In light of the overnutrition and vascular disease problems, however, it would appear advisable to add many of the remaining 800 to 1500 calories to the 1200 calories provided by the minimum servings in the guide by choosing more vegetable-fruit food group items and to avoid excesses of sweet and fatty foods by replacing them with more starches from the bread-cereal group.

The above plan for optimal nutrition would also tend to reduce between-meal eating and thereby benefit oral health.

Nutrient Excesses. Excesses of water-soluble vitamins are excreted as are electrolytes and the nitrogen of amino acids. Of course, a constant excess of salt maintains excessive body water. Excess energy is stored as fat and along with it the fat-soluble vitamins. Vitamins A and D can accumulate to toxic levels. Poisoning can result from the overenthusiastic use of "therapeutic" pharmaceutical preparations which provide several times the RDA of these vitamins when used as directed. There is growing pressure for dispensing these preparations only on a prescription basis. Good nutrition is best assured by the use of good foods but, if vitamins are supplemented, only those preparations providing maintenance dosages should be self-prescribed. For example, the currently popular megavitamin usage can lead to complications. Larger than RDA levels of vitamin E may protect against undesirable oxidative reactions in the body, especially if an excess of polyunsaturated fats is eaten. However, excess of the antioxidant vitamins E and C may also inhibit utilization of beta carotene and its storage as vitamin A in the liver. Reports of undesirable effects from megavitamin use are increasing. Predictably all excesses in nutrition eventually will be shown to have undesirable consequences.

Excesses of minerals can also be stored. Normally, an absorption barrier against excessive iron exists, but excessive use of pharmaceutical iron preparations has caused poisoning especially in children who have eaten candy-appearing iron-coated tablets. Like iron, calcium absorption is normally regulated so that calcium in body fluids, being under other homeostatic controls as well, is not readily influenced by dietary intake. Normally, body fluids contain enough calcium to form ectopic calcifications and calculi (stones) when various etiological factors, *e.g.*, infections, are present. Since excess dietary calcium is not a problem, the recommended servings from the dairy group need not be reduced because of high calcium content. This group along with the vegetable-fruit group contributes an alkaline effect, however, so the proper dietary change would be to combat urinary stones with a total dietary adjustment resulting in an acidic urine. Also, protein intake should be decreased. Recently, it has been shown that a lower but still RDA level of protein may decrease by half or more the presumed normal and obligatory urinary loss of 180 mg of calcium (Fig. 15–5). Protein excesses are common in this country and, like other nutrient excesses, are becoming suspect, especially with regard to carcinogenesis.

Overweight is not the only problem from excessive dietary fat. Recently, the excess bile required to digest our high fat diets has been associated with an alarming increase in cancer of the colon. Our decreased level of dietary fiber and a resultant slower movement of bowel contents are also associated with cancer. With increased "dwell time," colonic bacteria may convert excessive bile steroids to carcinogens. One consequence of our excessive sugar intake is its widespread use in breads and cereals where it dilutes the fiber of this food group.

In liver or kidney deficiencies or other medical disorders, excesses of certain foods or nutrients should be avoided. In such cases, the concern would be best directed toward providing a sound dietary plan with counseling to assure that it is understood and followed rather than to single out specific foods as harmful because they may produce certain effects. For example, when food allergies arise, even the smallest amount of specific foods is excessive. If the food has been important in the diet special care is necessary to make substitutions for it that will maintain good nutrition. Milk, egg, wheat, fish, nuts, strawberries, chicken, and pork are all nutrient-rich foods which commonly cause food allergies.

Metabolite Excesses. Inborn errors of metabolism are being increasingly recognized. When such exist, it is especially important not to overburden the enzyme deficient system with substrates it cannot metabolize. Zeal here needs to be tempered also, however. For example, the phenylketonuric infant should not be deprived of at least his minimal nutritional need for the essential amino acid phenylalanine. Too much phenylalanine may cause mental deficiency in such individuals but so can the lack of adequate protein nutrition.

In lactase deficiency, too much lactose (dairy foods) causes unpleasant symptoms. Since the defect is usually only partial, a simple solution is to distribute the dairy servings throughout the day. Protecting against metabolite excesses is usually a medical problem, but the dentist should be aware that some patients may be under dietary control because of allergies or metabolic deficiencies. The fact that a patient may be following dietary control measures should not inhibit inquiry into his nutrition, however, when his dental health shows any signs relating to nutritional causes. Neither the physician nor the dentist should look at only one aspect of a patient's health and make suggestions (*e.g.*, the elimination of milk or eggs from the diet) that ignore total nutritional needs having overall significance to systemic and oral health and to the conscious needs of the patient as a person.

Undernutrition

Deficiency Patterns. Undernutrition may be pictured as a series of levels of increasing nutritional deficiency of the tissues incurred at acute or chronic rates and accompanied by either specific or general symptoms (Table 15–8).

Table 15–8. Typical Patterns in Nutrient Deficiency

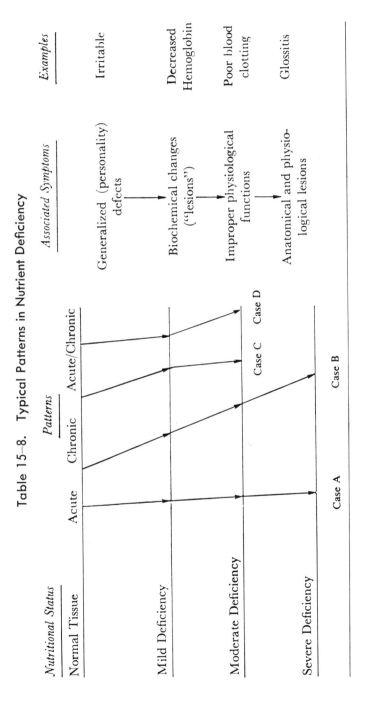

The reader can use this table along with medical, dental and dietary histories as an aid in assessing the nutritional status of patients. For example, some acute deficiencies (case A) may be expected to be reversed more quickly than chronic ones (case B), especially if the latter have become severe. The poor healing in case C may be the result of a developing chronic deficiency due to progressive loss of teeth and poor selection over many years and then suddenly appearing after an acute deprivation of nutrients due to influenza and high fever. Case D could be the result of food deprivation due to multiple tooth extractions followed by chronic failure to obtain adequate good-fitting dentures. Other cases may be drawn for nutritional changes associated with alcoholics, for those who have been on "fad" or "crash" diets and for those who have systemic ill health or psychological problems.

Moderate to Severe Deficiencies. The symptoms and confirmatory signs of nutritional deficiency are not specific. Tissues have only a limited variety of possible responses, and different nutrient deficiencies or non-nutritional factors may cause the same effects. It is important to recognize that tissues differ in their nutritional requirements and therefore in their susceptibility to deficiencies. For example, the tongue becomes painful and swollen early in a moderately severe niacin deficiency, yet thiamine deficiency is first indicated with neuritis effects in the lower limbs and probably never shows any typical effects in the tongue. There are many biochemical tests as well as physiological and anatomical observations used in determining nutritional status that are described in textbooks on clinical nutrition.

It is rare for the average dentist to encounter the classical symptoms such as the xerophthalmia of vitamin A deficiency, the stomatitis of pellagra, the angular cheilosis of ariboflavinosis, or the polyneuritis of beriberi, at least to the extent that he can classify them. It will suffice here to say that the dentist should develop skill at looking at the normal tissues with an eye toward detecting the abnormal. This is already being encouraged for detecting oral cancer. He can keep in mind that the head and neck region and especially the oral cavity are all prime areas for the manifestations of nutritional deficiency. He can be alert to the following effects:

stomatitis: generalized oral inflammation
glossitis: inflammation of the tongue (lingual swelling, papillary atrophy or hypertrophy, impaired taste, burning, pain, fissuring)
mucosa: pallor, reddening, ulceration
gingivae: hypertrophy, bleeding, secondary infection
salivation: xerostomia or ptyalism
cheilosis (cheilitis): inflammation of lips, secondary infection, especially at the angles of the mouth
osteoporosis: (not detectable even radiographically until about 25 to 30% of bone loss has occurred)
dermatitis: dry, itching, scaly, oily, secondary infection
eyes: dry, itching, reddened, secondary infection.

Subclinical to Mild Deficiencies. At the other end of the spectrum are the early, nearly subclinical mild symptoms. They resemble the effects produced when one has studied under nervous strain until late at night for several days. They were first used to describe early protein deficiency and may be classified as anorexia (loss of appetite), nervousness and fatigue. The general term neurasthenia best describes the condition. It is now generally agreed that most nutritional deficiencies first appear in this manner. Anorexia involves the gastrointestinal tract. The epithelial lining of this tract is replaced every 3 to 6 days so it has a very high nutrient demand. Two symptoms expected would be indigestion, due to lack of digestive enzymes and muscular tone for peristalsis, and abdominal discomfort followed perhaps by diarrhea. Poor appetite easily results in depressed growth and poor food selection habits. Infections are more common in the nutritionally deficient state and these often further inhibit proper food intake and compound the deficiency problem. Nervousness includes increased sensitivity to pain as well as paresthesia, headache, muscular pain, and psychic effects such as confusion, apprehension, depression, anxiety, and lack of concentration. Fatigue implies a generalized malaise or lassitude and weakness. The overall personality of such persons is affected and, as dental patients, they would be late for appointments, impatient with inconveniences, intolerant of dental procedures, difficult to accommodate, and disinterested in preventive programs including the nutritional guidance they need.

Moderate Deficiencies. In a moderate degree of deficiency, the problem of edema, especially prominent in protein and ascorbic acid deficiency, may make it difficult to fit dentures comfortably. A deficiency of either of these nutrients or niacin may make it difficult to prevent or cure gingival infection by periodontal therapy without treating the systemic deficiency also. Likewise, adequate wound-healing is especially dependent upon protein and ascorbic acid.

Prolonged inflammation and delayed wound healing may be the direct result of anoxia due to any of the nutritional anemias. Simple iron deficiency is most common in children, especially teenagers, and during reproduction. It notably exhibits the generalized symptoms listed above, especially fatigue. Dental patients suffering from the aforementioned moderate deficiencies and especially vitamin A deficiency would be expected to show high sensitivity to infection.

The blood-clotting phase of healing is inhibited by inadequate vitamin K. Vitamin K deficiency is not usually a problem except in the newborn in whom the intestinal flora are not yet developed for adequate synthesis of this vitamin. Because of the importance of intestinal synthesis of this vitamin and perhaps other vitamins, their lack may become critical in patients who have had extensive antibiotic treatment or have suffered prolonged diarrhea suffi-

Table 15–9. Availability of "Critical" Nutrients

Factors Influencing Availability†

"Critical" Nutrient*	Per Cent of US Families Receiving <RDA	Primary Deficiency Factors				Secondary	Main Food Group Source‡	Foods Commonly Fortified or Enriched
		Frequency of Eating	Limited Rich Food Sources	Expense	Processing or Storage Loss	Problem of Absorption		
Iron	30%	XX			XXX	X	All except DF	**
Calcium	30%	XX	XX	XX		XX	DF	
Ascorbic Acid	25%	XX	XX	X	XX		DF	Fruit Drinks
Vitamin A	20%	XX	X	X	X	X	VF	Margarine Milk
Thiamine	10%	XX			X		VF, BC, M	VF, DF, M
Riboflavin	10%	XX			X		All four esp. DF	**
Niacin	10%	XX			X		All four esp. M	**
Protein	10%	XX		XX			All except VF	Cereals Baby Foods

* Critical nutrients are those that are most frequently unavailable in the average US diet at recommended (RDA) levels.

† Number of X's indicates the probability of importance. More iron enrichment of foods is needed to compensate for processing losses (cf. Table 15–2, footnote h).

‡ DF = Dairy Foods (Milk Food Group); M = Meat Food Group; VF = Vegetable-Fruit Food Group; BC = Bread-Cereal Good Group. VF is the most "critical" group.

** Flours, breads, pastas, cornmeal, cereals and baby foods. Specific enrichment with critical nutrients does not necessarily convert non-food group items into food.

cient to upset intestinal synthesis. Physicians may administer vitamins parenterally as a precaution when oral antibiotics are prescribed.

Primary Deficiency. Assuring the availability of an adequate diet is the first step in overcoming nutritional deficiency. The nutrients most likely to be lacking in the average diet have been tabulated as "critical nutrients" in Table 15–9 along with the factors that influence availability. Obviously, improper food selection may result in too little of any of these nutrients. Prejudices, idiosyncrasies and, most often, ignorance of food values prevent proper selection. Selection is more difficult when there are few rich sources as with vitamins A and C and calcium. Selection is aided by specifically designating the food groups that serve as rich sources for these nutrients.

Enrichment also aids in the selection of quality foods. For example, diluted fruit juices such as grape juice enriched with ascorbic acid become valuable sources of this vitamin. In one study comparing breads from all over the world, white bread, enriched with the three major B-vitamins and iron, commonly sold in this country ranked very high nutritionally. More of such developments can be expected, *viz.* the baby food industry with formulas and cereals based directly on nutritional research. In addition to the nearly universal practice of fortifying milk with vitamin D, vitamin A fortification is also common. This provides an adequate supply of the vitamin to meet infant needs and modifies the large seasonal variations in the vitamin A content of milk. To compete with butter, margarine manufacturers have added these vitamins to their product.

Secondary Deficiency. Conditioned malnutrition, due to secondary or conditioning factors originating with the patient, may result from inability to *ingest*, perhaps from poor dental health or a lack of desire to eat. Malnutrition itself produces anorexia. Also, failure to digest, absorb, retain, or utilize nutrients may cause secondary deficiency. For these reasons, patients with acute or chronic infection or systemic diseases may also have nutritional problems. Fever, hyperthyroidism, drug treatments, and other stresses all may increase the turnover or destruction of nutrients and cause conditioned nutritional deficiency. Polyuria, diarrhea, excessive perspiration, loss of blood and exudate can also result in nutritional losses. Secondary malnutrition is more likely to occur than primary malnutrition in many dental patients, especially among older persons.

Deficiency and Dentistry. Preventing malnutrition, and specifically permitting proper food ingestion, is a prime biological purpose of dentistry. The ideal state of oral health allows for complete freedom in selecting foods for biting, mastication, and swallowing. Along with restorative work the patient needs guidance in choosing the foods necessary for good tissue tone, muscular strength, sensitive taste, and other physiological functions that make eating pleasurable. By not providing nutritional guidance, the primary value of oral rehabilitation may not be realized. Moreover, caries, gingival lesions, infections, and osteoporosis, all of which may involve nutritional considerations, can render useless even the finest of modern restorative therapy. Stomatitis may cause pain and discomfort with even the best dentures. Of practical interest are recent observations that protein supplements to denture patients decrease the amount of time required for additional appointments for adjustments by as much as one-half. Not only proteins but vitamins too may be associated with prosthesis-wearing patients. Patients select foods directly related to comfortable bite pressures; therefore firm foods such as salads and raw vegetables (high vitamin sources) are selected less often by denture wearers. This is true even for healthy young individuals so the situation could be expected to worsen with age.

Protein Deficiency. In the United States the probability that diets will contain less than the RDA intake of protein is less likely than that they have insufficient iron, calcium, ascorbic acid, and vitamin A. However, the protein requirement is so critical to dental health and so interrelated to the utilization of all other nutrients that special note should be made of the nature of protein deficiency beyond that already mentioned. Albumin, the most abundant plasma protein, contributes to the osmotic pressure of the blood, and when its concentration is decreased by protein deficiency, water moves into the tissues. The resulting edema produces effects characteristic of the tissue. In the intestines, diarrhea results, enhances nutrient loss and compounds the deficient state; in the lungs this results in susceptibility to pneumonia; in the mouth, inflammation of soft tissue is augmented due to decreased circulation caused by the edema and secondary infection then becomes a greater threat. In addition, vitamin A transport is impaired in hypoproteinemia. Since this vitamin is needed especially to prevent infection in mucosal linings, the resultant conditioned vitamin A deficiency further enhances the probability of infection and inflammation.

Moreover, antibodies supplying gamma globulin will be limited by protein deficiency. Beyond this, it is known that infection increases the protein turnover and depletes the amino acid pool to a degree beyond that attributable to the lesion itself. In acute periodontal disease the total lesion size can be 6 square inches or greater, and if accompanied by fever, many nutrients may be destroyed. For example, the ascorbic acid stores of the major endocrine glands may be depleted within hours. Protein depletion also causes vitamin loss in many cases, *viz.* the loss of riboflavin when flavoproteins are decreased.

In view of these critical roles for protein, periodontal patients, oral surgery candidates and those to be fitted with dentures, especially older persons, should be counseled prior to operative procedures involving blood loss or interference with food intake. They should be given appropriate food suggestions postoperatively to assure the best responses in decreasing inflammation and infection, while increasing blood clotting, wound healing, tissue metabolism, and underlying bone health. This also hastens a return to a normal diet. Acute needs can be readily provided by the commercially available liquid diets based on milk and fortified with ascorbic acid, iron, and other nutrients to make a balanced medium. However, once solid food is resumed, most patients could profit in oral and general health from nutritional counseling in the four food group plan of eating which assures a high intake of complete proteins as well as other valuable nutrients.

FURTHER APPLICATIONS OF NUTRITION TO DENTISTRY

Caries Prevention

The simple plan that follows incorporates many general procedures that would apply in giving nutritional guidance for anyone.

Etiological Factors. Caries results when susceptible teeth are exposed to cariogenic diets. It is not currently feasible to decrease the population of cariogenic microorganisms significantly, but their effect of producing acid from fermentable carbohydrate can be reduced by eliminating these carbohydrates from the diet. Carbohydrate elimination is neither desirable nor possible on a long-term basis. A youngster simply cannot "cut down on the carbohydrate" as is often suggested offhand and still meet energy demands— nor would this benefit him.

Carbohydrate Factor. A number of studies, including the famous Vipeholm experiments by Gustafsson and co-workers in Sweden, have indicated the quantity of sugar consumed per day is not the major factor. As much as 300 grams of sugar added to liquids or 50 grams of sugar consumed in breads *at mealtime* did not appreciably affect caries. Only two exposures between meals to smaller amounts of sweets, such as toffees or caramels, significantly increased caries. Despite many variables inherent in human caries studies and the resultant large experimental error, it was possible to show that four such exposures to sticky candy caused significantly more caries than two exposures.

Similarly, Weiss and Trithart in this country studied 783 children between 5 and $6\frac{1}{2}$ years of age and found a correlation between frequency of exposure to sweet items between meals and DEF ratings (the number of teeth decayed, extracted, or filled due to caries). As the number of exposures increased from 0 to 1.75 to 4 or more, the DEF was 3.3, 5.9 and 9.8, respectively.

Frequency. From these studies and others, it seems valid to conclude that one factor primarily needs to be controlled, namely, the *frequency of exposure* of the mouth to fermentable carbohydrates. Since it is not feasible to control all such carbohydrate, it seems reasonable to allow it at mealtime only and advise that it be eaten at the table. Perhaps a child would often prefer his candy or other sweets in place of the dessert being served. He can then be instructed to practice immediate oral hygiene.

Similarly, the detrimental effects of sweet items in the lunch may be reduced by inclusion of a "detergent" food. Even sufficient accessible water fountains in lunch rooms or near candy machines and the routine serving of water at the family table may be valuable in helping to remove oral residues of fermentable carbohydrates.

Oral hygiene, as usually practiced, is only partially effective even with guidance. Some acid production can occur within minutes after sugar reaches areas of dental plaque so that oral hygiene can never be rapid enough to combat a high frequency of carbohydrates. Also the average probability of practicing oral hygiene three times a day after meals is slight. The patient should be counseled to plan non-cariogenic *meals* for times when routine brushing afterwards is impossible such as at lunchtime. This seems simple enough but it is often overlooked. As a practical compromise, such counseling can be made with full recognition that some meals must be cariogenic and that sometimes brushing will not be done.

Retention. The Vipeholm studies showed that oral retention or stickiness was directly related to cariogenicity of carbohydrates. Volker showed, on the basis of oral retention of reducing sugars, that in each of 3 items with the same amount of sugar, the effect of gum was retained twice as long as cake and a wafer was retained twice as long as gum. Obviously a less retentive sweet such as the cake would become more hazardous if consumed more frequently. Total cariogenicity of a food appears to be a function of both frequency and retention. Unfortunately, there is as yet no satisfactory ranking of foods based on their cariogenicity, and it seems impractical to attempt control of fermentable carbohydrate on only a partial basis. The best plan then is to eliminate all known and suspected carbohydrates from between-meal eating whether they are highly retentive or not.

Patient Counseling

Control of the frequency factor may be achieved in two ways. Ideally, the patient is counseled to avoid all between-meal eating in favor of balanced meals. This will automatically limit frequency of exposures to fermentable carbohydrates. If this is impossible, the patient is instructed to replace all cariogenic between-meal items with non-cariogenic foods.

Initial Steps. This approach, as does any nutritional guidance, demands knowledge of the patient's diet and eating habits. Inform the patient that eating habits may cause oral health problems and suggest the possibility that what he eats may have something to do with his oral health. Ask him to provide a complete and accurate 5-day record of his normal eating habits. It is best to give no dietary guidance at this time. He should understand that unless the record is pertinent to his normal habits, it would all be a waste of effort. The record is an educational experience in itself for the patient, and how well it is done informs the dentist of the patient's interest.

12

Follow-up. When the record is returned, the dentist can determine the general eating habits such as the presence of meals and frequency of eating. He may note all cariogenic items to educate the patient with regard to such items. The frequent occurrence of fermentable carbohydrate in meals shows the patient that these items, such as sugar on cereal, syrup on pancakes, sweet dessert items, chocolate milk, etc., often are unavoidable. One can then write the word "Brush" after each meal and also after each cariogenic between-meal exposure. The impracticality of such frequent brushing may lead him to conclude that he must either eliminate between-meal eating or substitute non-cariogenic items. It is usually desirable to make daily tallies, or even more impressively a weekly tally, of all between-meal exposures to fermentable carbohydrates to introduce the discussion of the frequency factor.

If caries is even moderate, it is most likely that the frequency factor is involved, but this often is not apparent from the record. Careful questioning may bring out that gum is not listed, that candy is frequently or routinely kept in the house, that the children like sweets, etc. Often some omissions are due to the fact that the person did not consider the item a significant part of the diet so did not record it. Further questioning about certain exposures may also be necessary to find if, for example, the three cookies and soft drink listed as a snack were really eaten at one time or constituted two or even four exposures. Such questioning also allows emphasis of the frequency factor.

If the patient wishes to eliminate all between-meal eating when he sees it as undesirable, it may be necessary to help him satisfy his caloric needs more efficiently at mealtime. Additional milk and meat food group items may be useful because of their fat content. He may prefer, however, merely to transfer many of the cariogenic items into the mealtime, and this is the battle we are willing to lose in order to win the war against caries. The additional sugar at mealtime has not been shown to be a critical caries factor.

Although it is known that children may be weaned from their physiological desire for sweets, this may be undesirable. Mealtime exposures often fill this desire without between-meal eating.

Snack Lists. Often single or multiple snacks throughout the day are part of the eating pattern and these cannot be successfully eliminated. In such cases the counselor should help the patient prepare an *individualized* snack list. This is more considerate, useful, and likely to succeed than handing out a pre-printed snack list.

Snack ideas may be obtained from the 5-day record which includes many of the patient's food preferences, if the patient considers the items suitable, is willing to buy them regularly and keeps them easily available. As a main principle, it should be at least as easy for the patient to use items from the snack list as to use cariogenic items. Use the food guide for planning snacking habits (Table 15–10).

Manual for Nutrition Surveys, 2nd Ed., Inter-departmental Committee on Nutrition for National Defence, National Institute of Health, Bethesda, Md., U.S.G.P.O., Washington, D.C., 1963.

NIZEL, A. E. (Ed.): *The Science of Nutrition and its Application to Clinical Dentistry*, 2nd Ed., Philadelphia, W. B. Saunders Co., 1966.

NIZEL, A. E.: *Nutrition in Preventive Dentistry: Science and Practice*, Philadelphia, W. B. Saunders Co., 1972.

PIKE, R. L. and BROWN, M. L.: *Nutrition: An Integrated Approach*, 2nd Ed., New York, John Wiley & Sons, Inc., 1975.

Present Knowledge in Nutrition, New York, The Nutrition Foundation, Inc., 1967.

Recommended Dietary Allowances, 8th ed., Food and Nutrition Board, National Research Council, National Academy of Sciences, Washington, D.C., 1974.

Chapter 16

Inflammation

EDWARD H. MONTGOMERY, Ph.D.
ROBERT R. WHITE, Ph.D.

Most oral diseases are inflammatory, or at least inflammation occurs as part of their sequelae. This is understandable, because by definition inflammation is the normal response of living tissue to a sublethal injury. Specific biochemical and physiological alterations are characteristic of the inflammatory reaction which occurs at the site of injury as a defense against microbial invaders and/or noxious substances or stimuli. The cardinal signs of inflammation (redness, swelling, heat, pain, and loss of function) have been known and described for many centuries; however, the vascular and cellular alterations have been studied only within the last century.

Grossly, the acute inflammatory process occurs in the following stages:

1. Sublethal tissue injury that initiates the inflammatory process
2. Hyperemia resulting from dilatation of arterioles, capillaries, and venules
3. Increased vascular permeability and edema
4. Extravasation of polymorphonuclear leukocytes, macrophages, and lymphocytes
5. Dilution, neutralization, and destruction of the noxious substance
6. Limiting of the inflammation by circumscribing the area with new fibrous connective tissue
7. Beginning of repair

External noxious stimuli can cause cell injury and a resultant inflammatory reaction. In addition, activation of various endogenous systems by the stimulus, for example, complement activation, can lead to cellular self-injury. In such instances, the intended defense may become more harmful than the noxious stimulus that originated the reaction. Acute inflammation, a defense mechanism that attempts to remove the noxious stimulus, may progress to a chronic inflammatory reaction owing to extended triggering of the inflammatory response. Thus, the physiological acute inflammatory reaction becomes a pathological chronic inflammation resulting in permanent damage to the involved tissue.

As a physiologic defense mechanism acute inflammation may be viewed as the first step in healing. Healing and repair are mainly responses of the connective tissue. Appearance of macrophages, which digest fibrin and phagocytize debris, is one of the earliest signs of healing. Next, capillaries invade the area accompanied by fibroblasts, which lay down new connective tissue. Lymphatics follow the course of blood vessels. Within 3 to 4 weeks the area is vascularized, firm bundles of collagen are present, and the process of repair and healing has been completed.

In summary, (1) the inflammatory reaction is a physiological defense mechanism functioning to dilute, remove, and inactivate the noxious agent (stimulus) and to prepare the site for healing; (2) tissue injury may occur by the direct effects of a noxious stimulus; other stimuli that do not directly damage tissue may cause an inflammatory reaction indirectly by activation of endogenous systems; (3) regardless of the type of stimulus, the characteristic symptoms or observable events of the inflammatory process are stereotyped and are produced by the activation of endogenous compounds called *mediators*.

CHARACTERISTICS OF ACUTE INFLAMMATION

The acute inflammatory reaction is characterized by two basic events: (1) vascular alterations occurring early in the inflammatory process, and (2) cellular phenomena that usually appear later and progress more slowly. Each event may be mediated by different endogenous compounds.

Normal Microcirculation

The terminal vascular bed, that is, the microcirculation, consists of arterioles and venules and their direct intercommunications, the metarterioles (thoroughfare channels). Numerous true capillaries arise from both the metarterioles and the terminal arterioles. Normally fluid leaves the blood vessel at the precapillary end of the terminal vascular bed and enters the interstitial spaces. Fluid reenters the vasculature through the postcapillary vessels owing to their lower intraluminal pressure and the high osmotic pressure exerted by the plasma proteins.

The walls of both capillaries and venules are composed of a mosaic of flattened endothelial cells. Intercellular junctions of 150 to 200 Å occur and are filled with a mucoprotein which serves as both an intercellular cement and a differential filter to materials. These endothelial cells contain pinocytotic vesicles both at the luminal surface and at the surface adjacent to the basement membrane. Substances normally leave the vessels by two processes: (1) diffusion of low molecular weight substances through the intercellular junctions, and (2) transport of large molecules across the endothelial cells by pinocytosis.

Vascular Alterations in Inflammation

The earliest visible vascular alterations in the acute inflammatory reaction consist of a transient arteriolar vasoconstriction, rapidly followed by a prolonged vasodilatation of the arterioles, metarterioles, and venules. Venular dilatation lags behind arteriolar dilatation, resulting in an increased hydrostatic pressure in the vascular bed. In response to endogenous mediators, capillaries become engorged with blood, and the endothelial cells, mainly of venules, become spherical so that large gaps occur at the intercellular junctions (increased vascular permeability). Extravasation of fluid and protein occurs mainly by this increased vascular permeability; however, the increased hydrostatic pressure also contributes. The result is observable as swelling (edema). Blood flow, which was initially increased by the vasodilatation, becomes sluggish and finally static owing to the increased viscosity of the blood. These alterations occur for the most part as a result of the action of activated endogenous substances on the microvasculature.

Acute gingival inflammation serves as a good model for the study of the increased vascular permeability response, because the extravasated fluid emanates from the subcrevicular vessels into the gingival crevice as crevicular fluid, and can be collected, quantitated, and studied for various biochemical products. This fluid contains proteins, immunoglobulins, complement, other plasma components, inflammatory mediators, inflammatory cells, lysosomal enzymes, and other products. The quantity of crevicular fluid emanating through the crevicular epithelium into the sulcus is directly proportional to the severity of gingival inflammation. The increase in crevicular fluid is due to the increased permeability of the subcrevicular vessels, most of which appear to be venules. The venules are the vessels most susceptible to injury and also to the action of endogenous mediators. In chronically inflamed gingiva, the plexus of subcrevicular vessels in normal gingiva is replaced by tufts of looping vessels which occur between crevicular epithelial projections into the connective tissue. In addition, the overall number of vessels also appears to be increased as compared to that in healthy gingiva.

In summary, there are two major features regarding the vascular alterations of acute inflammation: (1) a brief transient vasoconstriction of arterioles, followed by a prolonged vasodilatation of all vessels in the terminal vascular bed, augmented blood flow and engorgement of these vessels with blood, and (2) widening of the gaps between endothelial cells, mainly of the venules, which results in increased vascular permeability and loss of fluid and protein from the intravascular compartment. The increased viscosity of the blood leads to a stasis of blood flow and thrombosis in the area of injury.

Cellular Phenomena

Changes occurring at the site of injury cause white blood cells to marginate and stick to the wall of the venules. The polymorphonuclear (PMN) leukocytes are the first white cells to migrate through the gaps between the venular endothelial cells and accumulate in the tissue at the area of injury. Accumulation of these cells in the interstitial tissue is indicative of the acute inflammatory reaction. The PMN leukocytes have the capability of phagocytizing foreign materials, such as bacteria, and contain a number of organelles called *lysosomes* which contain hydrolytic and proteolytic enzymes. The phagocytized material is digested by release of the lysosomal enzymes into the phagocytic vesicle within these cells. Substances that attract leukocytes, such as bacteria, antigen-antibody complexes, and other chemical materials are said to be chemotactic.

Migration of monocytes from the blood stream into the interstitial tissue at the site of injury apparently begins at the same time as does migration of the PMN leukocytes. The monocytes, which are large, mononuclear, phagocytic cells, are present in smaller numbers in the blood stream in comparison to the PMN leukocytes. In the interstitital tissue the monocytes undergo transformation into cells which are referred to as *macrophages*. Inflammatory exudates during early stages of the acute inflammatory reaction contain predominantly PMN leukocytes, whereas exudates obtained from late stages of acute and from chronic inflammatory lesions contain predominantly macrophages. The reason for this difference in cell types in acute versus chronic inflammatory sites is due to the fact that the PMN leukocyte has a relatively short life span (approximately 2 days) and does not undergo division; in contrast, the macrophage can undergo mitotic division and has a much longer life span than the PMN leukocyte. Like the PMN leukocyte, the macrophage is capable of phagocytizing bacteria and cellular debris and also contains lysosomal enzymes which function similarly to those of the PMN leukocyte. Lysosomal enzymes from both macrophages and PMN leukocytes, which are released into the tissue, are capable of enhancing and continuing the inflammatory reaction. These enzymes are involved in the degenerative changes occurring at the site of injury. In addition, PMN leukocytes have the ability to produce a kinin-like peptide that may function as an endogenous inflammatory mediator during the later phases of the acute inflammatory reaction.

As the severity of the gingival inflammatory reaction increases, the number of PMN leukocytes in both the gingival tissue and the gingival crevice also increases proportionately. The chemotactic properties of plaque may account for the increase in PMN leukocytes in the areas of chronically inflamed gingiva. A definite correlation between the number of leukocytes and the quantity of lysosomal-type enzymes in the inflamed gingival crevice suggests that these cells are releasing lysosomal enzymes in areas of inflamed gingiva. In addition, plaque bacteria also produce enzymes similar to those found in lysosomes. Enzymes from either source would contribute to the inflammatory reaction and destructive tissue changes occurring in gingival inflammatory diseases.

Several other cell types are associated with inflammation. The *eosinophilic leukocytes*, in contrast to the neutrophilic leukocytes (PMN leukocytes), are present in the blood stream in lesser numbers and may function in hypersensitivity reactions. However, the exact role of these cells in inflammatory reactions presently is not completely elucidated. *Lymphocytes* usually are present in inflammatory exudates from sites of chronic inflammation and are present in chronically inflamed tissue. Although lymphocytes are generally associated with the chronic inflammatory reaction, they may appear in the connective tissue early in the inflammatory reaction. The major role of these cells is to mediate the immune response; their role in inflammation will be discussed subsequently. *Plasma cells* are a major type of cell appearing in chronically inflamed tissue; they comprise a major source of antibody production. In chronically inflamed gingiva a large number of plasma cells are seen in the subcrevicular connective tissue beneath the gingival pocket. *Mast cells* are tissue cells which normally are present near the blood vessels. The mast cell is believed to play a major role in the acute inflammatory reaction. Mast cell granules contain several biologically active compounds,

Table 16–1. Some Biologically Active Substances Present in Mast Cells

Granular Fraction:
Histamine
5-Hydroxytryptamine (not present in
human mast cells)
Dopamine
Heparin
Proteases (chymotrypsin, fibrinolysin,
leucine aminopeptidase)
Phosphatidase A (or in cell membrane)
Glucuronidase
Acidic phosphatase
Alkaline phosphatase
ATPase

Particulate Fraction:
Succinic dehydrogenase
Amine oxidase
Fumarase

Nonparticulate Fraction:
Dopa decarboxylase
Histidine decarboxylase
5-Hydroxytryptophane (5-HTP)
decarboxylase
Heparin-forming enzymes (sulfurylase,
APS-kinase, sulfakinase)

Smooth Muscle-Stimulating
Compounds Associated with
Histamine Release:
Lipids
Slow-reacting substance

for example, histamine. A list of some of the active substances in mast cells is shown in Table 16–1. The role of some of these agents as inflammatory mediators will be discussed later in this chapter.

A number of biochemical changes occur, both extracellularly and intracellularly, in the area of tissue injury. Changes in metabolic pathways, changes in the intracellular and extracellular pH toward the acidotic range, and other changes in intracellular metabolic activity are important in influencing the phagocytic function of PMN leukocytes and macrophages.

The changes in cellular metabolic activity and tissue pH also may alter the enzymatic activities involved in the activation and/or destruction of endogenous compounds which may act as inflammatory mediators. In some cases, the acidic pH occurring in inflamed tissue prevents the enzymatic breakdown of certain compounds which may mediate the inflammatory reaction.

During the acute inflammatory reaction, alterations leading to fibrin formation both extravascularly and intravascularly occur. Platelets adhere to the vessel walls in the area of injury and eventually thrombi are formed within the affected vessels as a result of platelet aggregation and formation of fibrin. If this reaction is sufficiently severe, it leads to ischemia, tissue anoxia, acidosis, and finally necrosis of the involved vessels and tissue.

Lymphatics

Lymph capillaries, which are blind sacs returning fluid from the interstitial spaces to the vasculature, play an important part in inflammation. Large spaces (1500 to 2000 Å) occur between the endothelial cells of lymph capillaries, thereby allowing the entrance of large molecular weight proteins, blood cells, and macrophages. During inflammation lymphatic flow is increased as a result of the increase in interstitial fluid. Certain inflammatory mediators are present in the lymph draining from an inflamed area.

If the defense reaction of the tissue, that is, the acute inflammatory response, is successful in removing the noxious stimuli, the characteristic events of acute inflammation subside and healing results. Thus, the acute inflammatory reaction is a defense mechanism and is a prerequisite for tissue repair and healing. The acute inflammatory reaction should not be completely inhibited by therapeutic agents but should be controlled pharmacologically in such a manner as to prevent its progression to a chronic inflammatory reaction and permanent tissue damage.

ENDOGENOUS CHEMICAL MEDIATORS OF INFLAMMATION

The noxious stimuli may produce two types of injury: (1) a direct damaging effect on vessels from the stimuli, and (2) indirect effects on the vessels by activation and release of endogenous compounds which mediate the vascular and cellular events described previously. Obviously, direct injury of the vasculature will result in leakage of fluid, protein, and cells from the vessels.

However, in many types of injuries and in areas adjacent to direct injury, endogenous compounds mediate the vascular and cellular events. Endogenous compounds capable of producing the characteristic events of the inflammatory reaction may be categorized into the following groups:

1. *Vasoactive amines.* Histamine, 5-hydroxytryptamine (in some species except man), and the natural liberators of these compounds; enzymes that inactivate normally occurring vasoconstrictor substances.
2. *Proteases.* Plasmin, kallikrein, Hageman factor, various permeability factors, and enzymes of the complement sequence.
3. *Polypeptides.* Bradykinin, kallidin, other kinin peptides, and other basic and acid polypeptides.
4. *Nucleic acids and derivatives.* Lymph node permeability factor (LNPF).
5. *Lipid-soluble acids.* Lysolecithin, slow-reacting substance of anaphylaxis (SRS-A), and prostaglandins.
6. *Lysosome contents.* Lysosomal enzymes, proteases, and other constituents.
7. *Lymphokines.* Intracellular proteins from stimulated lymphocytes.

Vasoactive Amines

Considerable evidence indicates that histamine mediates the early phase of the permeability response of the acute inflammatory reaction in man. Histamine is formed by the action of the enzyme histidine decarboxylase on the amino acid histidine; it is inactivated by the enzyme histaminase. These reactions are shown in Figure 16–1. The major storage sites for histamine are the granules of mast cells in various tissues and the basophils in the circulation (see Table 16–1). Also, large quantities of histamine are present in some of the cells lining the stomach. Mast cell histamine can be released by injurious stimuli, by antigen-antibody reactions, and by certain

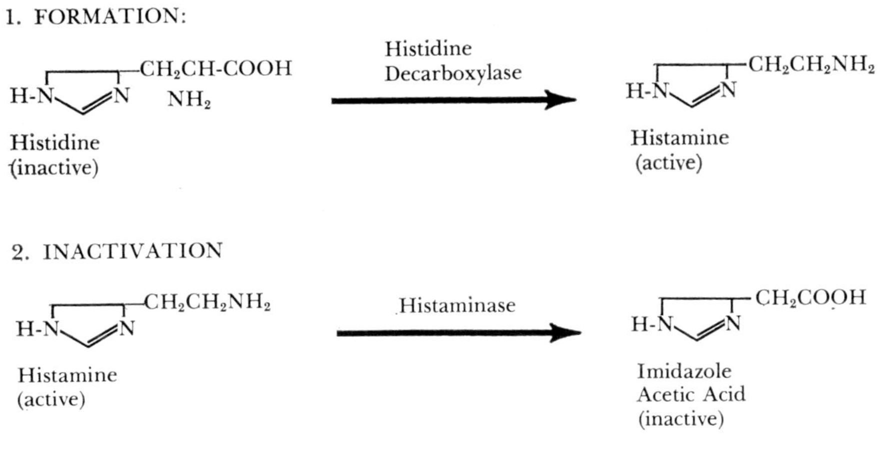

1. FORMATION:

2. INACTIVATION

FIG. 16–1. Formation and inactivation of histamine.

drugs and other chemical agents. Degranulation of the mast cell and release of histamine can occur without cell lysis. Histamine directly affects the microvasculature causing vasodilatation of arterioles, metarterioles, and venules, and engorgement of capillaries. Its direct effects on the venular endothelial cells result in formation of gaps at the intercellular junctions and in vascular leakage of fluid and plasma proteins. Histamine mediates the early vascular changes, but it is not involved with the more prolonged late changes in vascular permeability; likewise, it does not mediate the cellular aspects of acute inflammation.

Human gingiva contains a relatively large number of mast cells whose number is inversely related to the severity of gingival inflammation. Therefore, it seems probable that histamine is involved in mediating the early vascular changes occurring in acute gingival inflammation. The acute gingival inflammatory response, experimentally induced by topical application of endotoxin, can be inhibited by pharmacological agents that deplete mast cell histamine. However, actual measurement of the histamine content of healthy gingiva or changes in histamine content at various stages of gingival inflammation have not been reported. It is likely that histamine plays a sequential role in transiently increasing vascular permeability, thereby allowing the extravasation of plasma components such as protease enzymes which become activated and mediate subsequent gingival inflammatory changes.

Protease Enzymes and Polypeptide Products

Increased proteolytic activity, evident at the site of tissue inury, occurs by activation of existent, but inactive, protease enzymes present intracellularly or intravascularly. In this regard, the acute inflammatory reaction may be considered as a sequence of events resulting from release of intracellular and/or intravascular protease and esterase enzyme systems into the extracellular and extravascular compartments. Enzymatic action on specific substrates results in the formation of biologically active products which mediate the observable events of the inflammatory response. The kallikrein-kinin system is an example of a protease system which mediates certain aspects of the prolonged late phase of acute inflammation. The process of activation of this system and its interrelationships with other endogenous biochemical pathways are illustrated in Figure 16–2. Kallikrein enzymes from various sources act on substrates (kininogens) present in the α_2-globulin fraction of plasma proteins or substrates in tissues to form at least four distinctly different vasoactive polypeptides known as kinins. One of these polypeptides, bradykinin, is formed by the action of plasma kallikrein on the α_2-globulin fraction of plasma proteins. The structure of this active nonapeptide is shown in Figure 16–3. These polypeptides are among the most potent compounds known for producing some of the classic signs of acute inflammation. A few nanograms of these peptides can cause vasodilatation, increased vascular permeability, and pain. Kallikrein exhibits chem-

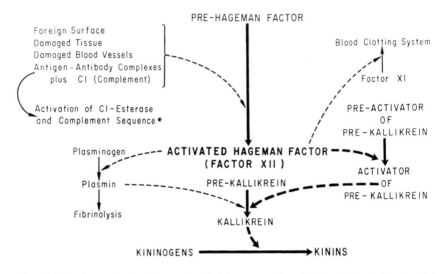

FIG. 16–2. Interrelationships and probable means of activation of the kallikrein-kinin system, complement sequence, fibrinolysis, and blood clotting system. Dashed arrows signify activation of or influence on the system indicated by solid arrows. The pathway for kinin formation is shown by heavy dashed and solid arrows. The asterisk (*) refers to Fig. 16–7. (The term Hageman factor refers to a serum protein found originally in the blood of a patient by the name of Hageman. This factor starts the intrinsic clotting mechanism.) (Modified by E. H. Montgomery, University of Texas Dental Branch, Houston, Texas, from Movat, H. Z.: *Inflammation, Immunity and Hypersensitivity.* New York, Harper & Row, 1971.)

otactic activity resulting in the migration of PMN leukocytes to the injured area where it has been activated.

The kinins such as bradykinin are inactivated by removal of the C-terminal arginine by carboxypeptidase-type enzymes known as kininases (Fig. 16–3). The activity of these enzymes is inhibited by the slightly acidic pH (6.0 to 6.5) in inflamed tissue. Therefore, kinin activity is increased at inflammatory sites owing to both increased formation and decreased inactivation of these peptides. These polypeptides apparently are involved with the late, prolonged phase of acute inflammation, because inhibition of kallikrein prevents the increased vascular permeability response occurring during this phase. A sequential release of histamine, followed by kinin activation and lastly by prostaglandin release, has been shown for some experimentally induced inflammatory reactions. Each compound mediates a specific phase of the acute inflammatory reaction. Some of the

H-ARG-PRO-PRO-GLY-PHE-SER-PRO-PHE-ARG-OH

1   2   3   4   5   6   7   8 ↑ 9

FIG. 16–3. Structure of the bradykinin nonapeptide. The arrow indicates the cleavage point of kininase inactivation.

anti-inflammatory actions of drugs may occur by preventing the formation of endogenous inflammatory mediators.

Several investigations have shown that the kallikrein-kinin system mediates certain aspects of acute gingival inflammation. Fluid taken from the gingival pockets of patients with periodontal disease contains kallikrein and kinin activities; the degree of gingival inflammation, assessed histologically, is directly related to the presence of kinin activity in the gingival tissue. An acute gingival inflammatory response, characterized by an increase in vascular permeability (*i.e.*, increased crevicular fluid flow), can be induced experimentally by the topical application of human plaque extracts or bacterial endotoxins to clinically healthy gingiva; the increase in crevicular fluid corresponds directly to the kallikrein-kinin activities present in this exudate. Furthermore, this acute gingival inflammatory response can be inhibited by compounds that interfere with the formation of the kinin peptides. Evidence indicates that both histamine and kinin-like peptides play important roles in mediating at least the acute stages of gingival inflammation induced by products of plaque bacteria.

Lipid-soluble Acids: Prostaglandins and Slow-Reacting Substance of Anaphylaxis (SRS-A)

The importance of prostaglandins in the inflammatory response has recently become apparent. These compounds are present naturally in seminal fluid and various mammalian tissues. They are partially unsaturated long chain fatty acids containing a saturated cyclopentane ring. They are derivatives of prostanoic acid and are formed by the action of lipid oxidase on polyunsaturated aliphatic acids such as arachidonic acid. Lysosomal enzymes may have a role in forming these compounds by splitting suitable fatty acids from the lecithin present in cell membranes. Four series of prostaglandins occur naturally, namely, the E, F, A, and B series; these differ structurally with regard to the number of double bonds and type of substitutions at specific carbon atoms of the aliphatic chain and/or cyclopentane ring. They also differ in physiological and pharmacological actions. Prostaglandins of the E-series, particularly prostaglandin E_2 (PGE_2), produce effects characteristic of the inflammatory reaction and may act as inflammatory mediators (see Fig. 11–5). In contrast, certain prostaglandins of the F-series exhibit anti-inflammatory activity. Complex interrelationships occur between these compounds as mediators and/or modulators of acute inflammation. Some of their effects may be related to their actions in altering cellular levels of cyclic adenosine monophosphate (cAMP) and cyclic guanosine monophosphate (cGMP). One of the nonsteroidal anti-inflammatory agents, indomethacin, may exert its pharmacologic effects by inhibiting the synthesis of prostaglandins. Levels of PGE are elevated in experimentally induced and spontaneously occurring inflammatory reactions. Exudates taken from periodontal pockets and inflamed human gingival tissue show increased levels of prostaglandin E_2. These levels are within the range of the levels necessary to stimulate bone resorption *in vitro*. Therefore, these compounds may contribute to the clinical manifestations of periodontal inflammation and the bone loss characteristic of periodontitis.

Slow-reacting substance of anaphylaxis (SRS-A) is a lipid soluble compound released during Type I reactions such as anaphylaxis (see page 370). The exact biochemical nature of this substance presently is unknown. It may be released from either PMN leukocytes or mast cells, depending on the species and type of immunoglobulin involved in the antigen-antibody reaction. This compound can cause vasodilatation, increased vascular permeability, and bronchoconstriction. This agent is probably one of the major bronchiolar constrictor substances acting during anaphylactic shock or other types of immediate hypersensitivity reactions, and accounts in part for the lack of effectiveness of antihistaminic drugs in treating this aspect of these immunologic reactions.

Lysosomal Enzymes

A number of tissue active substances, including proteases and other enzymes, are present in subcellular organelles called *lysosomes*. Lysosomes in PMN leukocytes, macrophages, and possibly other cells such as mast cells are involved in the production of some of the changes seen in acute inflammation. Lysosomal enzymes can release or activate inflammatory mediators. In addition, they may damage tissue directly because they degrade proteins and carbohydrates. A partial list of enzymatic and nonenzymatic sudstances present in the lysosome is given in Table 16–2. Enzymes similar to those found in lysosomes have been demonstrated in gingival debris, suggesting that lysosomal enzymes such as collagenase, proteases, hyaluronidase, acid phosphatase, and beta-glucuronidase are released in the area of inflamed gingiva. Lysosomal enzymes may be released during phagocytosis without cell lysis or they may be released when PMN leukocytes and macrophages undergo lysis. Lysosomal enzymes can be released from macrophages and PMN leukocytes without lysis when these cells are incubated with plaque extracts or oral bacteria. Enzymes similar to those found in lysosomes also may be produced by plaque bacteria. Therefore, both plaque bacteria and inflammatory cells can release enzymes which serve to cause inflammatory changes and produce the destructive tissue changes seen in periodontal disease. The tissue damage and necrosis occurring in certain immunologic reactions such as the Arthus and Shwartzman reactions are believed to be caused by the release of lysosomal enzymes.

Lysosomal and extralysosomal fractions of PMN leukocytes contain enzymes for both the formation and degradation of kinin-like peptides. By this mechanism, leukocytes migrating to the inflamed area can contribute to the formation and/or destruction of inflammatory mediators.

Table 16-2. Some Enzymatic and Nonenzymatic Substances Present in Lysosomes

Enzymatic Substances	Nonenzymatic Substances
Alkaline phosphatase	Anticoagulant substance
Acid lipase	Cationic proteins
Acid ribonuclease	Anionic substances
Acid deoxyribonuclease	Chemotactic factor
Acid phosphatase	Phagocytin
Beta-Glucuronidase	Plasminogen activator
Beta-Galactosidase	Mucopolysaccharides and glyco-
Beta-N-Acetylglucosaminidase	proteins
Cathepsins	Hemolysin
Kininogenase	Endogenous pyrogen
Collagenase	
Alpha-N-Acetylgalactosaminidase	
Alpha-N-Acetylglucosaminidase	
Alpha-L-Fucosidase	
Alpha-1-4-Glucosidase	
Alpha-Mannosidase	
Arylsulfatases A and B	
Hyaluronidase	
Esterases	
Phosphatidic acid phosphatase	
Phosphoprotein phosphatase	
Phospholipases (acid, alkaline)	
Proteases	
Lysozyme	

INITIATORS OF THE INFLAMMATORY REACTION

Any stimuli that can elicit tissue injury can result in an inflammatory reaction. The stimuli may be mechanical, traumatic, thermal, chemical, or biological in nature. Chemical stimuli that produce inflammation are of particular interest, because many spontaneously occurring inflammatory reactions result either from the direct toxic effects of chemical substances or as a result of their ability to activate endogenous systems.

Certain chemical substances used in dentistry may cause an acute and/or chronic inflammatory reaction when these are used improperly. For example, certain materials such as zinc phosphate cements, silicate cements, and silicates contain high quantities of phosphoric acid. If these acidic materials are allowed to contact the pulp directly or reach the pulp by diffusion through the dentinal tubules, the acid causes an acute, followed by a chronic, pulpal inflammation. Certain resinous materials contain high amounts of a monomer, methyl methacrylate, which may cause inflammation of the oral tissues when these materials are placed directly on vital tissue. Even zinc oxide-eugenol can produce pulpal inflammation if placed directly on vital tissue, for example, exposed pulpal tissue. Usually, various protective agents are used to protect the oral tissues from the irritant effects of these chemical agents and to prevent an inflammatory reaction which may become chronic and deleterious to the involved tissue.

The initiation of gingival inflammation exemplifies the role played by biochemical stimuli in producing an inflammatory reaction. By-products released by plaque bacteria may be directly toxic or may activate endogenous mediator systems and/or immune mechanisms. Cytotoxic substances produced by plaque bacteria may directly injure the crevicular epithelial barrier, thereby enhancing the entrance of other noxious substances. Bacterial lipopolysaccharides, that is, endotoxins, are multipotential initiators of gingival inflammation exhibiting (1) primary toxicity, (2) the ability to activate complement beginning at the C3 component, and (3) the ability to serve as an antigen. Enzymes produced by plaque bacteria comprise another group of biochemical agents which can initiate inflammation. These enzymes include hyaluronidase, collagenase, chondroitin sulfatase, elastase, proteases, and proteolytic enzymes which activate endogenous mediator systems.

Immunological Initiators

The body reacts to a foreign cell or molecule with a response, the immune response, designed to localize and eventually remove the invader. This response culminates in differing degrees of inflammation mediated by different endogenous compounds depending on the immunologic components involved. The susceptibility to infectious diseases and the abbreviated life spans of individuals with immunologic deficiencies leaves little doubt as to the protective nature of the immune response. However, the initiating stimulus may or may not be toxic to the host, it may or may not be biologically active, and it even may be a part of the host's own tissues. Regardless, the immune system responds with an inflammatory reaction which may in time destroy not only the invader but also injure the host's own tissues, injuries that may be much more severe than any produced by the stimulus alone. Thus, as an initiator of inflammation the immune system continues the paradox that characterizes the inflammatory response; it can play either a beneficial or a harmful role.

Three major components are directly involved in the immune response: antigens, antigen reactive lymphocytes, and antibodies. Antigens are foreign substances that induce the formation of the latter two components by lymphocytes. The immune response is divided into cell-mediated immunity and humoral immunity. Cell-mediated immunity (CMI) is mediated by the antigen reactive lymphocytes. These cells have been modified or activated by antigenic stimulation to produce several biologically active compounds and to react more vigorously with their specific antigens. Humoral immunity is mediated by antibodies that are soluble glycoprotein molecules. They also will react specifically with antigens which induced their formation.

The specificity of the reactants is probably the most unique characteristic of the immune response and it is of prime importance. Antigen reactive cells and antibodies will react only with the same antigen or with antigens similar to those that induced their formation. It is this specific reaction that initiates the events which may lead to an inflammatory response.

Antigens. An antigen is a substance that induces the formation of antibodies and antigen reactive lymphocytes, and reacts specifically with these immune components on subsequent exposure. Antigens are large molecules usually over 10,000 molecular weight. They are protein or polysaccharide or combinations of these with each other or with lipids or nucleic acids. They must be biodegradable and they are usually foreign to the tissue of the respondent. An individual does not normally mount an immune response to his own or "self" antigens. This differentiation of self from not self is an initial and critical function of the immune system. Occasionally, the impairment of this basic mechanism does result in autoimmunity, the induction of an immune response against one's own antigens.

An important exception to the rule that substances must be of a large molecular weight to be antigenic occurs with some small compounds, which when injected into the body are capable of adsorbing to the body's own proteins. These complexes, called conjugated antigens, may stimulate an immune response, because the small compound, or hapten, furnishes the foreignness, while the body protein, or carrier, provides the bulk required for an immune response. Thus, both a normal complete antigen or a hapten conjugated to a carrier protein may elicit formation of immune components or react with previously formed immune components.

Examples of the many different types of antigens are microbial cell walls, membranes, enzymes, and toxins. Likewise, plant and animal cells and cellular products make good antigens. In this context it should be noted that the determinant of foreignness may be a simple matter of minor genetic differences within a species. Thus, the normal components of one human being may appear as antigens to another.

In addition, self antigens may be made to evoke an immune response. Modification of the body's tissue by infectious microbes, by conjugation with haptens, or possibly even by hydrolytic enzymes released during an inflammatory response may render self antigens foreign to the host, and capable of eliciting an autoimmune response.

Lymphocytes. The immune response is a function of the lymphoid tissues, and lymphocytes are responsible for the reactions associated with immunity. Lymphocytes, which initially originate as stem cells in the bone marrow, have been divided into two groups with different but interrelated immunologic functions (Fig. 16–4). One group of lymphocytes becomes immuno-

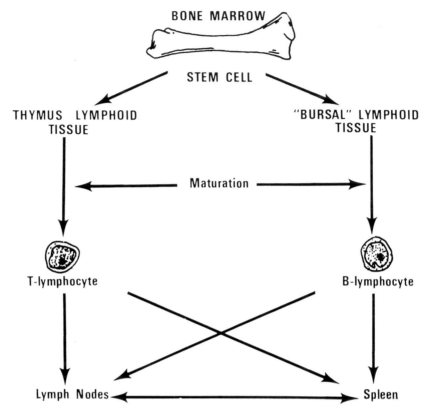

F<small>IG</small>. 16–4. The two component system of immunologic maturation. Stem cells from the bone marrow are induced by thymic or bursal factors to become mature T- or B-lymphocytes, which eventually populate the peripheral lymphoid tissues.

logically mature, that is, immunocompetent, as a result of alteration by the thymus gland. The thymic factor involved may be a humoral substance, possibly a hormone, called *thymosin*. These lymphocytes, called *thymic-derived* or *T-lymphocytes*, are the mediators of cell mediated immunity (CMI). Antigen reactive lymphocytes are derived from these T-lymphocytes. In addition, T cells function as a major regulatory mechanism in the immune response.

A second group of lymphocytes has been given the designation *bursa-derived* or *B-lymphocytes* because their maturation was initially discovered to be a function of a chicken lymphoid organ known as the bursa of Fabricius. A similar organ is not present in mammals, but bone marrow and the fetal liver have been suggested as mammalian lymphoid tissues homologous to the bursa. B-lymphocytes produce antibodies, the molecules responsible for humoral immunity.

After differentiation into T or B cells, lymphocytes pass through the circulation to populate lymphoid tissues such as lymph nodes and spleen where they await stimulation by an antigen (Fig. 16–4).

The Immune Response. The immune response is initiated by the entrance of an antigen into the tissues of the body. Entrance may be by any number of routes including infection, injection, or inhalation. Within the body the antigen is carried to a lymph node where with the assistance of a macrophage it is presented to a T- or B-lymphocyte capable of reacting to it. These are not random cells, but specific lymphocytes genetically programmed to react with the specific antigen. Once an antigen reaches the lymphocyte the cell is induced to proliferate and differentiate into at least two major functional populations of cells (Fig. 16–5). One consists of relatively short lived cells, the effector cells, which produce soluble biologically active molecules which mediate the effects that will be described later. These molecules are the lymphokines and antibodies produced by T-lymphocytes and B-lymphocytes, respectively. Effector cells themselves may also carry out activities related to the events displayed during the reaction. The second population of cells are the memory cells, which may survive for the life of the individual. When

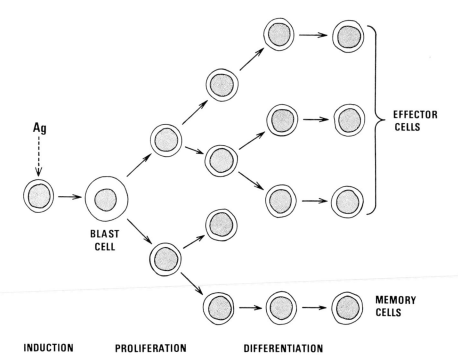

Fig. 16–5. Cellular events occurring in the immune response, either humoral or cell mediated. The effector cells in cell-mediated immunity are killer lymphocytes and lymphocytes that produce lymphokines. The effector cells in humoral immunity are plasma cells that produce antibody. On secondary stimulation, memory cells become blast cells and repeat the process. Ag = antigen.

exposed to antigen, memory cells will proliferate and differentiate into two populations as did the original lymphocytes. The population of memory cells produced during the initial or primary response usually is more numerous than the original population of reacting lymphocytes, and this results in an enhanced response on subsequent antigenic stimulation.

The response of the memory cell to the second and subsequent exposures to the same antigen, the secondary or booster response, varies from the primary in terms of the quantity of antigen necessary for induction, rapidity and magnitude of the response, and reactivity of the immune components. It takes less antigen to induce a more rapid and greater production of lymphokines, antibodies and/or antigen reactive cells, and the antibodies and lymphocytes are much more active in their reactions. Thus, the immune reaction to an antigen and, if present, the accompanying inflammatory reactions are usually much greater following secondary antigenic stimulation. Although we describe the primary and secondary responses as separate events, it is possible under certain circumstances that the primary may overlap the secondary with no apparent separation. Thus, in the presence of large amounts of antigen, or when an animal is subjected to an extended antigenic stimulation as in chronic diseases, the dichotomy of the responses may not be apparent.

The basic cellular phenomena of CMI and humoral immunity are similar. Induction, proliferation, differentiation, and the production of active molecules and memory cells occur in both cases. They vary with respect to the activities of the effector cells and the types of active molecules produced by these cells.

Cell-mediated Immunity. Although CMI responses appear to be predominantly a function of T cells, there is increasing evidence that B cells are also involved in similar, but not necessarily identical, activities. CMI effector cell activities include the direct actions of sensitized lymphocytes on antigen-carrying target cells and the production of lymphokines.

Lymphokines are biologically active molecules released by stimulated lymphocytes during the proliferation phase of a CMI response. Unlike antibodies, they are not immunologically specific. The same lymphokines are produced as a result of stimulation by different antigens, but they do not react with the antigen. They act on cells and tissues of the host. Lymphokines are proteins of about 20,000 to 80,000 molecular weight. Although they were originally reported to be products of reactive T-lymphocytes, they since have been also shown to be produced by B cells and even some non-lymphoid cells. Several lymphokine activities have been reported, but each activity may not be a function of a different molecule.

Some of the lymphokines are

1. Skin reactive factor: causes increased vascular permeability with accompanying swelling and reddening of the tissue.

2. Mitogenic factors: produced by specifically stimulated cells, induce the proliferation of nonspecific lymphocytes and increase the number of cells producing lymphokines.
3. Chemotactic factors: attract leukocytes to the area of the reaction. Factors for macrophages, polymorphonuclear leukocytes, eosinophils, and lymphocytes have been reported.
4. Migration inhibitory factor: inhibits the migration of macrophages, causing accumulation of these cells at the site of the CMI response.
5. Macrophage-activating factor: induces an enhancement of the ability of macrophages to phagocytize and kill microorganisms. These activated macrophages possess increased metabolic respiratory and hydrolytic capacities.
6. Cytotoxic or lymphotoxic factor: kills living cells in tissue culture.
7. Osteoclast-activating factor: induces the resorption of bone.

These lymphokines are produced and released into the surrounding tissue by antigen reactive lymphocytes stimulated by their specific antigens. In addition, CMI killer cells are capable of destroying antigen-bearing cells without the assistance of the lymphokines. They have been demonstrated to kill cells in tissue culture and are of importance in tumor and graft rejection. The cytocidal mechanism is unknown. It is apparent that lymphokines and killer cells can induce and amplify an inflammatory response. Although they are generated as a result of a specific immune reaction, they are nonspecific in their activity and this often results in injurious inflammatory reactions.

Humoral Immunity. The mediators of humoral immunity and the major products of B cells are antibodies. These are glycoproteins produced by plasma cells, effector cells derived from antigen-stimulated B-lymphocytes. Antibodies are gamma globulins and the name *immunoglobulins* has been coined to describe them. There are five classes of immunoglobulins with different biologic and biochemical properties. Some of these properties are listed in Table 16-3. The five classes have been assigned the letters A, D, E, G, and M. Originally they were designated by the prefix gamma (*e.g.,* gamma A, gamma D, gamma E), but this has been replaced by immunoglobulin and they are now called immunoglobulin A, immunoglobulin D, immunoglobulin E, and so forth. For brevity they are usually referred to as IgA, IgD, IgE, IgG, and IgM.

The basic antibody molecule is composed of four polypeptide chains: two identical light (L) chains of 20,000 molecular weight, and two identical heavy (H) chains of 50,000 molecular weight (Fig. 16-6). There are two major types of L chains and five major types of H chains. The latter determine the class of immunoglobulin. Amino acid sequence studies of these peptides have revealed that a certain definite portion of each type of chain is constant and another portion is variable. The constant portions of the H

Table 16-3. Some Properties of the Immunoglobulins

	Serum Conc. mg%	Percent of Serum Ig	Mol. Wt.	Valence	Placental Transfer	Complement-activating	Type of Allergy
IgG	600–1800	80	160,000	2	+	+	II & III
IgM	50–200	6	900,000	5	–	+	II & III
IgA (serum)	150–400	13	170,000	2	–	–	?
IgA (secretory)	elevated in secretions		400,000	4	–	–	?
IgD	1–5	1	200,000	2	–	–	?
IgE	0.01–0.05	0.002	200,000	2	–	–	I

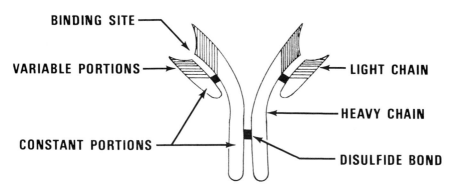

Fɪɢ. 16–6. Immunoglobulin model showing the arrangement of the polypeptide chains. The antigen binding site is formed by the variable portions of light and heavy chains. The biologic and chemical properties unique to each class of immunoglobulin are determined by the constant portions of the heavy chains.

chains of the molecule impart the properties unique to the class. For example, the constant portions of the H chains of IgG are responsible for its transplacental passage, its antigenicity, its activation of complement, and its participation in different hypersensitivity reactions. The two types of L chains are shared by all classes.

The variable portions of the L and H chains of an immunoglobulin molecule form the reactive site that is specific for the particular antigen. This is the part of the antibody molecule that reacts with the antigen. The basic immunoglobulin molecule contains two antigen binding sites; it has a valence of two. Those immunoglobulins composed of more than one of these basic units have greater valences (Table 16–3).

During formation of an immune complex it is the variable parts of the L and H chains that react with the antigen. Once within the immune complex the biologic activities of the immunoglobulin may be expressed. These activities, such as complement activation in the case of IgG and mast cell degranulation in the case of IgE, result from alterations in the molecular configuration of the constant portions of the H chains. Although the variable portions of all four chains initiate the immune reactions, the constant portions of the H chains mediate the events leading to an inflammatory response.

IgG is found in the highest concentration in the circulation and in most interstitial fluids. Because most antibodies are IgG, it is of major significance in protective immunity. It is also the mediator of types II and III hypersensitivities. The concentration of IgG in whole saliva varies with the oral health of the individual. It is the predominant immunoglobulin in crevicular fluids, and as the gingival index increases the concentration of IgG in whole saliva increases in proportion to the crevicular flow.

IgM is a polymer of five of the type of structures shown in Figure 16–6. Because of its large size it is called *macroglobulin*. It shares many of the biologic activites of IgG, but is of less significance because of its lower concentration. Its presence in the saliva is also primarily the result of passage through the gingival crevice.

IgA is second highest in concentration in the plasma. It is probably involved in protective immunity within the body, but it has not been shown to be involved in any hypersensitivity reactions. It is the principal immunoglobulin found in external secretions such as salivary, respiratory, gastrointestinal, and genitourinary fluids. This *secretory IgA* varies from serum IgA in that it is always at least a dimer possessing an additional peptide, secretory piece. Secretory IgA is a major defense mechanism at the mucous membrane level where it prevents entrance and adherence of microorganisms.

IgE is found in only minute amounts in the body. Although there is some evidence that it serves a protective function in the respiratory tract, its major significance is as the mediator of the type I hypersensitivities, anaphylaxis and atopy. It has not been demonstrated in saliva or gingival fluid, but it is present in gingival tissues.

IgD has not been found to be associated with any protective or harmful reactions and its significance is unknown.

Complement. Within plasma there is a group of substances that when activated amplify the effects of the antigen-antibody reaction through the formation of biologically active compounds. This amplifying mechanism, which may be either harmful or beneficial and plays a major role in the inflamma-

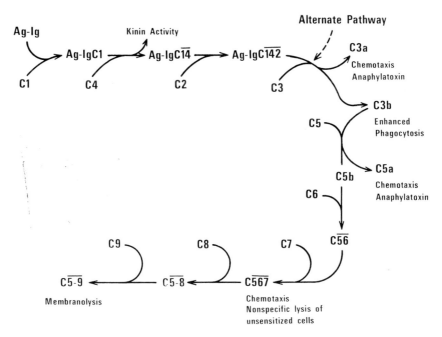

F‍ɪɢ. 16–7. The complement cascade. The classic pathway is initiated by immune complexes (Ag-Ig) acting on C1. The alternate pathway may be initiated by nonimmunologic components acting on C3.

tory response, is called *complement*. There are 11 components of complement which are activated in a sequence of reactions called the *complement cascade* (Fig. 16–7). Complement is usually abbreviated as C′, and the individual components as C1, C2, C3, and so forth.

Biologically active factors appearing as a result of C′ activation include *C-kinin*, which has properties similar to other kinins, *anaphylatoxins*, which induce the release of histamine from mast cells, *chemotaxins*, which attract polymorphonuclear leukocytes, *opsonins*, which enhance the phagocytic activities of leukocytes, and *membranolysins*, which disrupt cell membranes, of both bacterial and animal origin.

Many of these activities are integral parts of the inflammatory response, and as more information is obtained, it is becoming increasingly apparent that C′ is of major significance in inflammation. The initiation of the C′ cascade through C1 by an immune complex is called the *classic pathway*. Initiation of the cascade through C1 is a function of IgG and IgM, because only the H chains of these antibodies contain C′ activation sites. Reaction of one of these immunoglobulins with its specific antigen in the presence of C′ initiates the cascade, resulting in formation of the inflammatory by-products.

Another nonimmune mechanism of activation, the *alternate pathway*, has been discovered. Compounds such as endotoxin, lysosomal enzymes, and polysaccharides can activate the cascade beginning at C3. This is carried out through an enzyme complex called the *C3 proactivator system*. The complement cascade also may be activated by Hageman factor and plasmin at C1, by plasmin at C3, and by direct effects of proteases at C3 and C5. Because most of the inflammatory functions of C′ appear in the cascade after C3 activation, the alternate pathway and these other mechanisms serve as effective means of including C′ in inflammatory responses of nonimmunologic origin.

Hypersensitivity Reactions. In the event that an infectious microorganism invades the body, its presence stimulates the mobilization of the immune components described above. If it is a primary exposure the immune response may or may not be of sufficient magnitude to produce demonstrable symptoms. This will depend on the concentration and duration of exposure. If it is a second exposure to these antigens, memory cells are induced to proliferate and differentiate into effector cell and lymphocytes, and polymorphonuclear leukocytes and macrophages are attracted and stimulated by lymphokines or complement products. This is a beneficial response when undertaken in moderation against an invading microorganism; when carried to excess or in response to an inert agent, it can result in injurious inflammatory reactions, the hypersensitivity reactions. These may range from minute microscopic inflammatory foci to larger macroscopic lesions or even to systemic, fatal reactions.

Originally the hypersensitivity reactions were divided into delayed and immediate hypersensitivity. The former referred to the fact that visually

Table 16–4. Mediators of the Hypersensitivity Reactions

Type	Name	Mediators
I	Anaphylactic, atopic	IgE
II	Cytotoxic, antitissue	IgG, IgM
III	Immune complex, Arthus, serum sickness	IgG, IgM
IV	Cell-mediated, delayed hypersensitivity	Antigen reactive lymphocytes

demonstrable effects were manifested 24 to 72 hours after exposure to an antigen, whereas in immediate hypersensitivities the effects appeared much earlier, sometimes within minutes after exposure to antigen. The mechanisms mediating these reactions have been elucidated further and four types of allergies or hypersensitivities have been differentiated. These are shown with their mediators and clinical names in Table 16–4.

Type I Hypersensitivity. Type I hypersensitivity reactions are the classic immediate hypersensitivities, anaphylaxis and atopy. Anaphylaxis is the systemic shock syndrome, and atopy is the localized reaction commonly manifested as respiratory distress or urticaria. The basic mechanisms are similar; the differences are in the relative dissemination of the reaction and the accompanying severity. The determination of whether the effects will be local or systemic can be a function of the antigen, the dose, the portal of entry, and the particular sensitivity of the different tissues.

These reactions are characterized by dilatation of the capillaries and small vessels, increased vascular permeability, and smooth muscle constriction. Atopy is typified by the wheal and flare reaction in cutaneous tissues, and edema and increased secretory activities in mucous membranes such as those of the gastrointestinal or respiratory tract. Asthma, hay fever, and food allergies are the most common atopic hypersensitivities. Anaphylaxis is characterized by a generalized loss of blood pressure and often fatal systemic shock syndrome. It may be accompanied by bronchial constriction and pulmonary edema, resulting in severe respiratory distress. These reactions are initiated within minutes after the antigen enters the tissues of a primed individual.

Type I hypersensitivity reactions are mediated by IgE. The reaction of IgE with its specific antigen results in the release of several pharmacologically active agents including histamine, kinins, prostaglandins, slow-reacting substance of anaphylaxis (SRS-A) and an eosinophil chemotactic factor (ECF). Many of these agents are vasodilators and smooth muscle constrictors. All have been demonstrated to play some role in the development of the Type I reaction in different species, but all are not involved to the same extent in human beings.

The agent that appears to be the most important in Type I hypersensitivity reactions is histamine, because many of the effects of anaphylaxis and atopy may be prevented with antihistamines. Release of histamine is accomplished through the formation of immune complexes on the membranes of mast cells or basophils. Once IgE is formed as a result of an antigenic stimulus, it diffuses from the site of synthesis until it contacts a mast cell or basophil. On contact it attaches to the cell membrane through special receptors on its heavy chain and it remains in a dormant state. On reappearance of the antigen, the formation of an immune complex of IgE and the specific antigen causes degranulation of the mast cells and release of histamine.

SRS-A also is thought to play an important role in Type I reactions in man. Its source is not known but it also may be a product of the mast cell, and the mechanisms of its release into the circulation may be similar to those of histamine. Kinins and prostaglandins also have been shown to be present during these reactions, but again neither their source nor their mechanisms of release during this allergic reaction have been discovered. Although the release of ECF has been demonstrated during the anaphylactic reaction, and there is an increase in the number of eosinophils in local areas displaying chronic atopic reactions, the role, if any, of ECF during the actual reaction is not understood.

These hypersensitive reactions are usually short-lived, and except in the case of fatal anaphylaxis, recovery occurs within minutes after the reaction. However, in situations in which there is a constant antigen insult, as in hay fever, a chronic inflammation may develop.

Type I hypersensitivities are induced by a number of different antigens. Most clinical allergens such as procaine and penicillin are haptens. The most common natural allergens causing Type I hypersensitivity reactions include pollen, insect venoms, and foods such as eggs and milk. Within the oral cavity the severity of gingivitis has been shown to be correlated with the presence of Type I hypersensitivity to certain dental plaque bacteria.

Type II Hypersensitivity. Type II reactions are called *cytotoxic* or *antitissue reactions.* They cause direct injury to cells, either fixed or circulating, and involve the reaction of antibody with an antigen on the cell membrane, a complex ultimately leading to the death of the cell. The antigen may be a part of the cell membrane or it may be another antigen or a hapten adsorbed to the surface of the cell. Type II hypersensitivities directed against circulating cells are manifested as abnormally decreased numbers of these cells such as in hemolytic anemias. Where target cells are fixed such as in the kidney, there is localized destruction, especially of the basement membranes of these organs.

IgG and IgM are the mediators of this hypersensitivity, and complement, which is activated by these immunoglobulins, is usually involved. The opsonic and membranolytic activities of complement are especially significant in Type II hypersensitivities. The specific immunoglobulin reacts with membrane-bound antigens, complement is activated, and the cell is destroyed by phagocytosis or membranolysis. Phagocytosis may be carried out by polymorphonuclear leukocytes or by fixed or wandering macrophages whose activities are enhanced by the opsonic activity of immunoglobulins and complement. Membranolysis results from the activation of the complement cascade. It has been demonstrated that cells of the lymphoreticular system which do not appear to be typical T- or B-lymphocytes also may be active in the cytotoxic reaction. These cells, which have been designated killer or K cells, react with the H chain of immunoglobulins complexed to the target cell membrane and kill the cell to which they are attached. It should be noted that because IgG and C′ are involved in this reaction, as in Type III reactions, many of the injurious effects found in Type III reactions will also occur in Type II.

Some examples of Type II reactions are transfusion reactions, Rh disease, and certain organ transplant rejections. Many drug-induced hemolytic anemias or thrombocytopenias are cytotoxic reactions. In these cases the drug, a hapten, adsorbs to the red blood cells or platelets and the immune system produces antibodies directed against the conjugate. These antibodies do not usually react with normal cells or platelets in the absence of the drug. Several autoimmune diseases including hemolytic anemias, thyroiditis, and glomerulonephritis are caused by Type II hypersensitivities. Any mechanism that can induce rearrangement of the molecular configuration of self antigens has the capacity to induce an autoimmune Type II reaction. This may be an acute, relatively short-lived effect, or it may be a permanent or semipermanent (chronic) condition.

Type III Hypersensitivity. Type III hypersensitivities occur as a result of activation of C′ by an antigen-antibody complex. These are called *antigen-antibody* or *immune complex* hypersensitivities and may be of two types, local or systemic. The local reaction is called the *Arthus reaction*, after the investigator who first described it. The systemic reaction was named after the syndrome with which it was previously associated, *serum sickness*. The molecular and cellular mechanisms in either type are similar; the location of the reaction is dependent on the route of antigen entrance and the quantity of antibody present. Immune complex reactions are characterized by increased vascular permeability and edema, a marked infiltration of polymorphonuclear leukocytes, and vasculitis with hemorrhage and thrombosis.

The major components associated with these hypersensitivities are antigen, antibody, complement, and polymorphonuclear leukocytes, Platelets also play a role. Almost any antigen, including conjugated antigens, can elicit immune complex allergies. The antibodies mediating the reaction are IgG and IgM, and their involvement is the result of their ability to activate complement. Once activated, complement, through its anaphylatoxic and chemotactic activities, induces an influx of PMNs into the area of the immune complex. The opsonic effects of C′ and immunoglobulins encourage phagocytosis of the immune complexes. During the phagocytic process lysosomal enzymes are released into the area and these hydrolases produce the vasculitis. The significance of the role that these enzymes play in this reaction is easily demonstrated by injecting lysosomes or the contents of these granules into a target tissue. A typical Type III lesion will occur.

If there is a high concentration of antibody present, the immune complex will precipitate at the point of antigen entrance and a local or Arthus reaction, which takes a maximum of 2 to 5 hours to develop, will ensue. The reaction may simply be a mild local inflammation or it may progress to a necrotic lesion. The severity of the reaction will vary with the concentration of the antibody.

If there is no or little antibody present the antigen will reach the vascular system and remain in the circulation until sufficient antibody is produced in response to the antigenic stimulation. As antibody is formed, it will complex with the circulating antigen and these small complexes may be filtered out in the walls of the vessels or in the glomeruli of the kidneys. Minute foci of vascular inflammation occur wherever these complexes localize. Symptoms include fever, joint pains, swollen lymph nodes, and glomerulonephritis.

Local or Arthus immune complex hypersensitivity reactions are not common. However, systemic vasculitis resembling that seen in serum sickness may follow large injections of serums or penicillin and other drugs. The inflammation of rheumatoid arthritis appears to be of an immune complex derivation, and glomerulonephritis of a Type III origin has been demonstrated with some chronic viral infections, as a sequel to streptococcal infections, and in association with systemic lupus erythematosus. Although it is not an immune complex reaction, many aspects of the Shwartzman reaction, an inflammatory response produced by bacterial endotoxins, are essentially those of a complement-mediated hypersensitivity; one initiated through the alternate pathway.

Type IV Hypersensitivities. When antigen is injected into the tissues of an individual who has sensitive lymphocytes specific for that antigen, an indurated nodule, which reaches a maximal size in about 24 to 48 hours, may develop. Histologically this is characterized by a dense mononuclear cell infiltrate composed of lymphocytes and macrophages. This is the Type IV or delayed hypersensitivity reaction mediated by antigen reactive lymphocytes.

The tuberculin reaction is the classic Type IV hypersensitivity. Twenty-four to seventy-two hours after intradermal injection of tubercle bacillus antigens into a hypersensitive individual, a slowly developing indurated swelling reaches maximal size and then regresses. In severe reactions a necrotic lesion may develop. Tuberculin hypersensitivity may be passed from a sensitive subject to a normal individual by antigen reactive lymphocytes, but not by serum, indicating that it is a CMI response.

The presence of these mononuclear infiltrates and the accompanying inflammatory injury may be explained on the basis of the release of lymphokines by antigen reactive lymphocytes. When exposed to their specific antigen these lymphocytes are induced to proliferate and produce lymphokines.

Skin reactive factor causes an increase in vascular permeability and facilitates the influx of cells into the area. Macrophage chemotactic, migration inhibitory, and activating factors attract, hold and enhance the activity of these phagocytes. Chemotactic factors also attract polymorphs and monocytes. Infiltrating lymphocytes that are not sensitive to a specific antigen are nevertheless susceptible to blastogenic lymphokines, and these induce their proliferation with additional lymphokine release. Thus, within the area of the immune reaction there is an accumulation of inflammatory cells, and an amplification of the response as a result of nonspecific stimulations of lymcytes in the inflammatory infiltrate.

In addition to the aforementioned effects, tissue cells in the immediate area of the immune response may be killed or injured as a result of the nonspecific actions of cytotoxins and the direct cytocidal effect of sensitized lymphocytes. Furthermore, as tissues are injured or killed, and as the cells in the infiltrate carry out phagocytosis, release of lysosomal enzymes and other intracellular components may add to the inflammation and injury.

Delayed hypersensitivity reactions are the cause of graft rejections, of the granulomatous lesions characterizing many bacterial, viral, and fungal infections, and of many autoimmune diseases. Contact sensitivity is the result of a dermatitis in which haptens such as mercury bind to skin proteins and induce a local CMI hypersensitivity reaction. Within the oral cavity, CMI reactions have been associated with chronic periodontal disease.

The systemic effects of allergic reactions are the most dramatic. However, the basic mechanisms of these systemic reactions are the same as those producing local immunologic reactions. These local effects, minute hypersensitivity reactions, are sufficient to initiate an inflammatory response capable of protecting or injuring the host.

Because of their nature the injurious effects of immunologically induced inflammatory reactions stand out. However, the basic function is that of protection. For example, although IgE is notorious as the mediator of anaphylaxis, it also has been found that individuals with a congenital deficiency of IgE suffer from chronic respiratory infections. In order to gain a true perspective of the role of IgE, it might be better to consider the relative absence of such chronic infections as opposed to the prevalence of anaphylaxis. Similar consideration should be given to other immunologic initiators of inflammation.

The four types of hypersensitivity reactions have been described as individual processes. However, because the immune response usually results in the formation of both immunoglobulins and antigen reactive cells, it is doubtful whether under natural conditions they ever occur as completely isolated inflammatory responses. Probably a combination of reactions occur simultaneously, with the predominant one giving the characteristics of that type of reaction to the total response. This would be especially so in the case of gingivitis or periodontal disease induced by dental plaque, which contains a multitude of antigens capable of eliciting any of these reactions.

SELECTED REFERENCES

BELLANTI, J. A.: *Immunology.* Philadelphia, W. B. Saunders Co., 1971.

CIMASONI, G.: The crevicular fluid. In H. M. Meyers (Ed.): *Monographs in Oral Science,* Vol. 3, New York, S. Karger, 1974.

GELL, P. G. H., and COOMBS, R. R. A. (Eds.).: *Clinical Aspects of Immunology,* 3rd ed. Philadelphia, Lippincott, 1975.

HOUCK, J. C.: A personal overview of inflammation. In B. K. Forscher (Ed.): *Chemical Biology of Inflammation.* New York, Pergamon Press, 1968.

KEARNY, J. F.: T and B lymphocytes, J. Oral Pathol., *3(4),* 151, 1974.

LEHNER, T.: Cell mediated immune responses in oral disease: A review, J. Oral Pathol., *1(1),* 39, 1972.

MERGENHAGEN, S. E., and SCHERP, H. W. (Eds.): *Comparative Immunology of the Oral Cavity.* Bethesda, Md., U.S. Dept. of Health, Education and Welfare, 1973.

MOVAT, H. Z.: *Inflammation, Immunity and Hypersensitivity.* New York, Harper & Row, 1971.

ROCHA E SILVA, M., and LEME, G.: *Chemical Mediators of the Acute Inflammatory Reaction.* New York, Pergamon Press, 1972.

SPRAGG, J.: The plasma kinin-forming system. In G. Weissman (Ed.): *Mediators of Inflammation.* New York, Plenum Press, 1974.

TAICHMAN, N. S.: Mediation of inflammation by the polymorphonuclear leukocyte as a sequela of immune reactions, J. Periodontol., *41,* 228, 1970.

WAKSMAN, B. H.: *Atlas of Experimental Immunobiology and Immunopathology.* New Haven, Yale University Press, 1970.

WEISSMAN, G.: Introduction. In G. Weissman (Ed.): *Mediators of Inflammation.* New York, Plenum Press, 1974.

WILLOUGHBY, D. A.: Recent advances in inflammation. In J. E. Eastoe, D. C. A. Picton, and A. G. Alexander (Eds.): *The Prevention of Periodontal Disease.* London, Henry Kimpton Publishers, 1971.

ZURIER, R. B.: Prostaglandins. In G. Weissman (Ed.): *Mediators of Inflammation.* New York, Plenum Press, 1974.

ZWEIFACH, B. W.: Microvascular aspects of tissue injury. In B. W. Zweifach, L. Grant, and R. T. McCluskey (Eds.): *The Inflammatory Process,* 2nd ed., Vol. II. New York, Academic Press, Inc., 1973.

Index